Manual of
GYNAECOLOGY

MANUAL OF GYNAECOLOGY

Compiled and edited

by

Dr. Saritha Shamsunder MD, MRCOG (London)

Senior Medical Officer,
Department of Obstetrics and Gyanaecology
Vardhmaan Mahavir Medical College &
Safdarjung Hospital, New Delhi

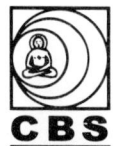

CBS

CBS PUBLISHERS & DISTRIBUTORS PVT. LTD.

NEW DELHI • BANGALORE • PUNE • COCHIN • CHENNAI (INDIA)

MANUAL OF GYNAEOCOLOGY

ISBN : 81-239-1446-6

First Edition : 2007
Reprint : 2010

Published by Satish Kumar Jain and produced by V.K. Jain for
CBS Publishers & Distributors Pvt. Ltd.,
CBS Plaza, 4819/XI Prahlad Street, 24 Ansari Road, Daryaganj,
New Delhi - 110002, India.
e-mail: cbspubs@vsnl.com, cbspubs@airtelmail.in, delhi@cbspd.com
Website: www.cbspd.com

Branches:
- *Bangalore:* Seema House, 2975, 17th Cross, K.R. Road,
  Bansankari 2nd Stage, Bangalore - 560070
  Fax: 080-26771680 • e-mail: bangalore@cbspd.com
- *Pune:* Shaan Brahmha Complex, 631/632, Basement, Appa Balwant
  Chowk, Budhwar Peth, Next to Ratan Talkies, Pune - 411002
  Fax: 020-24464059 • e-mail: pune@cbspd.com
- *Cochin:* 36/14, Kalluvilakam, Lissie Hospital Road,
  Cochin - 682018, Kerala • e-mail: cochin@cbspd.com
- *Chennai:* 20, West Park Road, Shenoy Nagar,
  Chennai - 600030 • e-mail: chennai@cbspd.com

Printed at :
Swastik Packagings, Delhi

Dedicated to my family, without whose support this task would have been impossible.

Foreword

Gynaecology, like all other fields in medicine is advancing rapidly. Advancements in reproductive endocrinology, gynaecological endoscopy, assisted reproductive technologies, molecular biology, oncology, to name a few, are taking place everyday. To integrate the basics of gynaecology with the recent advances and yet, keep the book simple and interesting for a medical student is a challenging task which this book has been able to achieve. A student of gynaecology needs to be given in depth knowledge of the subject without compromising on clarity. The comprehensive text given in points with flow charts and illustrations make the contents of this book easy to grasp and retain. I congratulate Dr. Saritha Shamsunder for writing this beautiful book with inputs from eminent teachers of gynaecology. I am sure this book will prove to be very useful for not only the undergraduates and postgraduates but also for the practising gynaecologists.

Dr. Shubha Sagar Trivedi
Director Professor and Head
Dept. of Obstetrics and Gynaecology
Lady Hardinge Medical College,
New Delhi 110001, India

Қ

Preface

There has long been a need to have a comprehensive handbook for use by students of obstetrics and gynaecology. This "Manual of Gynaecology" is written mainly for use of undergraduate students of medicine, but can be used by trainees and residents in obstetrics and gynaecology. Each topic has been written by experts in the field incorporating the latest knowledge in evidence based management. Figures and tables have been added to facilitate understanding of the subject and reproducibility in exams. The format of the text is designed for easy reading and rapid revision of facts. The chapter on FAQs (Frequently Asked Questions) incorporates questions from past papers of MBBS exams from medical colleges all over the country.

I hope medical students all over the country find the book useful either alone or as a supplement to other text books.

I am indebted to all my seniors and colleagues who have contributed chapters for this book; my juniors Shweta, Hanika, Surveen and Satyavrat for their invaluable help in proofreading and giving a feedback. My sincere thanks to Mr. Rajiv Vohra, Mr. Praveen Sharma for the illustrations, Mrs. Nishi Sharma for patiently type-setting and editing the text and lastly, CBS Publishers & Distributors for bringing out this book.

Saritha Shamsunder

List of Contributors

Dr. Shubha Sagar Trivedi Director & Professor of Obstetrics and Gynaecology, Lady Hardinge Medical College and Smt. Sucheta Kriplani Hospital, New Delhi

Dr. Sudha Salhan Consultant Obstetrician & Gynaecologist, Vardhmaan Mahavir Medical College & Safdarjung Hospital, New Delhi

Dr. Bharti Minocha Consultant Gynaecologist, Vardhmaan Mahavir Medical College & Safdarjung Hospital, New Delhi

Mr. Issac Manyonda Consultant Gynaecologist, St. George's Hospital & Medical School, London

Dr. Sunesh Jain Professor of Obstetrics and Gynaecology, AIIMS, New Delhi

Dr. Shashi Prateek Consultant Gynaecologist, Vardhmaan Mahavir Medical College & Safdarjung Hospital, New Delhi

Dr. Raksha Arora Professor of Obstetrics and Gynaecology, Maulana Azad Medical College, New Delhi

Dr. Urvashi Jha Consultant Gynaecologist, Apollo Hospital, New Delhi

Dr. Lalit Kumar Additional Professor of Medical Oncology, Institute Rotary Cancer Hospital, AIIMS, New Delhi

Dr. Mohanty Consultant Urologist, Vardhmaan Mahavir Medical College & Safdarjung Hospital, New Delhi

Dr. Manjula Sharma Specialist in Obstetrics and Gynaecology, Vardhmaan Mahavir Medical College & Safdarjung Hospital, New Delhi

Dr. J.B. Sharma Assistant Professor of Obstetrics and Gynaecology, AIIMS, New Delhi

Dr. Binod K Khaitaan Associate Professor of Dermatology & Venereology, AIIMS, New Delhi

Dr. S.N. Basu Specialist in Radiotherapy, Vardhmaan Mahavir Medical College & Safdarjung Hospital, Delhi

Dr. Bipin Sethi Consultant Endocrinologist, Care Hospital, Hyderabad (A.P)

Dr. Sridhar Chitruri Endocrinologist, PGIMER, Chandigarh

Dr. Leena Wadhwa Pool Officer in Dept. of Obstetrics and Gynaecology, Maulana Azad Medical College, New Delhi

Dr. Naseera Banu Ragistrar in Obstetrics and Gynaecology, St. George's Hospital, London

Dr. Shivani Agarwal Senior Research Associate, Human Research and Reproduction Council, Indian Council of Medical Research, New Delhi

Dr. Sunita Seth Research Officer, Dept. of Obstetrics and Gynaecology, Safdarjung Hospital, New Delhi

Dr. Monika Gupta Resident in Obstetrics and Gynaecology, Safdarjung Hospital, New Delhi

Dr. Shilpa Monga Resident in Obstetrics and Gynaecology, Safdarjung Hospital, New Delhi

Dr. Monica Madaan & Sharda Patra Residents in Obstetrics and Gynaecology, Lady Hardinge Medical College, New Delhi

Dr. Suchitra Berge Research Officer in Medical Oncology, Institute Rotary Cancer Hospital, AIIMS, New Delhi

Dr. Deepa Janga Research Officer in Gynaecology Oncology, Institute Rotary Cancer Hospital, AIIMS, New Delhi

Dr. Shalini Malhotra–Medical Officer, Dept. of Radiotherapy, Vardhmaan Mahavir Medical College & Safdarjung Hospital, New Delhi

Dr. Trilokraj Tejasvi & Dr. Radhakrishna Bhat Registrars in Dept. of Dermatology and Venereology, AIIMS, New Delhi

Dr. Garima Luthra Resident in Obstetrics and Gynaecology, Vardhmaan Mahavir Medical College & Safdarjung Hospital, New Delhi

Dr. Renu Bansal Registrar in Obstetrics and Gynaecology, Vardhmaan Mahavir Medical College & Safdarjung Hospital, New Delhi

Dr. Swasti Clinical Assistant, Dept. of Obstetrics and Gynaecology, Indraprastha, Apollo Hospital, New Delhi, India

Dr. Shweta Rajani Resident in Obstetrics and Gynaecology, Safdarjung Hospital, New Delhi

Contents

Section III
Gynaecological Cancers

Section IV
Contraception and Medical Termination of Pregnancy

Section V
Disorders of the Pelvic Floor and Urinary Tract

Section VI
Operative Gynaecology

Section VII
Frequently Asked Questions (FAQ)

Section I
The Basics of Gynaecology

Anatomy of the Female Genital Tract

The genital tract comprises of the external genitalia (commonly known as the vulva) and the internal genitalia comprising of the vagina, uterus, uterine appendages and the ovaries. The organs in close relation are the bladder, urethra, rectum, anus and the sigmoid colon.

THE VULVA

The vulva is an ill defined area comprising of the following (Fig. 1.1):

1. Mons pubis
2. Labia majora
3. Labia minora
4. Clitoris
5. Vestibule
6. Bartholin's glands

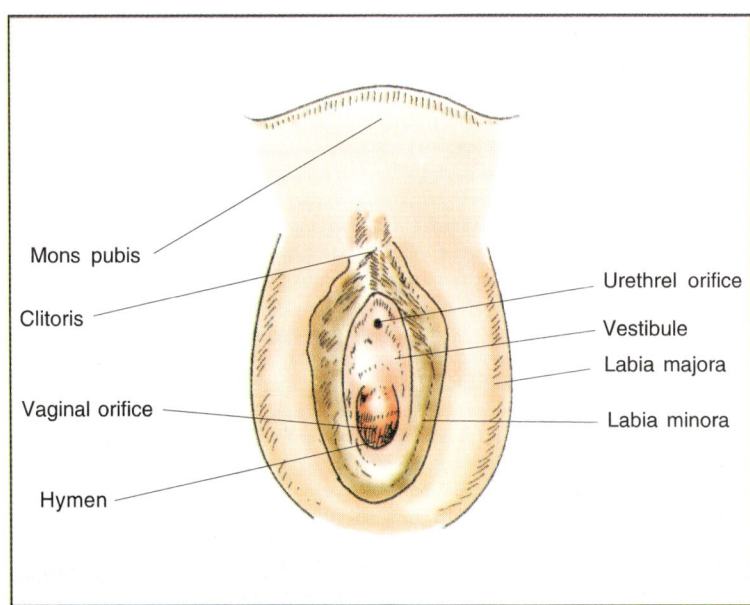

Fig. 1.1. Parts of the vulva

3

1. **Mons pubis** mainly has subcutaneous fat. Pudendal hair appears at puberty.

2. **Labia majora** (analogous to the scrotum in males) consist of folds of skin with variable amounts of fat. It has two ends, the anterior and posterior commissure, which are maximally developed in reproductive age. In children and post-menopausal women, the amount of subcutaneous fat is small, hence the interlabial cleft is conspicuous. The outer surface of the labia majora has hair and glands; whilst the inner surface has no hair. They are covered by squamous epithelium containing specialised apocrine glands. A tumour arising from these glands is called a *hidradenoma*.

3. **Labia-minora** are made up of two thin folds of skin with no fat. Anteriorly they enclose the clitoris forming a prepuce at it's upper end and a frenulum at the lower end. Posteriorly they join to form the *fourchette*, which has no glands, or hair follicles. *Fossa navicularis* is a small hollow between the hymen and the fourchette.

4. **Clitoris** consists of erectile tissue with abundant nerve supply. The body of the clitoris, '*corpus cavernosum*' is highly vascular, corresponds to the penis in males and contributes to female orgasm.

5. **Vestibule** is the cleft between the labia minora which contains
   - the external urethral meatus
   - the orifices of the paraurethral (Skene's) glands
   - the vaginal orifice with hymen
   - the orifices of bartholin's glands

6. **Bartholin's glands** are small, pea-sized glands situated posterolaterally in relation to the vaginal orifice, at the junction of mid and posterior third of the labia-majora
   - Their function is to secrete lubricatory mucus during coitus.
   - They are normally impalpable when healthy but can be readily palpated between the finger and the thumb when inflamed.
   - The gland and its duct are inflamed in acute gonorrhoea.

Blood supply of the vulva

- *Arteries*   Arterial supply is via branches of the internal pudendal artery (branch of internal iliac) and femoral artery

- *Veins*   Drain into the internal pudendal, vesical or vaginal venous plexus and long saphaenous vein.

Nerve supply   The nerve supply is derived mainly from $S_{2,3,4}$ segments of the spinal cord. The anterosuperior part receives it's nerve supply from the $L_{1,2}$ segments.

Lymphatic drainage These mainly drain into the superficial inguinal lymph nodes which then drain into the deep inguinal and femoral lymph nodes.

Development of the external genitalia (also see chapter 4 and 5)

- The clitoris is developed from the genital tubercle
- The labia minora develop from the genital folds
- Labia majora develop from the labioscrotal swellings
- The vestibule develops from the urogenital sinus.

VAGINA

- Muscular organ which connects the external orifice to the uterus. Its walls are thrown into various rugosities.
- The posterior wall is 11 cm long and anterior is 9 cm.
- The vaginal vault has four fornices–posterior, anterior and two lateral.
- In transverse section, the mid-vagina appears as a transverse slit and the lower vagina is H-shaped.

Histology It has a *mucosal layer*, a *submucosa* and a *muscularis*. The mucosa is made of stratified squamous non-keratinized epithelium with no gland openings into it. In the neonate the vagina is lined by transitional epithelium.

Vaginal secretions are derived partly from the mucous discharge of the cervix and partly from transudation through the vaginal epithelium. It is normally small in amount, it also contains squamous cells shed from the vaginal epithelium and Doderlein's bacilli (gram positive anaerobic rods). *Normal vaginal pH* before puberty is 7, after puberty the pH falls to 4.5 due to lactic acid produced by the action of Doderlein's bacilli on the glycogen of the vaginal epithelium.

Relations of the vagina (Fig 1.2)

Anterior Upper half – bladder
    Lower half – urethra and paraurethral glands

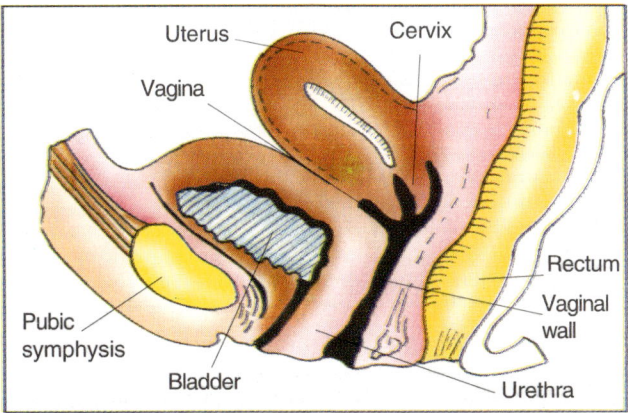

Fig. 1.2. Sagittal section of the female pelvis showing the relations of the vagina

Posterior Upper third – anterior wall of pouch of douglas (site of colpocentesis: used to diagnose a ruptured ectopic pregnancy).

Middle third – rectum

Lower third – perineal body

Perineal body is a fibromuscular mass occupying the area between the vagina and anal canal. It supports the lower part of the vagina.

Superior Cervix forms four fornices–anterior, posterior and two lateral. The posterior fornix is the deepest.

Lateral From below upwards are the cavernous tissue of the vestibule, superficial muscles of the perineum, levator ani, the endopelvic fascia and their condensations i.e., the mackendrodt ligaments (Fig. 1.3).

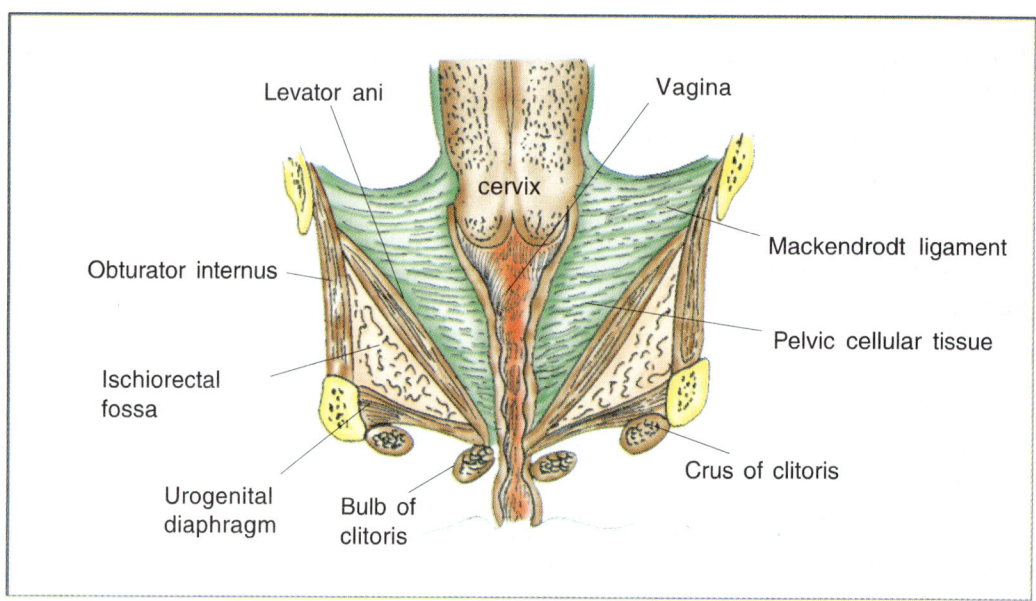

Fig. 1.3. Coronal section of the pelvis showing the relationship of vagina and pelvic floor

UTERUS

It is the child bearing organ in females. It is shaped like an inverted pear and measures 9x6.5x3.5cm [3x2x1 inches]

Parts of uterus are as follows: (Fig. 1.4)

1. Body (corpus)
2. Cervix

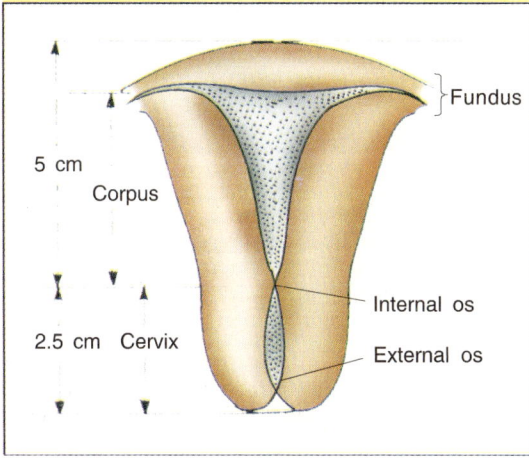

Fig. 1.4. Parts of the uterus

The line of division corresponds to the level of the *internal os*. It is also an important landmark for the following changes to take place.

- The peritoneum on the front of the uterus gets reflected on to the bladder.
- The uterine artery reaches the uterus and runs up vertically along the lateral wall.

The *fundus* of the uterus is the part of the corpus that lies above the insertion of the fallopian tubes.

Walls of the uterus   The uterine wall is made up of three layers:

a) *Perimetrium* is the peritoneum covering the uterus which anteriorly covers the entire uterus upto the level of the internal os and posteriorly, the whole of the uterine body.

b) *Myometrium* is the thickest layer made of muscle fibres arranged in three layers; external longitudinal, where the fibres run longitudinally over the uterus from the cervix; middle layer is made of interlacing bundles which serve as living ligaments for control of bleeding after separation of the placenta. The inner circular layer is well developed at the level of the internal os and openings of the fallopian tubes.

c) *Endometrium* is the mucous membrane lining the uterus. It is normally 1-5 mm thick and has two phases–

  Proliferative phase–due to the effect of oestrogens

  Secretory phase–due to the effect of oestrogens and progesterone.

The *isthmus* is the intermediate zone which lies between the endometrium of the body and the mucous membrane of the cervical canal and forms the lower uterine segment in late pregnancy.

Position and angulation   Normally the uterus is ante-flexed and anteverted (Fig. 1.5).

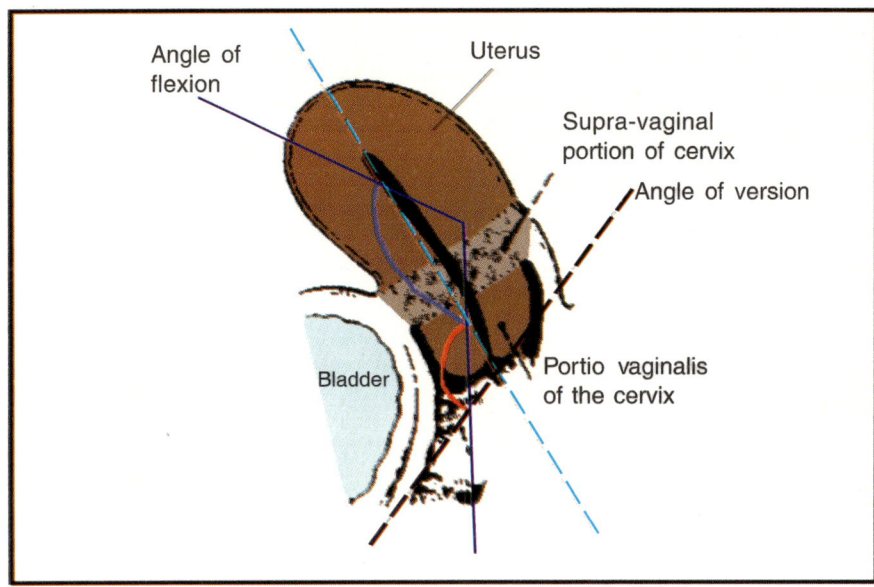

Fig. 1.5.   Position and angulation of uterus

- **Flexion** indicates the angulation of the body of the uterus and cervix, ante-flexed means the forward bending of the body of the uterus on the cervix which is normally 120°.

- **Version** indicates the relation of the long axis of the uterus with the long axis of the vagina. Ante-version means the forward bending of the uterus in relation to the vagina and is normally 90°.

Cervix It extends from the internal to the external os. It is 2.5 cm long and lined by ciliated columnar epithelium with racemose glands. The cervical secretion is alkaline and contains fructose which renders it attractive to the ascending sperms. The secretion collects as a plug in the cervical canal and possibly hinders ascending infection. In nulliparous women, the external os is circular, but in parous women it is transverse (Fig. 1.6).

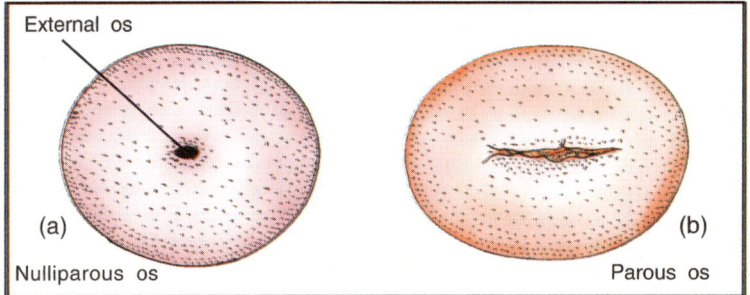

Fig. 1.6ab.   The external os in (a) Nulliparous and (b) Multiparous women

Cervix-corpus ratio The size of the cervix and body of uterus changes during the life of the woman (Fig. 1.7). The cervix: corpus ratio at various stages in the reproductive life of the woman are:

- Before puberty 2:1
- At puberty 1:2
- Reproductive years 1:3
- After menopause, the uterus and cervix become atrophic and ratio becomes 1:1.

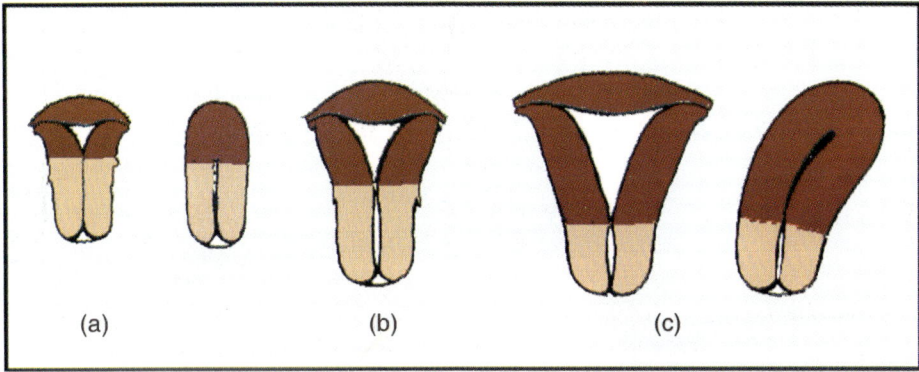

(a)   (b)   (c)

Fig. 1.7. Changes in the uterus with age (a) Before puberty (b) At puberty (c) Reproductive years

Blood supply of the uterus

- ***Arterial supply*** Mainly from the uterine and ovarian arteries. The Uterine artery arises from the anterior division of the internal iliac and runs downwards and forwards until it reaches the uterus at the level of the internal os. It then runs up along the lateral wall giving out the *arcuate arteries* which run transversely along the myometrium. *Radial arteries* arise from the arcuate arteries and reach the basal layers of the endometrium. The *vaginal branch* arises before the uterine artery runs up vertically and reaches the vagina in the region of the lateral fornix. There is extensive anastomosis between both the sides, the least vascular portion being the midline.

- ***Venous drainage*** The veins drain into the uterine vein which finally drains into the internal iliac vein.

Lymphatic drainage

- ***The fundus*** of the uterus drains via the round ligament to the superficial inguinal lymph nodes and along the ovarian ligament to the para-aortic group of lymph-nodes.

- ***Body of the uterus*** drains to the external iliac lymph nodes.

- ***Cervix*** drains to the external and internal iliac, obturator nodes and sacral nodes.

FALLOPIAN TUBE

Embryologically the fallopian tube represents the cranial end of the mullerian duct. It is made up of four **parts** (Fig. 1.8):

1. *Intramural:* This is the narrowest and innermost part being 1mm in diameter and the shortest (18 mm).

2. *Isthmic:* Comprises the mid 1/3, is 35 mm long and 2 mm in diameter.

3. *Ampullary:* Lateral 2/3 and is the widest and longest part, being 60-75 mm in length 4 mm in diameter. The mucosa is arborescent with many complex folds.

4. *Infundibulum:* This is the fimbriated end of the fallopian tube, is 3 mm in diameter and has an abdominal ostium opening into the peritoneal cavity. It resembles a sea-anemone as the fimbriae are motile with a considerable degree of movement.

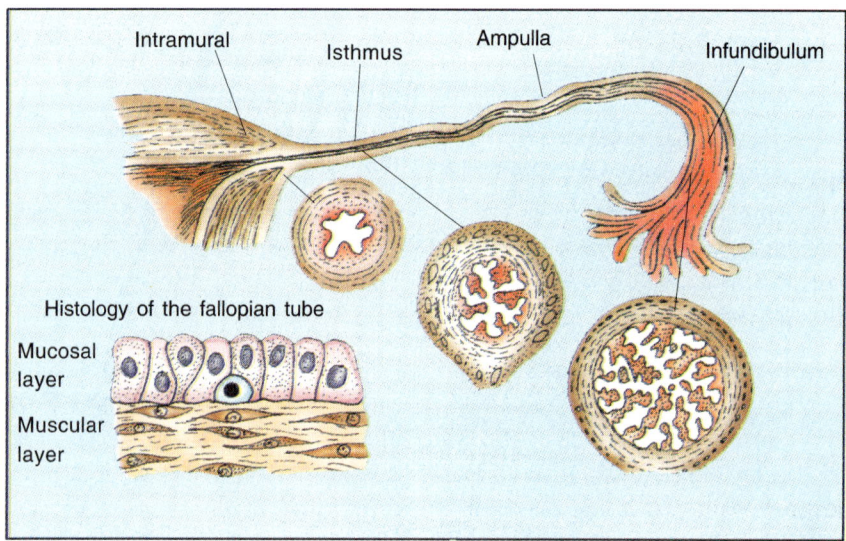

Fig. 1.8.   Parts of the fallopian tube

Blood supply Uterine and ovarian artery.

Lymphatics Drain into the para-aortic and superficial inguinal lymph nodes.

Histology The wall of the fallopian tube is made up of three layers:

1. **Serous**–this is the peritoneal covering which covers all the areas of the tube except inferiorly where it is attached to the broad ligament.

2. **Muscular**–has two layers, outer longitudinal and inner circular layer.

3. **Mucosa**–made up of three types of cells:

   • *Ciliated columnar cells* The cilia propel the fluid current towards the uterus to transport the inert ovum

- *Peg cells* purpose unknown
- *Goblet cells* their main function is lubrication.

OVARIES

They are 3x2x1 cm in size and almond shaped.

They are attached to the broad ligament by the mesovarium.

They are the only intra-abdominal structures not covered by peritoneum.

Relations

- Inferiorly–the ovarian ligament which attaches it to the uterus.
- Superiorly–the suspensory ligament attaches it to the pelvis.
- Laterally–it is related to the fossa below the bifurcation of the common iliac artery and the ureter.
- Medially are the tubal fimbriae.

Vestigeal remnants (also see chapter on sexual differentiation)–Vestigeal remnants of the mesonephic duct run parallel to and below the fallopian tube. *Epoophoron* (organ of rosenmuller) represents the cranial end of the wolffian body. A cyst developing in the caudal part of the Wolffian duct remnant is called a *Gartner's cyst*. *Paroophoron* represents the caudal end of the wolffian body.

THE URINARY TRACT

The urinary tract in the pelvis comprises

1. The pelvic part of the ureter
2. The urinary bladder
3. The urethra

1. The Ureter

- The ureter runs half of its course in the abdomen and half in the pelvis.
- It is 25-30 cm long, with a diameter of 3 mm.
- It has three layers, outer fibrous, middle muscular and inner mucosal layer lined with transitional epithelium.
- Course and relations: (Fig. 1.9) It enters the pelvis anterior to the sacroiliac joint crossing the bifurcation of the common iliac artery. It passes along the posterolateral aspect in front and below the internal iliac artery and it's anterior division. It then runs lateral to the cervix through the base of the broad ligament and is crossed

superiorly from lateral to medial side by the uterine artery (***water under the bridge***). It enters the bladder 1.5 cm lateral to the cervix. ***Importance:*** The ureter can be damaged accidentally at any point in the pelvis during a difficult Caesarean section or hysterectomy.

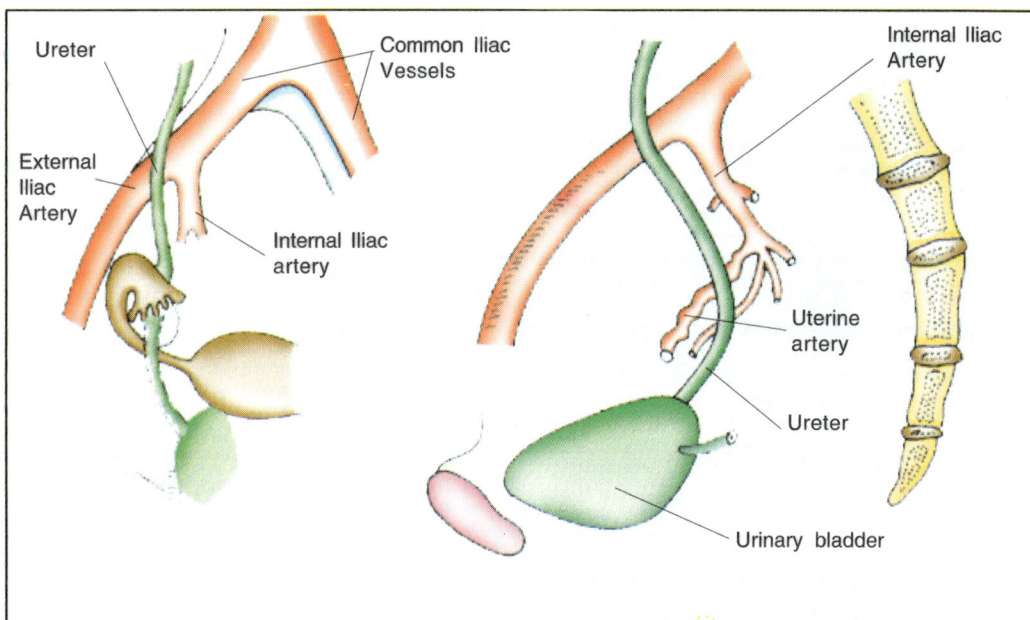

Fig. 1.9. Course of the ureter

2. The Urinary bladder: (diag cross section of pelvis Fig. 1.10)

- It is a muscular extraperitoneal structure lying behind the symphysis pubis.

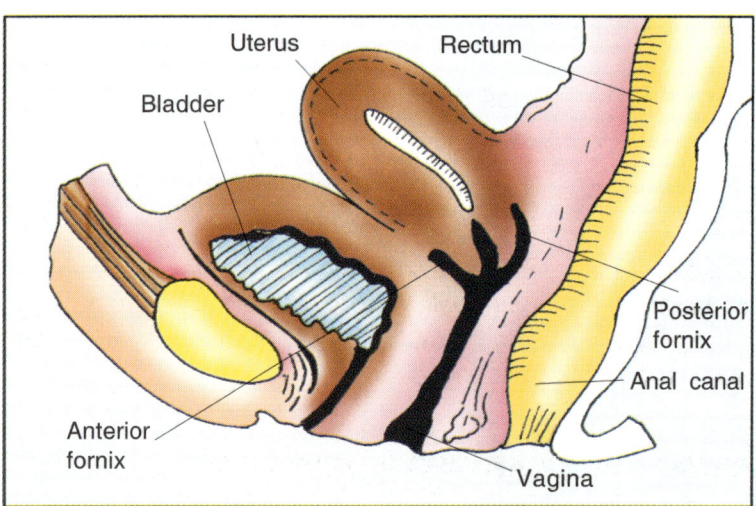

Fig. 1.10. Sagittal section of the pelvis showing the relations of the bladder and urethra

- Posteriorly, it's relations are from below upwards–the upper vagina, the supravaginal portion of the cervix and the peritoneal reflection of the uterovesical pouch.
- Normal bladder capacity is 300-600 mls.
- Importance–the bladder may be accidentally injured during a caesarean section, hysterectomy or surgery for prolapse.

3. Urethra

- It is 4 cm long and 6 mm in diameter, and lies in close relation to the symphysis pubis.
- It has no anatomical sphincters, the tone and elasticity of the involuntary muscle maintains it's closure. Circular muscle fibres 1 cm from it's lower end form the **external urethral sphincter**. The epithelium is transitional which gets converted to squamous epithelium near the external meatus.

THE RECTUM AND ANAL CANAL

The **Rectum** is 12 cm long, the lower end dilates to form the *ampulla*, which bulges into the posterior vaginal wall and continues as the anal canal.

- It has no sacculations, appendices epiploicae or mesentery.
- It has no peritoneal covering in its lower third.
- *Relations*–Posteriorly, the lower three sacral vertebrae, the coccyx and the rectal vessels. Anteriorly, it is closely related to the upper vagina and pouch of douglas with it's contents above and the lower vagina below.

The Anal canal

- It is about 3 cm long and passes downwards and backwards from the rectum
- It is slit like when empty but distends greatly during defecation
- Anteriorly it is related to the perineal body and lower vagina and posteriorly to the anococcygeal body
- It has two sphincters–**Internal anal sphincter** which is involuntary and is a thickening of the circular muscle of the gut wall. The **external anal sphincter** is voluntary and composed of three layers of striated muscle. The external sphincter can be torn during child birth resulting in fecal incontinence.

PELVIC CELLULAR TISSUE AND PELVIC LIGAMENTS

The ligaments of importance in the pelvis are given below (Fig. 1.11). All of them except the broad ligament are condensations of pelvic cellular tissue; the broad ligaments are folds of peritoneum on either sides of the uterus.

- Round ligaments
- Broad ligaments
- Cardinal ligaments
- Uterosacral ligaments
- Ovarian ligaments

- **The round ligaments** are two narrow flat bands arising from the lateral angles of the uterus running laterally to the deep inguinal ring where they turn into the inguinal canal to end in the subcutaneous tissue of the labia-majora. Together with the uterosacral ligaments, they are believed to help the uterus remain anteverted and anteflexed.

- **The broad ligaments** are folds of peritoneum on either sides of the uterus which enclose the fallopian tubes at their upper end and loose cellular tissue of the pelvis i.e. the parametrium.

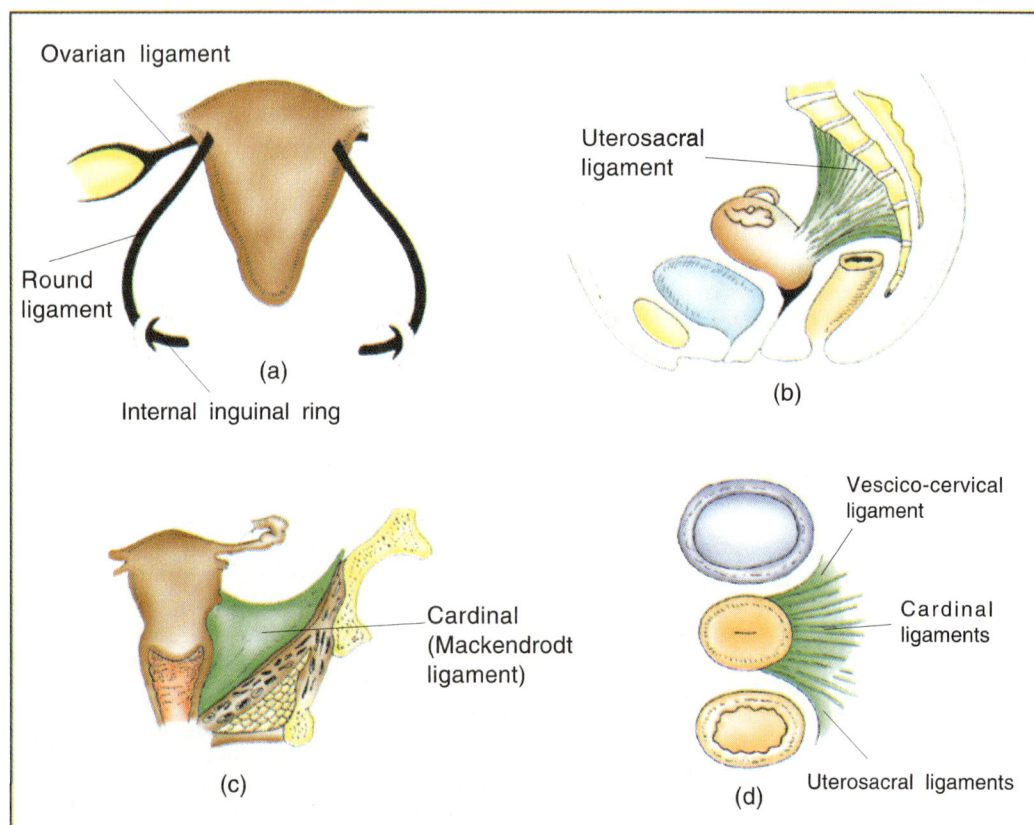

Fig. 1.11a-d. Ligaments of the pelvis

- **The cardinal ligaments** are condensations of pelvic fascia on the upper surface of the levator ani muscles. They are attached to the uterus at the level of the supravaginal part of the cervix and pass laterally upto the pelvic wall.

- **The uterosacral ligaments** arise as posterior condensations of the cardinal ligament around the lateral margins of the rectum and insert into the periosteum of the fourth sacral vertebra. They provide the major support to the uterus and prevent uterine descent. They also pull the uterus backwards, maintaining anteflexion.

- **The ovarian ligaments** are fibromuscular cords running from the cornu of the uterus to the medial border of the ovary. The round ligaments and ovarian ligaments together form the homologue of the gubernaculum testis of the male.

The cardinal and uterosacral ligaments are the strongest supports of the uterus and are called the **true supports**, while the round ligaments, broad ligaments and ovarian ligaments are mere condensations of fascia and are called *false supports*.

Blood supply of the pelvis

The main arterial supply is from the internal iliac artery and its branches (Fig. 1.12). The internal iliac is a division of the common iliac artery. Collateral circulation arises from the ovarian and external iliac vessels.

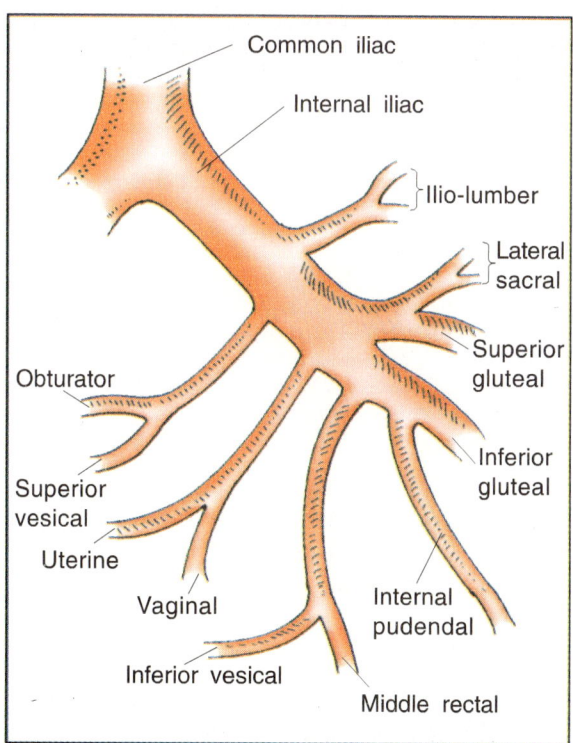

Fig. 1.12. The common iliac artery and its branches supplying the pelvis

Nerve supply of the pelvis

The pelvis is supplied by both sympathetic and parasympathetic nerves and somatic nerves.

Sympathetic fibres enter via the lumbosacral chain and form the *presacral nerve* at the bifurcation of the aorta. They pass along the uterosacral ligaments to reach the viscera and are known as the *Frankenhauser's plexus* or hypogastric plexus.

Parasympathetic nerves join the sympathetic fibres from sacral roots 2, 3 and 4.

Somatic nerves are derived from the lumbosacral plexus formed by the anterior primary rami of $L_{1,2,3}$ nerves and partly L_4 and T_{12} which lies on the surface of the psoas major and gives off a number of major branches–the ilioinguinal, iliohypogastric, genitofemoral, femoral, pudendal, saphaenous and obturator nerves.

PELVIC DIAPHRAGM

The levator ani and coccygeus muscles on either sides form the pelvic diaphragm separating the structures in the pelvis from the perineum and ischiorectal fossa.

Levator ani is a wide, thin curved sheet of muscle arising anteriorly form the pelvic surface of the body of the pubis, the ischial spine and the tendinous arch of the obturator fascia. It has three parts–

1.   Puborectalis–is the most medial part, encircles and supports the rectum and vagina.

2.   Pubococcygeus–the strongest part extending from the pubis to the coccyx.

3.   Iliococcygeus–is the most posterior and is also attached to the coccyx.

2 Physiology of Menstruation

Menstruation is the monthly bleeding from the uterus which occurs for 4-5 days every 28 days during the reproductive life of a woman, with an average loss of about 20 to 60 mls of blood. It has been observed that about two third of adult women have menstrual cycles lasting from 21 to 35 days. Knowledge of normal menstrual physiology will help in understanding abnormal menstrual situation and its management.

Control of monthly uterine bleeding is by co-ordination between the hypothalamus, pituitary and ovary forming a neurohormonal pathway. Thus menstruation consists of an *endocrine cycle*, an *ovarian cycle* and a *uterine cycle* (Fig. 2.1).

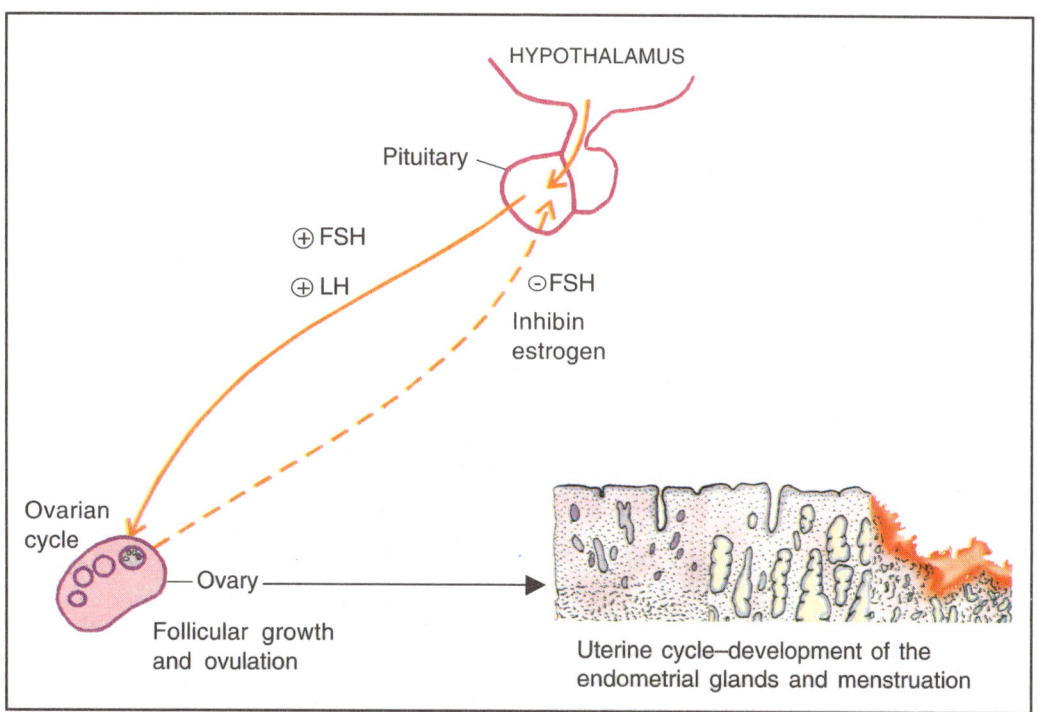

Fig. 2.1. Hypothalamo-pituitary ovarian uterine cycle

1. THE ENDOCRINE CYCLE

It is controlled by sex steroids and peptides produced in the ovulatory follicle. The organs involved are the hypothalamus, pituitary and the ovary.

Hypothalamus

Gonadotropin Releasing Hormone (GnRH), a neurohormone, is a decapeptide secreted by the peptidergic neurones in the median eminence and arcuate nucleus of the hypothalamus and delivered to the anterior pituitary by the portal vessels.

Pituitary

The gonadotropins, FSH (Follicular Stimulating Hormone) and LH (Luteinising Hormone) are produced by the anterior pituitary cells. The anterior pituitary has two types of secretory cells, acidophilic and basophilic, based on their staining with haematoxylin and eosin. The gonadotropins are secreted by the basophilic cells and are glycoprotein in structure.

Ovary

Ovarian function occurs in a cycle and has two phases *the follicular phase* and *the luteal phase.* Sex hormones like oestrogen, progesterone, some amount of androgens and peptides like inhibin and activin are released from the ovary and are responsible for normal menstruation. The cyclical changes in hormone levels in the different phases of ovarian cycle are shown in Fig. 2.2.

2. THE OVARIAN CYCLE

- At birth they become about 300,000 in number
- In the reproductive life of a woman about 400 follicles ovulate

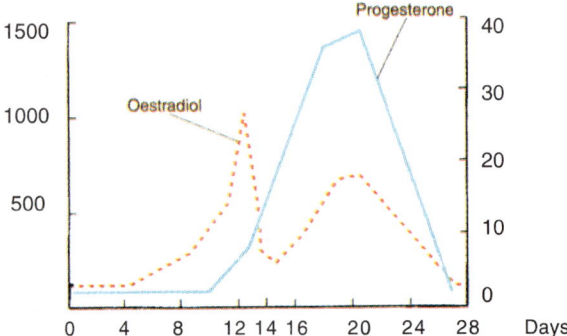

Fig. 2.2. Ovarian hormonal changes: The graph shows the oestrogen and progesterone levels during the two phases of the menstrual cycle

- At menopause the ovary has dense stromal tissue with only few follicles remaining.
  The ovarian cycle occurs in two phases, the follicular phase and the luteal phase.

Follicular phase

Starts at the end of menstruation when the levels of both the gonadotropins are low. In this phase a number of follicles mature but only one follicle becomes dominant and matures to ovulate. The mechanism for determining how many follicles will grow in one menstrual cycle is not known yet. The activity of FSH starts as menstruation is ceasing. FSH controls follicular differentiation and growth.

The ***primordial follicle*** consists of an oocyte and a single layer of spindle shaped cells known as the granulosa cells. As follicles mature, the size of the oocyte increases and the shape of the granulosa cells changes to cuboidal. With multiplication of cuboidal granulosa cells, the primordial follicle becomes a primary follicle. In the ***primary follicle*** the granulosa cells are separated by a basement membrane from the stromal cells. The stromal cells later differentiate into theca cells. As the follicle grows a fluid-filled cavity appears inside which secretes two peptides, inhibin and activin.

FSH influences the follicles to secrete oestrogen from the granulosa cells. A small amount of LH available in the early follicular phase stimulates the theca cells to produce androgens, which are later aromatized by the granulosa cells and get converted into oestrogen. Both the FSH and local oestrogens cause proliferation of granulosa cells resulting in increased oestrogen production. This brings about a ***proliferative change in the endometrium.***

By the 5th day FSH level reaches its peak, Selection of the dominant follicle is decided by days 5-7. The effect of FSH is most on this oestrogen dominant follicle. By day 7 oestrogen level starts rising. The rise in FSH also causes a rise in inhibin which causes a negative feed-back suppression of FSH. A rise in oestrogen helps in growth and maturation of the dominant follicle; a rise in inhibin suppresses FSH release preventing the growth of other follicles. A positive feed-back on LH causes a rise in LH levels.

Late follicular phase

There is a gradual rise in LH, and this increased level, along with the local oestrogen production in the follicle, influences the granulosa cells to produce some progesterone. Sufficient oestrogen level induces an LH surge. The peak oestrogen level is seen 48 hours before ovulation; the LH peak occurs about 24-36 hours before ovulation. Atresia of the unsuccessful primordial follicles occurs while one follicle becomes dominant.

With the LH surge, progesterone level starts rising, which has a negative feedback on LH. The fall in FSH brings about a reduction in the level of inhibin and a rise in the peptide activin in the pre-ovulatory follicle (graffian follicle). This results in a mid cycle rise in FSH and serves to free the oocyte from the follicular attachment.

Ovulation

There is a perforation in the follicular wall with slow release of the oocyte (Fig. 2.3).

Luteal phase

With the release of the oocyte, the follicle is now called the *corpus-luteum*. It derives its name from a yellow pigment called *lutein* which starts collecting in the pre-ovulatory stage. Luteal phase starts from ovulation and lasts for 14 days. In this phase, the oestrogen and progesterone levels rise, being secreted by the corpus-luteum. Some androgen production occurs in the theca cells of the unsuccessful follicles which are nearing atresia, which get aromatized by the granulosa cells.

A rise in progesterone and oestrogen brings about the secretory phase in the endometrium. Corpus luteum remains mature from day 19-26 and degenerates on day 27-28, if no pregnancy occurs in the concurrent menstrual cycle. The mechanism of degeneration of the corpus-luteum is still not known. This results in fall of progesterone and oestrogen

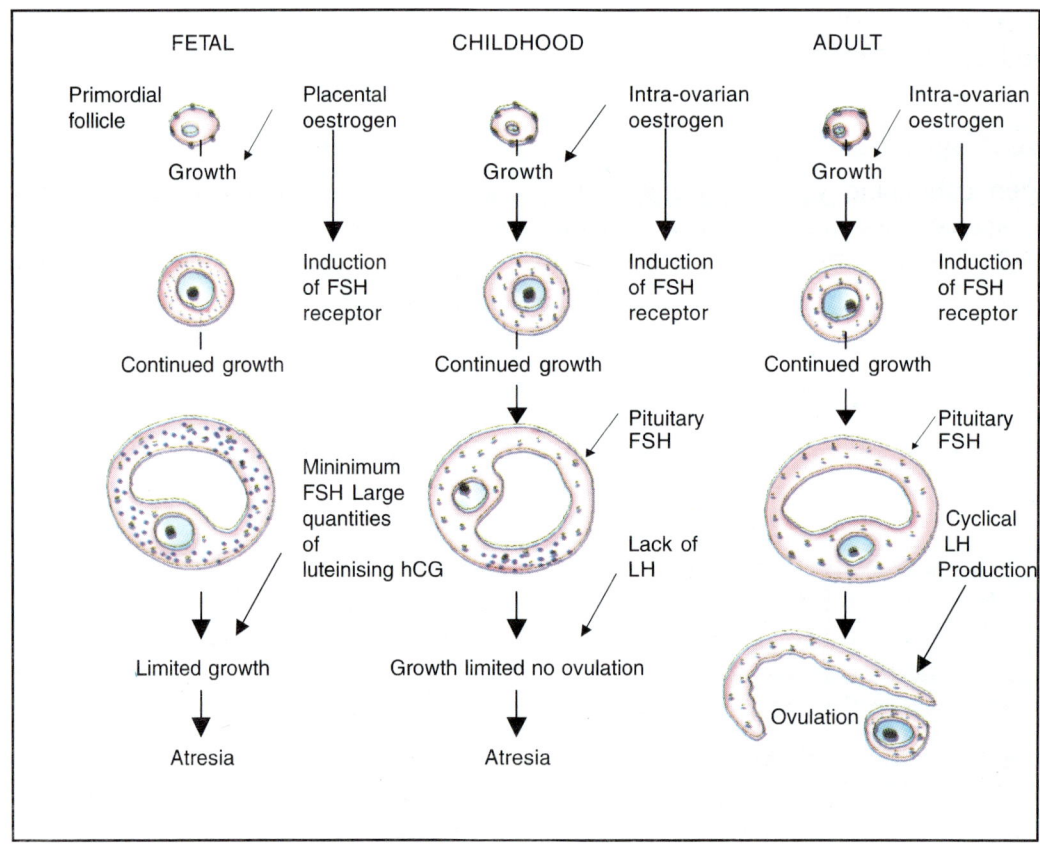

Fig. 2.3. Growth and development of follicle and ovulation

and menstruation takes place. A fall in these two hormones and also of inhibin results in a positive feedback mechanism and triggers the hypothalamus to release GnRH for the follicular phase of the next menstrual cycle.

3. UTERINE CYCLE

Changes occur in the endometrial glands and surrounding stroma in two phases namely **proliferative** and **secretory** under the effect of oestrogen and progesterone. The upper two third of the endometrium is shed during menstruation is called the **decidua-functionalis**, the lower or deep one third of the endometrium is called **decidua-basalis** from where the new endometrium regenerates for the next menstrual cycle if no pregnancy occurs.

Proliferative phase

The short and narrow endometrial glands become long and tortuous. The cells are in a low columnar pattern in the early proliferative period and changes to a pseudo-stratified pattern before ovulation. The stroma is now dense (Fig. 2.4a-b).

Secretory phase

Glycogen containing vacuoles appear in the cells of the endometrial glands. Initially these vacuoles are sub-nuclear; they then, progress towards the glandular lumen. By day 20-21, the secretory activity of the glands is maximum, the glands become crenated

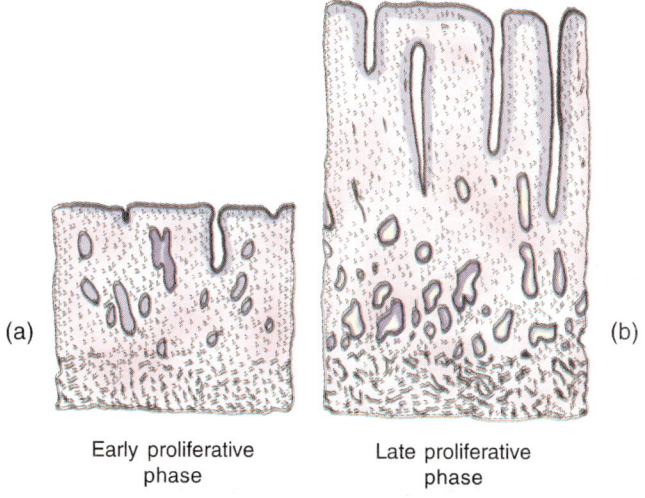

(a) (b)

Early proliferative phase Late proliferative phase

Fig. 2.4a-b. Uterine cycle–proliferative phase

and assume a corkscrew shape. The stroma becomes swollen and edematous. There is an increase in the length and coiling of the spiral arteries (Fig. 2.5a).

Menstruation

If pregnancy does not occur, glandular secretion stops and an irregular breakdown of the decidua functionalis occurs (Fig. 2.5b). There is shedding of this layer which is

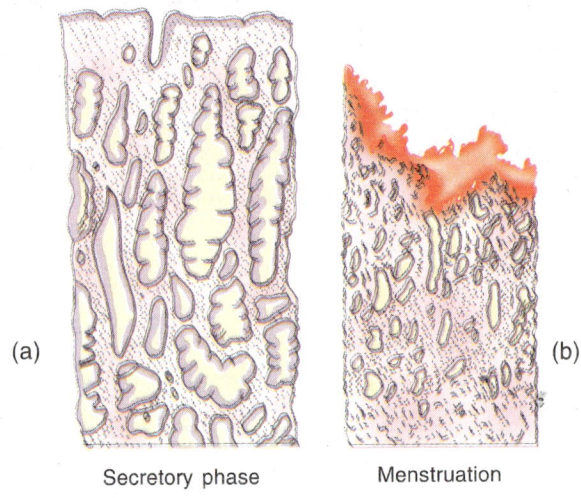

(a)   (b)

Secretory phase   Menstruation

Fig. 2.5a-b.   Uterine cycle (a) secretory phase and (b) menstruation

termed as **menses**. The corpus-luteum atrophies, sex steroids levels fall, with marked vascular spasm of the spiral arteries resulting in endometrial ischaemia. Prostaglandins produced throughout the menstrual cycle also bring about a similar change in the endometrium.

3

Making a Gynaecological Diagnosis

A proper gynaecological diagnosis can be made by taking a good history, carrying out a thorough clinical examination and conducting relevant investi-gations.

HISTORY

A brief introduction by the doctor establishes a good rapport with the woman and is helpful in obtaining a good history. It is important to note certain personal details regarding the age, occupation, educational status, marital status and residential address as they can influence the management. The history is then taken in the following order:

- **Presenting complaint** This is the problem for which the woman consults a doctor.

- **Menstrual history** Information regarding the age at menarche, regularity of cycles, and Last Menstrual Period (LMP) are noted.

- **Obstetric history** Information regarding the number of pregnancies (Gravidity), number of viable children delivered (Parity), number alive (L), the number of mis-carriages (A) and the age of the last child (LCB) are noted and abbreviated as GPLA, LCB.

- **Past medical history** History of medical problems eg. asthma, tuberculosis, diabetes, hypertension are essential as they could help in making a diagnosis and plan the management.

- **Past surgical history** History of abdominal surgery could influence the diagnosis eg. an appendicectomy done in the past could be the cause of infertility and pelvic pain. It is also helpful in planning the right management eg. a patient who has had abdominal surgery is at high risk of haemorrhage and bowel injury if repeat surgery or laparoscopy are needed, a conservative approach could be planned.

- **Family history** A family history of diabetes, hypertension and gynaecological cancer has a higher risk of the patient having similar problems.

23

- **Personal history** Information regarding the appetite, bowel habits and micturition are noted.
- **Drug history** Information regarding any drug intake either prescribed by a doctor or drug abuse are noted. A woman who is a drug abuser has a high risk of having HIV and hepatitis B.
- **History of allergies** Allergies to chemicals, food and drugs are noted as they can influence the chemicals and drugs used.

Presenting complaints   The types of complaints patients may present with are given in table 3.1. They could present with–

(a) Menstrual disorders

(b) Pain

(c) Vaginal discharge

(d) Abdominal lump

Table 3.1. Common Gynaecological complaints

Menstrual	– Menorrhagia
	Polymenorrhoea
	Metrorrhagia
	Continuous bleeding
	Post-coital bleeding
	Post-menopausal bleeding
	Amenorrhoea
Pain	– Dysmenorrhoea
	Abdominal pain
	Backache
Vaginal discharge	
Abdominal lump	

a) Menstrual disorders

- *Menorrhagia:* Regular cyclical bleeding of increased duration or increased flow as seen in fibroid uterus, pelvic inflammatory disease (PID) or endometrial hyperplasia.
- *Oligomenorrhoea:* Cycle is longer > 35 days or the duration of bleeding is reduced seen in hyperprolactinaemia and genital TB.
- *Polymenorrhoea:* Frequent regular cyclical bleeding occurring in less than 21 days seen in abnormalities of HPO axis.
- *Metrorrhagia:* Irregular acyclical bleeding seen in carcinoma cervix, cervical polyp or cervical erosion.

- *Continuous bleeding:* causes seen in miscarriage, ectopic pregnancy, carcinoma cervix or endometrium.

- *Contact bleeding* or *post-coital bleeding:* eg. cervical erosion, carcinoma cervix.

- *Post-menopausal bleeding:* Bleeding from the genital tract in any woman who has not had a period in the preceding six months or longer eg. malignancy of the genital tract.

- *Amenorrhoea:* Absence of menstruation, which could be primary or secondary.

  Primary amenorrhoea: is defined as failure of menstruation to begin by the age of 14; or in the presence of well developed secondary sex characters, menstruation does not start by the age of 16 yrs.

  Secondary amenorrhoea: A woman with previously normal menstrual function has no periods for 6 months or more.

  The causes of primary and secondary amenorrhoea are discussed separately.

b) Pain

Types of pain are as follows:

- *Dysmenorrhoea* Painful menstruation could be of two types–

  1. Spasmodic–when the pain develops on the first day of the menstrual cycle
  2. Congestive–pain develops a few days before the onset of menstrual flow and is relieved by the bleeding

- *Dyspareunia* Painful sexual intercourse; could be *superficial* due to any lesion at the introitus or *deep* due to endometriosis of the uterosacral ligaments or retroversion of the uterus.

- *Abdominal pain* not related to menstruation could be due to an ectopic pregnancy, acute PID, twisted ovarian cyst and torsion of a pedunculated sub-peritoneal fibroid. In tubal rupture the pain is severe and comparable to the pain of a perforated peptic ulcer. In tubal abortion, the pain is intermittent and colicky. In acute PID the pain is acute in onset but less dramatic. Uterine fibroids can cause continuous pain when they undergo red degeneration or torsion.

- *Back pain* lower than the first sacral vertebra could be due to a gynaecological cause eg. genital prolapse.

c) Vaginal discharge

Profuse foul smelling discharge with pruritus is pathological.

Physiological discharge contains mucus, desquamated epithelial cells and lactic acid and is very watery. It is apparent at—

- Ovulation when increased oestrogen levels induce the endocervical glands into excessive secretion
- Sexual stimulation—the main component is secretions from bartholin's glands
- Premenstrually due to premenstrual congestion
- During pregnancy due to increased congestion and transudation.

d) Abdominal lump

Could be due to unsuspected pregnancy, a full bladder, uterine or ovarian mass.

Menstrual history

The points to be noted are—

- Age at menarche—The usual age is 8-12 yrs. If the girl attains puberty before 8 yrs. it is termed as *Precocious puberty*. Puberty is termed as *delayed* if the girl does not attain menarche by the age of 16 yrs.
- Menstrual rhythm—Duration of menstruation and regularity of cycles is to be noted. The normal range is 28±3 days with the bleeding normally lasting 3-5 days.
- Amount of blood loss—Passage of clots, symptoms of anaemia are other indicators of excessive blood loss.
- Last Menstrual Period (LMP)—The date of the last normal menstrual period is noted.

Marital history   The following information needs to be recorded.

- Whether the woman is living with her husband eg. infertility could be due to non-cohabitance.
- Intercourse—frequency, any dyspareunia and achievement of orgasm should be noted.
- Contraception used in the past and present is to be noted.

Obstetric history History of previous deliveries, miscarriages needs to be recorded as the present problem could be secondary to the episode eg.

- Secondary infertility could be secondary to post-abortal or puerperal sepsis.
- Pain in the lower limbs could be related to a prolonged lithotomy position at delivery.

Past Iliness

- History of tuberculosis suggests possibility of genital tuberculosis.
- History of diabetes, asthma, cardiac disease, hypertension, thyroid disease needs to be taken as they should be controlled prior to surgery.

- History of blood transfusion.
- History of Sexually Transmitted Diseases (STD)–as they could be the cause of infertility.
- History of Pelvic Inflammatory Disease (PID)–as it may be the cause of menstrual disturbances, abdominal pain, dysmenorrhoea and infertility.
- Previous history of abdominal surgery may be the cause of abdominal pain, retroverted fixed uterus and infertility.

Family history

- History of tuberculosis indicates a possible diagnosis of pelvic tuberculosis.
- History of carcinoma ovary, breast, colon-cancer is important as gene positive cancers could be familial.

EXAMINATION

General examination

The following points are noted

- General condition: It is important to note if the patient looks well, ill and toxic (in sepsis) or cachexic and emaciated (in malignancies).
- Height and build are to be noted. Short stature is seen in Turner's syndrome and pituitary dwarfism.
- Weight: The woman may be emaciated due to anorexia nervosa, advanced malignancy or chronic illness like tuberculosis. An obese and overweight woman is a poor candidate for surgery.
- Pallor and icterus are noted by looking at the palpebral and bulbar conjunctivae respectively.
- Breasts should be examined in every patient, metastatic carcinoma of the breast may present as a Krukenberg's tumour.
- Thyroid gland: Any thyromegaly is noted as thyroid dysfunction could be the cause of menstrual dysfunction.
- Lymphadenopathy: The neck, axillae and groins are examined for any enlarged lymph nodes.
- Dependant edema in the feet or presacral area (in patients who are bed-ridden); unilateral pedal edema may be a sign of ovarian malignancy.
- Examination of the cardiovascular and respiratory systems.

Abdominal examination

The abdomen should be examined systematically in every patient by inspection, palpation, percussion and auscultation.

1. *Inspection*　The abdomen is inspected to note any

   • distension of abdomen–uniform in ascites, localized to the lower abdomen in pelvic tumours

   • scars of previous surgery

   • eversion of the umbilicus seen in ascites, large intra-abdominal tumours and pregnancy

   • cutaneous nodules–*Sister Marie Joseph's* nodules represent cutaneous deposits of ovarian carcinoma

   • *Cullen's sign* (periumbilical echymosis seen in chronic ectopic pregnancy) represents intra-peritoneal bleed

2. *Palpation*　The clinician should be standing on the right side of the patient, looting for hepatosplenomegaly and for any pelvic mass. In a pelvic mass upper and lateral margins can be felt, but the lower border cannot be reached.

   A *suprapubic lump* could be due to

   a) *Pregnancy* should be always kept in mind. Cervix appears bluish in pregnancy and the uterus feels soft.

   b) A *full bladder* may be distended upto the umbilicus if there is any mechanical obstruction to urine flow. Patient should always be asked to empty her bladder before examination. If she cannot empty her bladder, a catheter needs to be passed before examination.

   c) *Uterine neoplasms*　Uterine neoplasms are situated in the midline, with mobility restricted from side to side only. The causes of uterine enlargement are given in table 3.2.

Table 3.2. Causes of uterine enlargement

Benign	Malignant
Fibroid uterus	Endometrial carcinoma
Adenomyosis	Leiomyosarcoma

   d) *Ovarian neoplasms* These swellings are usually in one of the iliac regions, may be freely mobile, consistency may be fluctuant or firm to hard. The commonest cystic ovarian neoplasm is a dermoid cyst.

   e) *Tubo-ovarian mass (TO mass)* Seen in ectopic pregnancy or pelvic inflammatory disease. In chronic ectopic pregnancy, bleeding can occur into the peritoneal tissues and form adhesions with peritubal structures mimicking a pelvic tumour. Chronic PID may be associated with a hydro or pyosalpinx and present as a pelvic mass.

f)   *Haematometra and haematocolpos* Collection of blood within the uterine cavity due to a mechanical block in the cervix or vagina. This could be due to—Imperforate hymen (failure of canalization of the urogenital membrane) or Vaginal atresia (congenital aplasia of the vagina).

3.   *Percussion*   Large ovarian cysts occupy the peritoneal cavity, are dull to percussion, but the flanks are resonant (Fig. 3.1). Dullness in the flanks which shifts indicates the presence of free fluid in the peritoneal cavity or ascites; as seen in tuberculous peritonitis or ovarian malignancy.

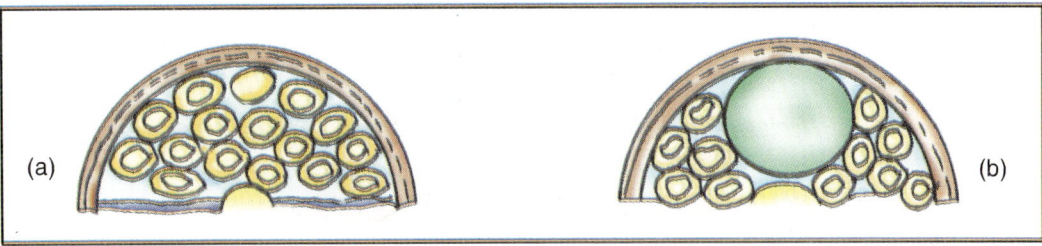

(a)   (b)

Fig. 3.1ab.   Differentiation of ascites and ovarian cyst on percussion (a) Ascites–dullness in the flanks, centre resonant, (b) Ovarian cyst–dullness in the centre, flanks resonant

4.   *Auscultation*   The points to be noted on auscultation are:

•   Bowel sounds–absence indicates peritonitis or paralytic ileus, exaggerated indicates bowel obstruction.

•   Souffle over a tumour indicates its vascularity. Uterine souffle is heard in pregnancy and large fibroids.

Pelvic examination

Includes examination of the external genitalia, bimanual and rectal examination. The prerequisites are a good light, a chaperone, gloves, and lubricant jelly.

1.   *Examination of the external genitalia*   The vulva is inspected for

•   Distribution of pubic hair

•   Any redness or swelling in the labia majora eg. bartholin's cyst is seen at the junction of anterior 2/3 and posterior 1/3 of labia majora.

•   Any prolapse or genital descent.

2.   *Speculum examination*   For visual inspection of the cervix and vagina. Two types of specula are available (Fig. 3.2).

(a) The Cuscoe's self retaining speculum facilitates taking a pap smear, collecting vaginal discharge from the posterior fornix for hanging drop/KOH, or for colposcopic examination.

(b) The Sims vaginal speculum requires an assistant to hold, is good for assessment of uterovaginal prolapse and for examination of vesicovaginal fistulas.

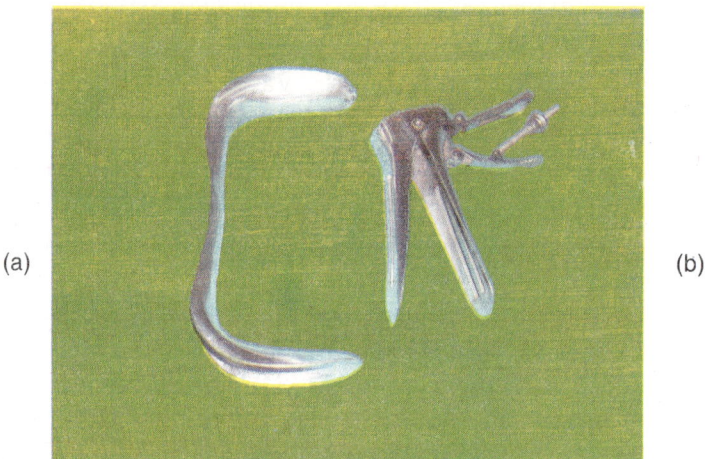

(a)   (b)

Fig. 3.2.   Types of vaginal speculum   (a) Sims speculum, (b) Cuscoe's speculum

3. *Bimanual examination*

The labia-minora are separated with the thumb and index fingers of the left hand. Two fingers (index and middle fingers) of the right hand are introduced (after lubrication) through the vaginal introitus. The direction of cervix and its consistency are noted, The cervix is then moved from side to side to see if it causes pain (*cervical excitation*) eg. ectopic pregnancy and acute PID.

The examining fingers now lift up the uterus which is brought within the reach of the abdominal hand for assessing its position, size, shape, mobility, or tenderness (Fig. 3.3a).

The tips of the examining fingers of the right hand are then introduced into the lateral fornices with the abdominal hand in the iliac fossae to feel for any adnexal mass (Fig. 3.3b). Normally the ovaries are not palpable.

The Pouch of Douglas (POD) is then examined, swellings in the POD could be due to a loaded rectum (commonest), a retroverted uterus, ovarian tumours, endometriotic nodules or secondaries from ovarian tumours.

4. *Rectal examination* is indicated in

• virgins for bimanual assessment of pelvic structures.

• carcinoma cervix to determine the extent of parametrial involvement.

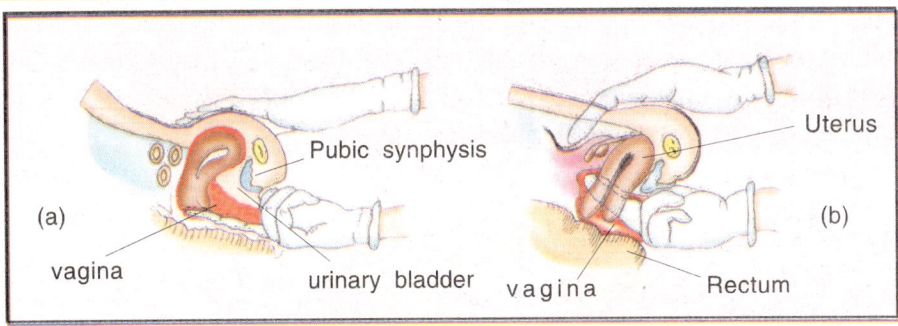

Fig. 3.3. Bimanual pelvic examination (a) Assessment of the uterine size, (b) Assessment of the adnexae

The points to be noted in the history and examination are given in table 3.3.

Table 3.3. Evaluation of a gynaecological patient

History	Examination
Presenting complaints	General condition
Menstrual history	Height and weight
Obstetric history	Pallor & icterus, edema, lymphadenopathy
Past medical history	Examination of breasts
Past surgical history	Thyomegaly
Family history	Abdominal examination
Personal history	Per-speculum examination
Drug history	Bimanual examination
History of allergies	Rectal examination

INVESTIGATIONS

General investigations These tests are carried out to determine the patient's fitness for surgery or to provide a baseline for future comparison. They include

1. *Full blood count* which includes haemoglobin percentage, total and differential white cell count.

2. *Urinalysis* Urine is tested for albumin, sugar and microscopy carried out for red cells, epithelial cells, casts and crystals. Urine culture is indicated if urine microscopy reveals >5 pus cells/hpf, or in women with urinary complaints.

3. *Blood sugar* A random blood sugar of <180mg/dl is taken as normal. Fasting and postprandial blood sugars are necessary in patient >40 yrs. old, or if the patient is known to be a diabetic or the random blood sugar value is ≥180mg/dl

4. *Blood urea and serum creatinine* to know the renal function.

5. *Liver function tests* serum bilirubin, amino-transferase and alkaline phosphatase levels are indicated in women with a previous history of jaundice and all women with malignancies of the genital tract.

6. *Hepatitis B surface antigen (HBsAg), HIV I and II* A patient who tests positive is potentially infectious. Special care needs to be taken by the health care professionals in the wards and operating theatres.

7. *Chest x-ray* Previous pulmonary kochs, chronic obstructive pulmonary disease (COPD) can be picked up.

8. *ECG* is indicated in women >50yrs. of age as undiagnosed angina may be present.

9. *Blood group and Rh type* for booking and cross-matching blood prior to surgery.

The investigations are summarized in table 3.4.

Table 3.4. Investigations in a gynae patient	
General –	Full blood count
	Urinalysis
	Blood sugar
	Blood urea and serum creatinine
	Liver function tests
	Chest x-ray
	ECG
	Blood group and Rh type
	HBsAg and HIV (in selected cases)
Specific –	Pap smear
	Colposcopy
	X-ray abdomen and pelvis
	Ultrasonography
	HSG
	CT scan
	MRI

Specific Investigations

Depend upon the underlying symptom. The investigations routinely carried out are:

1. Cervical cytology

The use of exfoliative cytology for screening of cervical cancer was introduced in 1928 by Papanicolau in New York and Babes in Bucharest. The use of cervical screening programmes has significantly reduced the mortality of cervical cancer in western countries. Exfoliative cytology of the cervix is indicated in all women of reproductive age between 20-60 yrs.

Taking a smear: The accuracy of the smear depends on the quality of material collected, the preparation of the smear and the stains used.

• Instruments needed (Fig. 3.4) Cuscoe's speculum and Ayre's or modified Aylesbury spatula. The cytobrush, though not a part of routine screening, is useful in post-menopausal women or when an endocervical lesion is suspected.

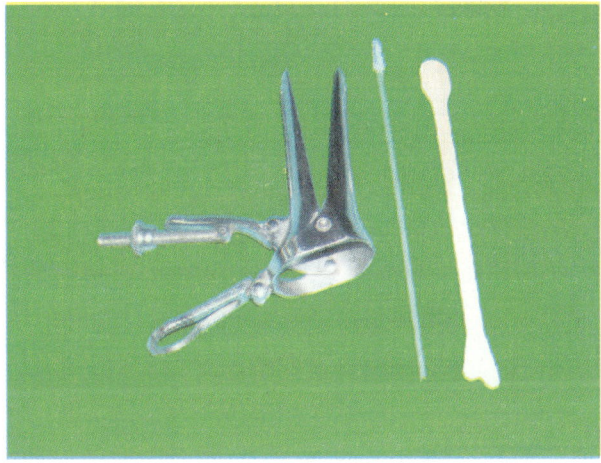

Fig. 3.4. Instruments for taking a pap smear (a) Cuscoe's speculum, (b) Cytobrush and (c) Ayre's spatula

• The spatula is applied to the external os with the long end inside the os and rotated 360° with the spatula firmly applied to the cervix. The endocervical brush is introduced into the canal until only the last row of bristles is just visible at the external os and then rotated through 180° only.

• The smear is made by spreading the sampler swiftly on a clean, pre-labelled glass slide. The cytobrush is rolled on to the slide with a firm rolling motion.

• The smear is fixed with formalin either dipped in solution or sprayed with cytospray.

Interpretation of cervical smears: The smear may be reported as Normal, Dyskaryotic or Inflammatory (Fig 3.5a-d).

1. Normal: A normal smear contains squamous cells shed from the ectocervix and some endocervical cells. The normal squamous cell has a small pyknotic nucleus and uniform cytoplasm.

2. Dyskaryosis: This is the cytological nuclear change associated with a histological diagnosis of cervical dysplasia (Cervical Intra-epithelial Neoplasia–CIN). The nuclear-cytoplasmic

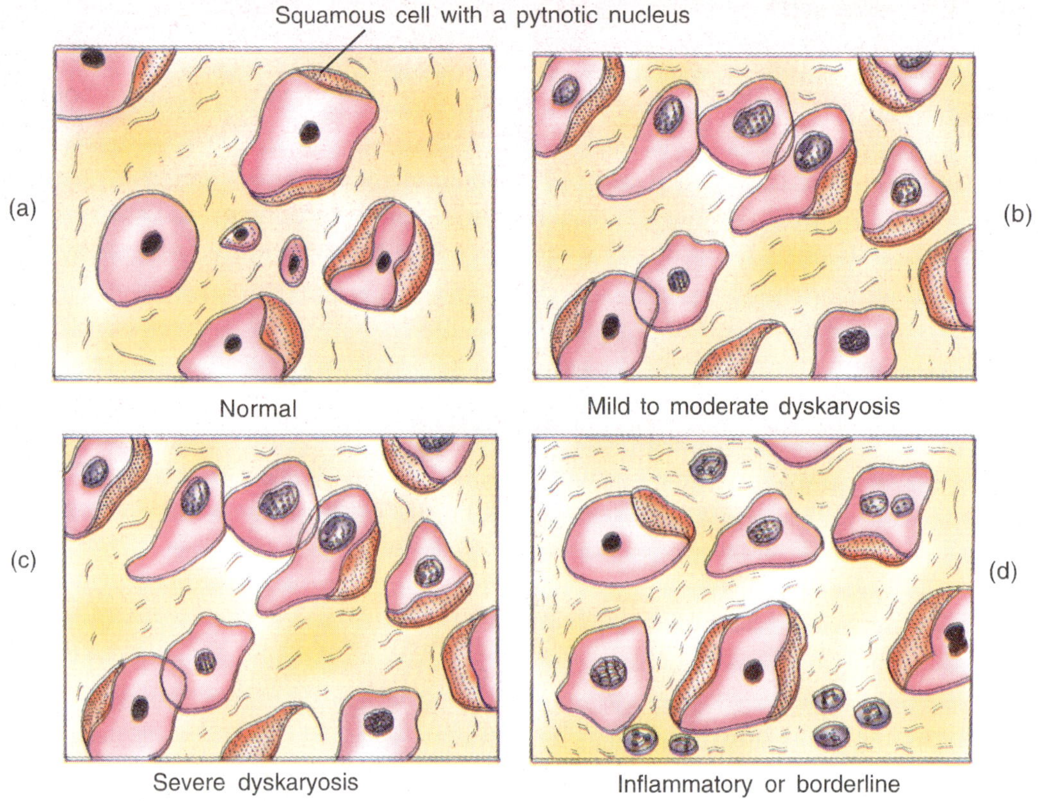

Squamous cell with a pytnotic nucleus

(a)   (b)

Normal   Mild to moderate dyskaryosis

(c)   (d)

Severe dyskaryosis   Inflammatory or borderline

Fig. 3.5a-d. Interpretation of cervical smears

ratio is increased corresponding to the severity of dysplasia of the squamous epithelium. Mild dyskaryosis usually corresponds to mild dysplasia; moderate to severe dyskaryosis indicates severe dysplasia.

3. Inflammatory: Trichomonas vaginalis, candida, actinomyces can cause changes in the cervical cells, which can be recognized by an experienced cytologist. They are considered as negative for dysplasia.

Late follicular phase
2. Colposcopy

The colposcope (Fig. 3.6) is a system which allows both magnification and illumination of the cervix. It was first introduced in 1925 by Hans Hinselmann. The magnification range is between 6 and 40 fold. The focal length varies between 200-300 mm. A green filter is usually provided with the standard colposcope which allows better definition of vascular architecture, as the green light absorbs the red colour of the blood vessels, which then appear black and prominent.

The colposcopic examination: With the patient comfortably lying on a couch, the cervix is exposed with a bi-valved cuscoe's speculum. A cervical smear if required is taken at this stage. Excess mucus is gently removed with a saline-soaked cotton wool ball. Acetic

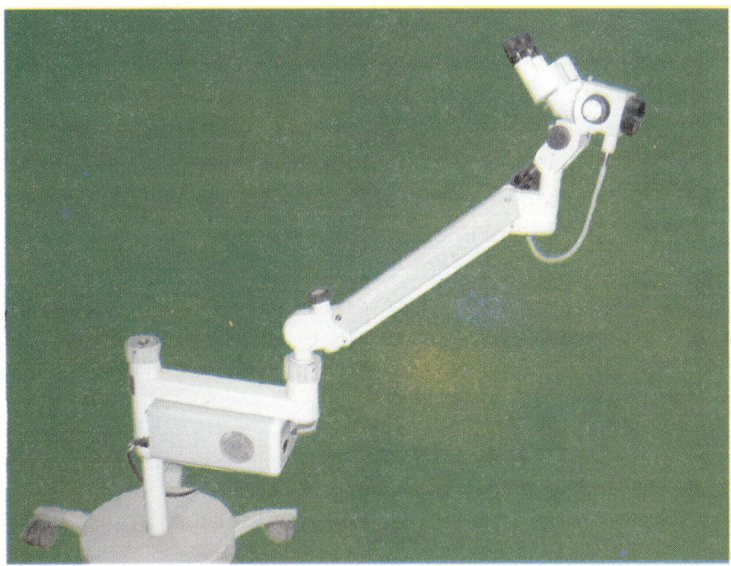

Fig. 3.6. The Colposcope

acid (3-5%) is gently applied to the cervix and upper vagina and left in-situ for 5-10 seconds. The acetic acid causes the columnar and abnormal squamous epithelium to appear white (acetowhite) and is easily distinguishable from the normal pink squamous epithelium. The cervix is next painted with Lugol's iodine. The types of appearances are

- Normal squamous epithelium contains glycogen and takes up the stain.
- Atypical squamous epithelium has no glycogen, does not take up the stain and appears iodine negative. The findings on colposcopy are documented with a diagram, or saved using a computer generated software attached with a camera to the colposcope.

Types of epithelium: An understanding of the colposcopic appearances is based on a thorough understanding of the anatomy and histology. The cervix has two fundamental types of epithelium, columnar and squamous meeting each other in an abrupt fashion at the original squamocolumnar (OSCJ) junction. Normally, the OSCJ is situated at the external os. The types of epithelium which can be seen are:

1. *Columnar epithelium:* This appears red to the unaided eye as the epithelium is very thin and the blood vessels give the villi a red colour. On colposcopic examination, this epithelium appears 'grapelike'.

2. *Squamous epithelium:* Two types of squamous epithelium may be recognized, the original squamous epithelium and the transformed or metaplastic squamous epithelium. The original squamous epithelium is formed during fetal development, covers a variable part of the ectocervix and is similar to the squamous epithelium of the vagina. On colposcopy, it appears pale pink in colour. Metaplastic squamous epithelium appears pale pink with openings of glands.

3. *Metaplastic squamous epithelium:* The squamocolumnar junction (SCJ) of the cervix is the point at which the endocervical columnar epithelium meets the ectocervical stratified squamous epithelium. Before puberty, the SCJ is located at or close to the external os of the cervix. Under the influence of increasing ovarian hormones, there is an increase in the size of the corpus and cervix which leads to eversion of the cervix. This is more marked anteriorly and posteriorly, the endocervical epithelium then comes to lie on the vaginal portion of the cervix. This zone of eversion is exposed to the acidic environment of the vagina, and changes to squamous epithelium by a process of squamous metaplasia. Thus, the *transformation zone* is an area of variable width and configuration lying between the columnar epithelium and the original squamous epithelium. This area contains areas of columnar epithelium and metaplastic squamous epithelium at various stages of maturity.

Cervical intraepithelial neoplasia (CIN) indicates abnormalities in the squamous epithelium which could be pre-malignant CIN is graded as I, II & III based on the thickness of epithelium involved as shown in Fig. 3.7a-d. Nuclear abnormalities are the most impor-

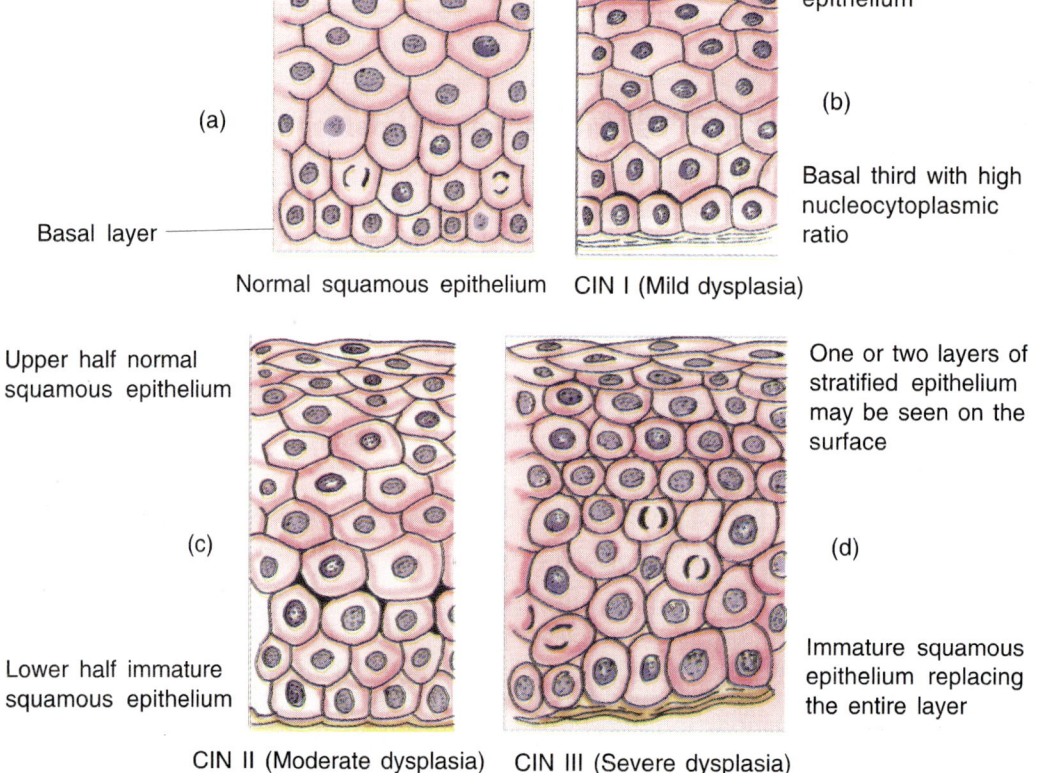

Squames at surface

Basal layer

Normal squamous epithelium   CIN I (Mild dysplasia)

Upper two thirds normal squamous epithelium

Basal third with high nucleocytoplasmic ratio

(a)   (b)

Upper half normal squamous epithelium

Lower half immature squamous epithelium

CIN II (Moderate dysplasia)   CIN III (Severe dysplasia)

One or two layers of stratified epithelium may be seen on the surface

Immature squamous epithelium replacing the entire layer

(c)   (d)

Fig. 3.7a-d.   (a) Normal squamous epithelium and (b-d) CIN I-III

tant factor in diagnosis, the nuclei become large hyperchromatic and show mitotic figures which is revealed in a pap smear.

Abnormal colposcopic appearances

1. Acetowhite epithelium: This is a transient phenomenon seen after application of acetic acid due to increased nuclear density, seen in CIN, HPV infection and dysplasia of the cervix.

2. Abnormal vascular pattern: The types of vessel patterns seen are

   • Mosaic–The capillaries appear parallel to the surface giving a *'crazy-pavement'* pattern and forming a mosaic.

   • Punctation–The stromal capillaries produce a stippled or punctate appearance within the epithelium.

   • Atypical vessels–The vessels are arranged in a haphazard way and demonstrate gross variation in calibre and branching.

3. Imaging of the genital tract

The types of imaging used to make a gynaecological diagnosis are:

• X-rays–plain and contrast enhanced
• Ultrasonography
• Computerised Axial Tomography (CAT Scan)
• Magnetic Resonance Imaging (MRI)

X-rays: Any x-rays in a woman of reproductive age should be performed within 10 days of her menstrual cycle. An x-ray of the pelvis is useful in–

• Locating a missing IUCD, to note calcifications in a dermoid cyst (Fig. 3.8).

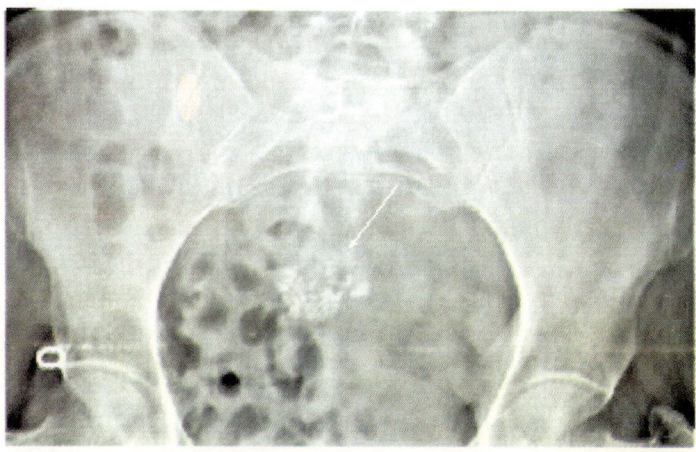

Fig. 3.8. X-ray pelvis showing calcifications in a dermoid cyst (courtesy: Mahajan Imaging centre)

- Hysterosalpingography: A radiographic contrast study of the uterine and tubal anatomy.

Hysterosalpingography

Indications

- To check tubal patency in patients with infertility
- To diagnose uterine anomalies
- To diagnose cervical incompetence

Technique

The procedure is done within 10 days of the menstrual cycle due to the fear of dislodging a fertilized ovum. An antispasmodic is given prior to the procedure to prevent tubal spasm. The patient is then asked to empty her bladder. She is placed in a dorsal position with buttocks at the edge of the table. The vulva and vagina are thoroughly cleaned with an antiseptic solution. A bimanual examination is performed to note the position of the uterus. A posterior vaginal speculum is introduced, the anterior lip of the cervix is held by an allis tissue holding forceps and a uterine sound is passed to note the length of the uterocervical canal. A water soluble radio-opaque dye (50% di-iodine with 6% polyvinyl alcohol in water) is then taken into a 20cc syringe. A Leish-wilkinson's cannula filled with the dye is introduced into the os and the dye pushed in slowly into the uterine cavity. The dye enters the uterus and spills out through both fallopian tubes. The passage of the dye is observed under fluoroscopy and a maximum of three films are taken. Normal fallopian tubes are seen as thin lines with spillage into the peritoneal cavity through the tubal ostia (Fig. 3.9). Fig. 3.10 shows hydrosalpinx.

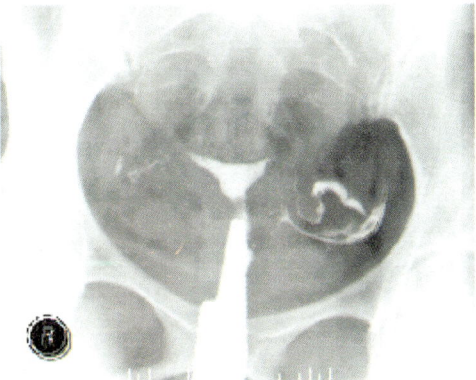

Fig. 3.9. HSG showing normal tubes with peritoneal spillage

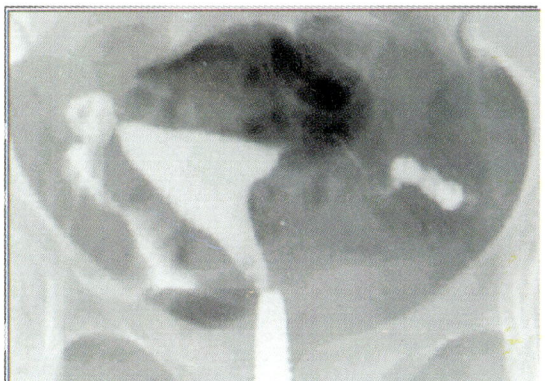

Fig. 3.10. HSG showing left hydrosalpinx (courtesy: Mahajan Imaging centre)

Complications

- Vasovagal syncope
- Peritoneal irritation and pelvic pain

- Flaring up of pelvic infection

- Intravasation of dye into the venous and lymphatic channels

- Allergic reaction to the dye

Ultrasound

The basics of ultrasound: Ultrasound waves are generated by a piezoelectric crystal mounted in a transducer, the whole construction being referred to as a *probe*. Peizo materials respond to an applied voltage by changing thickness and correspondingly, produce electrical signals of a few millivolts when compressed. The ultrasound pulse is then transmitted into the tissues and reflected back as an echo at an interface between tissues of different acoustic impedance. Homogenous materials such as clear fluids are echo free; low level echoes result from an interface between fibrous tissue (high impedance) and fatty tissue (low impedance); maximal echoes are given by interfaces between soft tissues and bone or gas, both of which are opaque to ultrasound. The choice of frequency of the probe is a compromise between the spatial resolution and the depth of penetration required. With higher frequencies, the resolution improves, but the depth of penetration is compromised. The frequency of the probe used for transabdominal (TA) scanning is 3.5 MHz and 5 MHz to 7 MHz for transvaginal scanning.

4D ultrasound (Fig. 3.11a) provides better resolution with 3 dimensional images obtained in real time. *Tomographic ultrasound imaging* (TUI) (Fig. 3.11b-c) (Fig. 3.12a-c) is a new development in ultrasound providing thin sections through the tissues; small lesions missed on conventional ultrasound can be picked up by this technique.

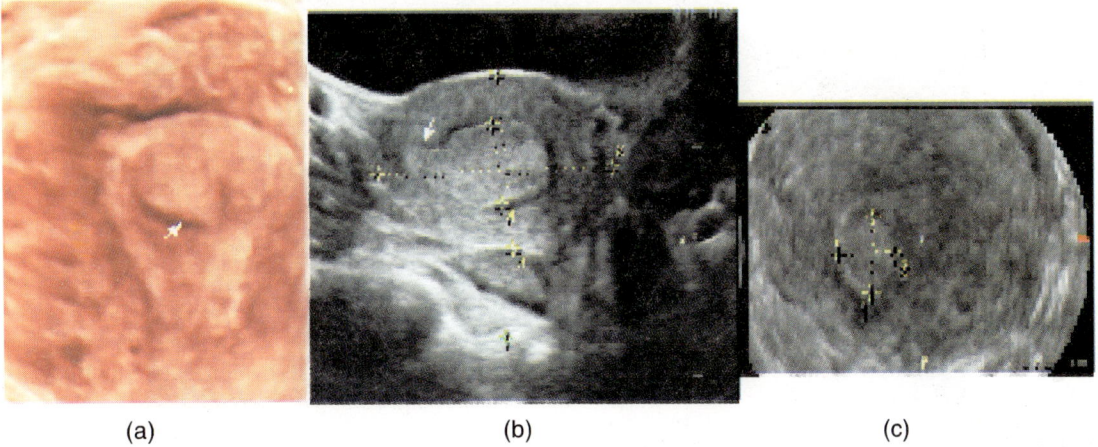

(a) (b) (c)

Fig. 3.11a-c. (a) Coronal section of an endometrial polyp on 4D ultrasound, (b-c) Tomographic ultrasound imaging (TUI) showing coronal section through the uterus with an endometrial polyp (courtesy: Mahajan Imaging centre)

Doppler ultrasound: Doppler operates by detecting a change in the frequency of ultrasound echoes caused by movement of the target. Doppler is used for fetal heart monitoring and to measure blood flow in pelvic vessels. In colour doppler the velocity signals are presented as a colour-coded overlay, superimposed on the real-time scan. An angiogram like map is provided which provides information on the morphological arrangement of the vascular tree.

Uses of ultrasound: The ultrasound has become an extension of the clinical examination though it should not be used as a replacement. It is indicated;

• For diagnosis of early pregnancy

• Differential diagnosis of a pelvic mass

• Diagnosis of ectopic pregnancy

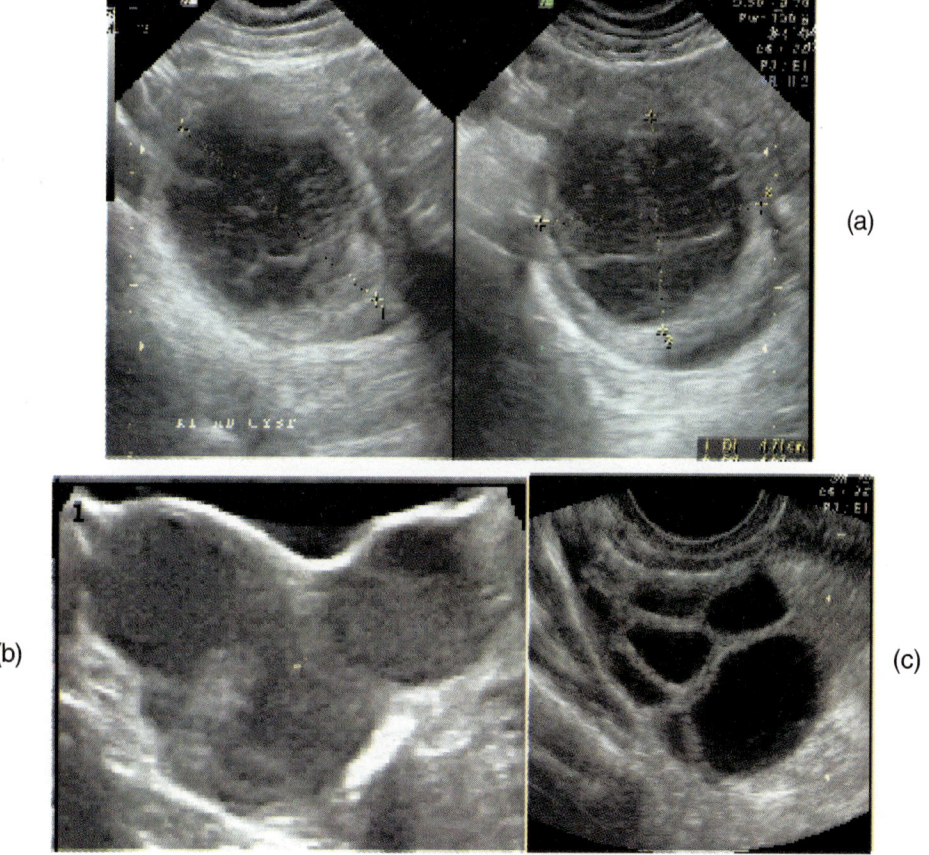

Fig. 3.12a-c. TUI pictures showing (a) ovarian cystadenoma with multiple loculations and internal echoes, (b) coronal section of the pelvis with an endometriotic cyst (Note the increased echogenicity due to haemorrhage), (c) hyperstimulated ovaries with multiple follicles (courtesy: Mahajan Imaging centre)

- Differential diagnosis of primary and secondary amenorrhoea
- Locating a 'missing' intrauterine contraceptive device
- Staging of cervical, ovarian and endometrial carcinoma
- Diagnosis of deep vein thrombosis (doppler ultrasound is used for this).

Computed Tomography (Fig. 3.13)

The attenuation of a finely collimated beam of radiation passing through the patient at multiple angles produces images of high quality. Though not used as a routine investigation, it is useful in

- Differential diagnosis of a pelvic mass, when ultrasound has not been helpful
- Carcinoma ovary with massive ascites–to look for omental caking and retroperitoneal lymph nodes

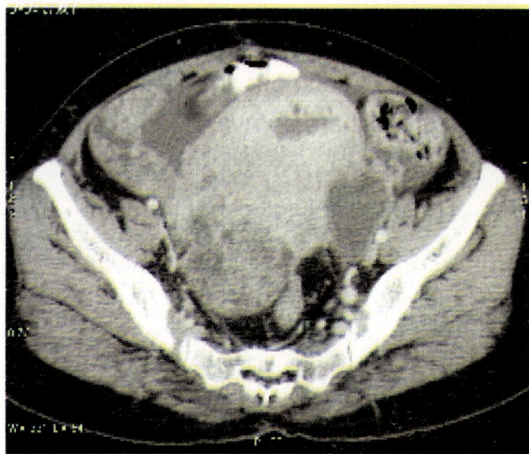

Fig. 3.13.   CT scan of the pelvis showing a large ovarian tumour (courtesy: Mahajan Imaging centre)

Magnetic Resonance Imaging (MRI)

MRI scan is a radiology technique that uses magnetism, radio waves, and a computer to produce images of body structures. The MRI scanner is a tube surrounded by a giant circular magnet. The patient is placed on a moveable bed which is inserted into the magnet. The magnet creates a strong magnetic field which aligns the protons of hydrogen atoms in the body, and they produce a faint signal that is detected by the receiver position of the MRI scanner. The receiver information is processed by a computer, and an image is then produced. The image and resolution produced by MRI is quite detailed and can detect tiny changes of structures within the body. Contrast agents such as gadolinium can be used to increase the accuracy of images. While CT provides good spatial resolution (ability to distinguish two structures at small distances from each other as separate), MRI provides comparable resolution (the ability to distinguish the differences between two arbitrarily similar, but not identical tissues)

MRI scanning is painless and does not involve x-ray radiation. Patients with cardiac pacemakers, metal implants cannot be scanned with MRI because of the effect of the magnet. However, claustrophobic sensation can occur with MRI scanning.

MRI is commonly used for the brain, it provides valuable information on glands and organs in the abdomen and pelvis (Fig 3.14a-c).

MRI is useful in gynaecology, mainly for staging of malignancies.

(a1) 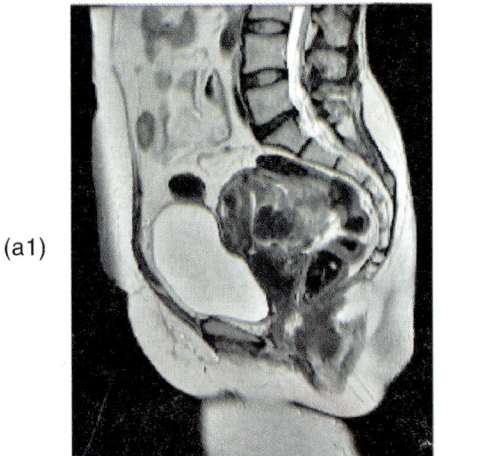 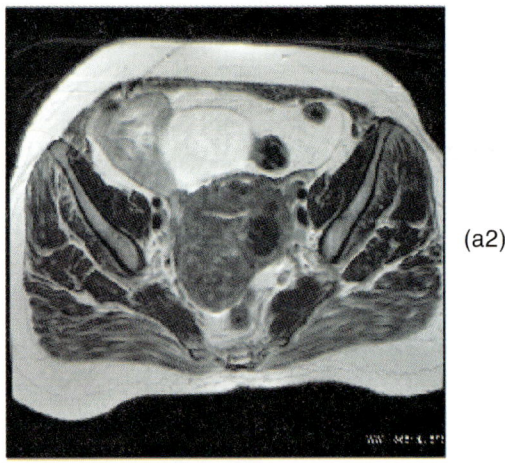 (a2)

Fig. 3.14a1-a2 MRI showing a sagittal and coronal sections of an enlarged uterus with a large posterior wall fibroid, smaller fibroids are seen on the anterior wall (courtesy: Mahajan Imaging centre)

(b) 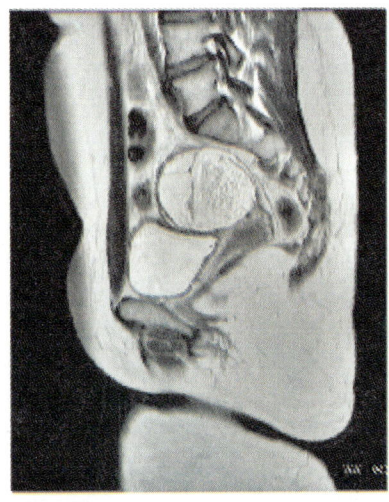 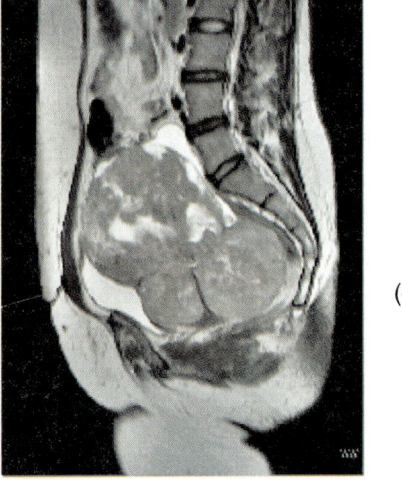 (c)

Fig. 3.14bc.   (b) MRI showing a dermoid cyst (c) sagittal section of the pelvis with large solid ovarian tumour (Note the compression and displacement of the bladder by the mass) (courtesy: Mahajan Imaging centre)

Section II

Benign disorders from Puberty to Menopause

4

The Female Reproductive Tract–Development and Congenital Anomalies

The female genital tract consists of the external genitalia, the reproductive tract and the ovaries. Embryologically these three differ in their origin and anomalies of the reproductive tract may not be associated with anomalies of ovaries and external genitalia. Reproductive tract comprises of the fallopian tubes, the uterus, cervix and the vagina.

DEVELOPMENT OF THE REPRODUCTIVE TRACT

The reproductive tract develops from the *mullerian* or the *paramesonephric* duct. The mullerian duct appears at about 37 days after fertilization just lateral to each wolffian duct, as an invagination of the dorsal coelomic epithelium (Fig. 4.1a). The two mullerian ducts grow caudally and fuse in the midline at the middle and caudal end to form the uterus and the upper part of the vagina. The free cranial end of the mullerian ducts form the fallopian tubes (Fig. 4.1b).

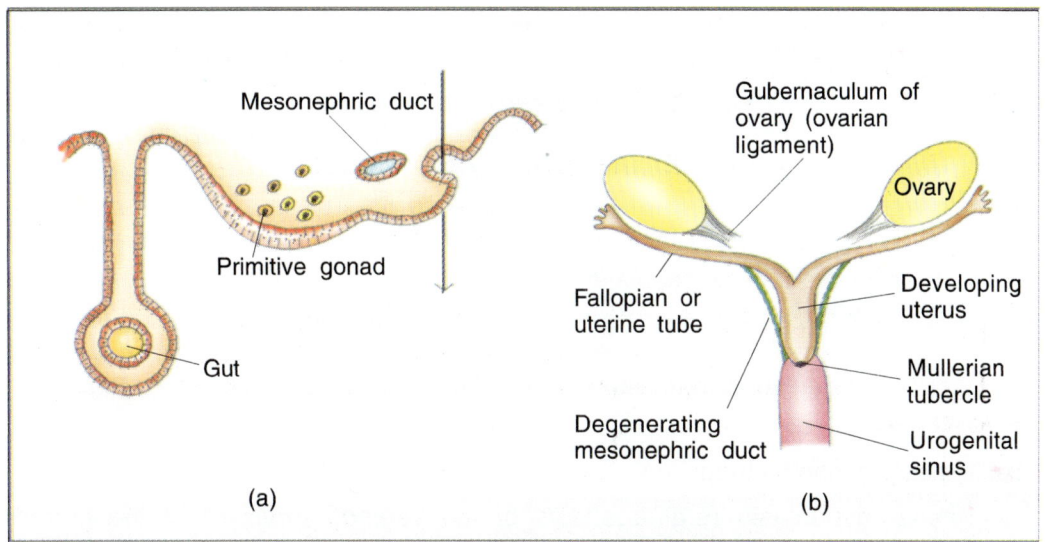

Fig. 4.1a-b. Development of the reproductive tract

The septum between the two fused mullerian ducts gradually disappears leaving a single uterovaginal canal. Failure of fusion of the two ducts results in varying degrees of double uterus; a complete failure resulting in **uterus didelphus,** failure of resorption of the septum between the two fused mullerian ducts results in a **septate uterus**.

The lower part of the vagina has a different origin from the vaginal plate of the urogenital sinus and joins the upper part derived from the mullerian duct (Fig. 4.2). A **transverse vaginal septum** can be present at the junction of the vagina developed from the caudal end of the fused mullerian ducts and the lower vagina developed from vaginal plate of the urogenital sinus. A large segment of the vagina may be atretic if the tissue between the caudal part of mullerian duct and vaginal plate is not absorbed or if fusion between the two components of vagina does not occur.

The hymen is not derived from the mullerian ducts. The distal portion of the sinovaginal bulbs proliferate to form the hymen, which becomes perforate before birth.

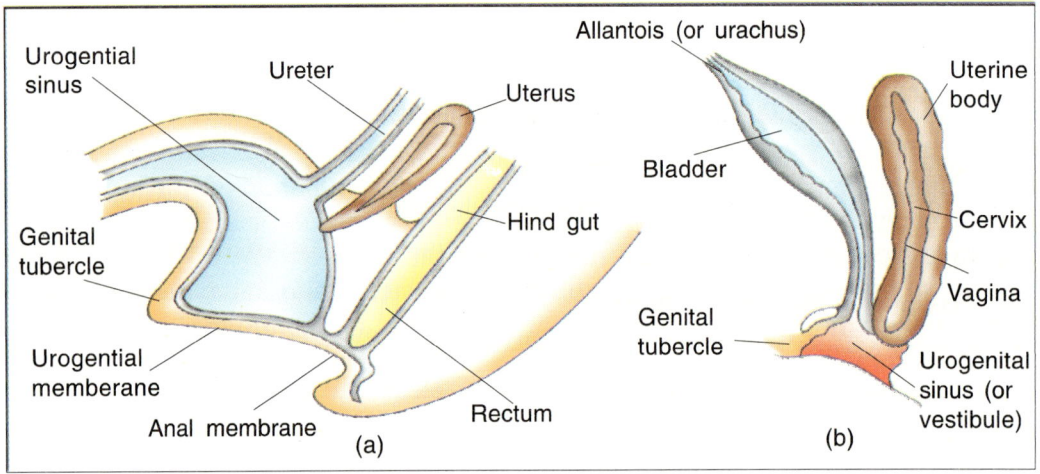

Fig. 4.2ab. Development of the vagina

MULLERIAN DUCT ANOMALIES

Incidence

- Seen in 1-3% of the female population
- Seen in 10% of women with recurrent pregnancy loss or infertility

Classification
Congenital anomalies of reproductive organs have been classified in various ways.

a) A basic classification includes

1. Agenesis / hypoplasia (e.g. agenesis of the vagina, cervix or of the complete reproductive duct)

2. Vertical fusion or canalization defects (e.g. transverse vaginal septum)

3. Lateral fusion defects (e.g. double or septate uterus)

b) American fertility society (AFS) classification of mullerian anomalies is given in table 4.1. A modification of this classification is sometimes used to describe these anomalies.

Table 4.1. AFS Classification of mullerian anomalies	
Class I	**Segmental mullerian agenesis/Hypoplasia** • Vaginal • Cervical • Fundal • Tubal • Combined anomalies

Class II	**Unicornuate uterus**
	• With rudimentary horn
	   – Communicating with endometrial cavity
	   – Non-communicating
	• Without rudimentary horn

Class III	**Uterus didelphus**
Class IV	**Bicornuate uterus** • Complete (division down to the internal os) • Partial
Class V	**Septate uterus** • Complete (septum upto the internal os) • Partial
Class VI	**Arcuate uterus**
Class VII	**Diethylstilbesterol related anomalies**

AFS Class I–Segmental mullerian agencies (Fig. 4.3)

This can be of three different types:

1. Congenital absence of the vagina and uterus with normal ovaries (*Mayer-Rokitansky-Kuster-Hauser syndrome*)

2. Transverse vaginal septum

3. Congenital absence or dysgenesis of the cervix

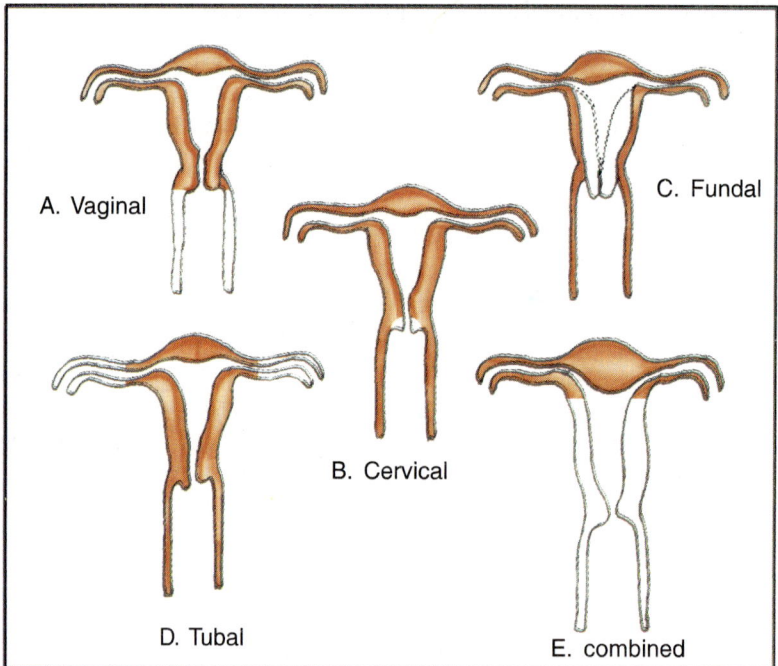

Fig. 4.3a-e.   AFS-Class I–Segmental Mullerian agencies

1. ***Congenital absence of vagina and uterus with normal ovaries (Mayer-Rokitansky-Kuster-Hauser syndrome)***

   - It is reported to occur in 1 in 4000 to 5000 females and is a common cause of primary amenorrhoea.
   - It may be associated with a variety of genetic, endocrine and other body systems anomalies.
   - Skeletal abnormalities are associated in approximately 12%, and urological in about 47%.
   - Chromosomal pattern is normal (46 XX) and secondary sex characters develop normally but menstruation does not occur.
   - Ovarian function including ovulation is present.
   - Fallopian tubes and rarely rudimentary uterine bulbs may be present.

   Management

   - Careful evaluation and counselling needed.
   - Thorough check-up and investigations including chromosomal analysis or buccal smear for chromatin body should be done to exclude chromosomal anomalies.
   - Tests to exclude other associated anomalies especially of the renal system are to

be performed. Ultrasound of pelvis and abdomen gives valuable information in this regard.

- Counselling is necessary, she should be explained that though ovulation is occurring, she cannot bear children as the uterus is not developed.

- Adoption or having conception in a surrogate mother is an option and should be explained to the patient. Vaginoplasty is carried out to establish coital function.

Vaginoplasty

1. *Non surgical technique*: Manual dilatation of the vagina.

   Frank described a non-surgical technique of vaginoplasty with good results. The patient is asked to apply manual pressure to the fourchette with a dilator twice a day for 15 min. Ingram (1981) advocated wearing of a small mould and sitting astride a special stool designed like a bicycle seat. Reasonable results have been reported with this method (Frank 1936, Dewhurst 1987).

2. *Mc-Indoe operation*

   - A transverse incision is given over the mucosa of the vaginal vestibule just behind the urethra, a space is created by blunt and sharp dissection between the bladder in front and the rectum behind.

   - A foam mould covered with a condom is made, a split skin graft obtained from the thigh or buttocks is sewn over it.

   - This mould is then placed in the neo-vagina for 7-10 days.

   - Once the graft has taken up, the patient is given instructions to remove, clean and re-insert the mould daily.

   - The cavity needs to be kept open with the mould till regular intercourse begins.

   - *Results* The results are excellent in uncomplicated cases and the neo-vagina functions like a normal vagina.

   - *Complications*

     The granulation tissue can cause pain, dyspareunia and leucorrhoea.

     Closure of the vagina due to scar tissue can occur unless persistent and regular dilatation is practised.

     Intra-operative damage to the bladder and rectum: Vesico or recto-vaginal fistula due to the pressure of the solid mould can occur. This can be reduced by using a soft sponge mould.

3. *Williams vulvo-vaginoplasty*

   A perineal pouch using the skin of labia-minora is created. It is a simple technique but the results are less satisfactory as the direction of the vagina is not normal. The advantages include the feasibility of this operation even after failure.

2. Transverse vaginal septum

- Failure of fusion or canalization of the urogenital sinus and the mullerian ducts.
- This is less common than mullerian agenesis.
- Septum may be present in the upper, mid or lower vagina. Upper vagina is involved in approximately 46% of cases, middle vagina in 40% and lower vagina in 14% (Lodi et al).
- Urological and other anomalies are encountered less often as compared to the Rokitansky syndrome but it may be associated with other anomalies like bicornuate uterus and imperforate anus.
- In a neonate *hydrocolpos* may develop leading to pressure effects on the surrounding organs and may require removal.
- A *haematocolpos* may develop after puberty. Sometimes a small tract opens in the septum and menstrual blood may escape.
- With a complete septum blood may collect in the uterus, fallopian tubes or peritoneum and haematocolpos and endometriosis can develop.
- Ultrasound and MRI should be done to locate the level and thickness of the septum.
- *Management:* Incision of the vaginal septum and anastomosis between the lower and upper vagina. Exploratory laparotomy may be necessary to guide a probe through the uterine fundus and cervix to assist in locating a high haematocolpos.

3. Congenital absence or dysgenesis of the cervix

- This is a relatively less common mullerian anomaly, often associated with absence of a part or whole of the cervix.
- When associated with a functioning uterus a haematometra occurs but the vagina does not distend as seen with a high transverse vaginal septum.
- Ultrasonography and MRI along with careful pelvic examination help in diagnosis of this condition.
- In the presence of a functioning uterus, a passage needs to be created through the fibrous tissue between the uterine cavity and vagina with placement of a stent to keep the tract open.
- Pregnancy is unlikely, as the uterovaginal tract closes from constriction by fibrous tissue giving rise to haematometra and sepsis.
- Many authors recommend hysterectomy in patients with functioning uterus and congenital absence of cervix and vagina as this eliminates cryptomenorrhoea,

sepsis, endometriosis and multiple operations. Cases have, however, been reported where a split thickness graft has been placed in the endocervical canal with good result and pregnancies have been reported.

AFS Class II–Unicornuate uterus (Fig. 4.4)

- Development of only one mullerian duct leads to a unicornuate uterus (hemiuterus) with one fallopian tube.

- **Incidence** of unicornuate uterus among all anomalies of mullerian ducts is around 14%. Clinical presentations of unicornuate uterus include infertility, recurrent abortions, intrauterine growth restriction, preterm deliveries and breech presentation.

- Fetal survival in unicornuate uterus is low and has been reported to be about 40%. Abnormal shape, insufficient muscle mass of the uterus, reduced volume of the uterine cavity and inability to expand are responsible for fetal loss.

- Unicornuate uterus, however, is often associated with a rudimentary horn, which may or may not communicate with the fully developed horn (Class IIA and IIB). 90% of the rudimentary horns are non-communicating (Leary et al).

- Haematometra can occur due to the functioning endometrium in a non-communicating rudimentary horn. Severe dysmenorrhoea can occur; cryptomenorrhoea may not be considered a diagnosis as patient continues to menstruate from the normal horn. Retrograde menstruation and pelvic endometriosis may develop if fallopian tubes are patent.

- Pregnancy in the rudimentary horn invariably results in rupture of the horn and has a high mortality.

- An early diagnosis and removal of the non-communicating rudimentary uterine horn with functioning endometrium will maintain the reproductive potential in the woman. The horn is usually connected by a fibromuscular band.

- Laparoscopic resection of the rudimentary uterine horn has been described (Glenn et al). The hospitalization time, the cost and the postoperative pain is less as compared to the classic abdominal approach.

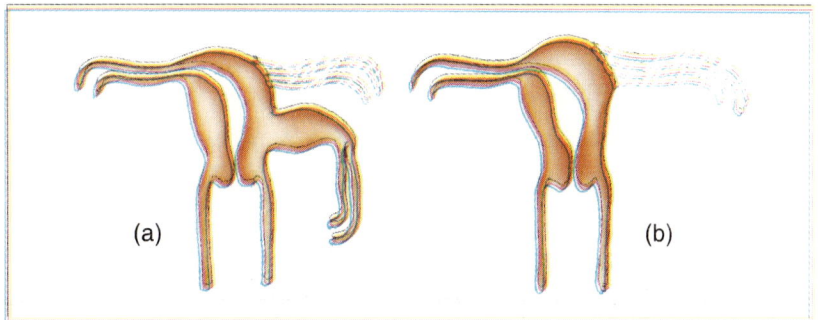

(a)   (b)

Fig. 4.4ab. AFS Class II–Unicornuate uterus (a) With rudimentary horn (b) Without a rudimentary horn

AFS Class III–Didelphus uterus (Fig. 4.5)

- Complete failure of medial fusion of mullerian ducts results in duplication of the vagina, cervix and the uterus.

- *Clinical presentation* includes history of dyspareunia, menorrhagia, abortions, intrauterine growth restriction, breech presentation and preterm births.

- *Diagnosis* can be made on pelvic examination when two vaginal cavities and two cervices can be seen and felt.

- The didelphic uterus has the best possibility of successful pregnancy among all uterine anomalies (except arcuate uterus). A 64% fetal survival is reported without metroplasty (Heinonen), however, the incidence of prematurity, malpresentation, caesarean section and perinatal mortality is higher.

- Unification operation is not advocated in a didelphic uterus as it is technically difficult. Unification of the cervix may lead to stenosis or cervical incompetence. Straussman metroplasty can be performed, however, improvement in reproductive performance has not been observed. A vertical vaginal septum may, however, be removed as it may lead to dyspareunia and difficulty during vaginal delivery.

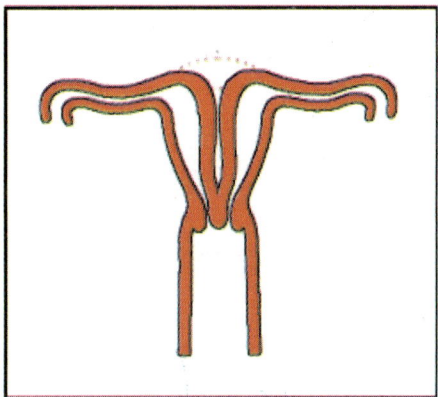

Fig. 4.5. AFS Class III–Didelphus uterus

AFS Class IV–Bicornuate uterus (Fig. 4.6)

- Partial fusion of the two uterine horns give rise to a bicornuate uterus.

- The two uterine cavities may be separate with two cervices (*uterus bicornis bicollis*) or there may be fusion of the two cornua in the lower part resulting in a single cervix (*uterus bicornis unicollis*).

- Bicornuate uterus is often asymptomatic and does not require any surgical treatment. According to Jones and Jones only one third of patients with a double uterus have reproductive problems.

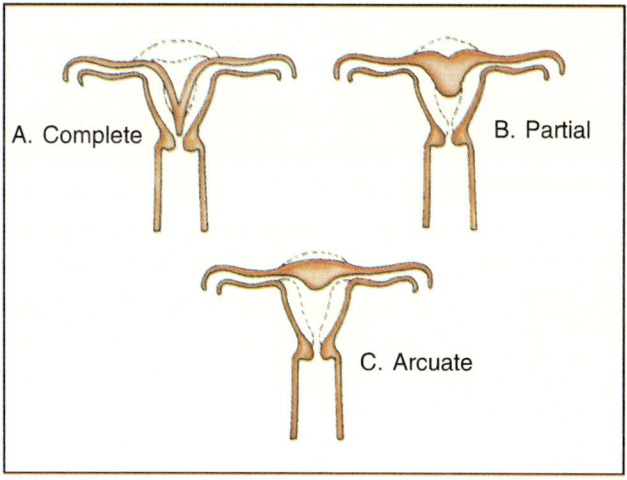

Fig. 4.6a-c. AFS Class IV–Bicornuate uterus

AFS Class V–Septate uterus (Fig. 4.7)

- This results due to failure of absorption of the uterine septum between the two fused mullerian ducts.

- The septum may be *partial* or *complete*. A complete septum may completely divide both the uterine cavity and endocervical canal into two equal or unequal components.

- *Clinical presentation* There may not be any symptoms and the condition may be diagnosed incidentally. A septum may be present in 2-3% of women with a normal reproductive history. Repeated abortions, preterm births (seen in 33%), abnormal fetal lie and an increased incidence of caesarean section are noted with a septate uterus.

- *Diagnosis*
  - Hysterosalpingogram–reveals a linear filling defect in the uterine cavity or two

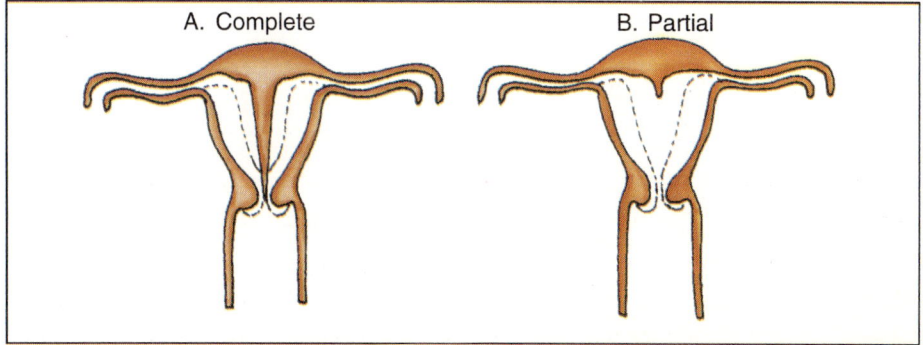

Fig. 4.7ab AFS Class V–Septate uterus

separate uterine cavities. An HSG, however, cannot distinguish between a septate and bicornuate uterus as both show two cavities.

- Hysteroscopy–is definitive and reveals the intrauterine septum.
- Diagnostic laparoscopy reveals the two cornua in a bicornuate uterus and one fundus in a septate uterus.

- *Management* Removal of the septum is indicated for repeated fetal loss if no other cause of habitual abortion can be demonstrated. The septum can be removed by hysteroscopy or by open surgery. The former is more popular. Hysteroscopically the septum is incised with scissors or with an electrosurgical knife, argon laser or Nd: YAG laser. Removal under laparoscopic guidance is associated with lower morbidity and shorter postoperative stay as compared to abdominal metroplasty. Caesarean section is mandatory after abdominal metroplasty. Vaginal delivery can be allowed after hysteroscopic removal of the septum, however there is a risk of uterine rupture.

AFS Class VI–Arcuate uterus

In this condition the fundus of the uterus is either flat or has a shallow concave depression. It is asymptomatic and does not affect the reproductive performance. No treatment is required.

AFS Class VII–Diethystibesterol related anomalies (Fig. 4.8)

Diethylstilbesterol was being used in many countries including USA and UK for abortions, IUGR, pregnancy induced hypertension and preterm labour when it was found that it was responsible for large number of uterine and vaginal defects besides causing

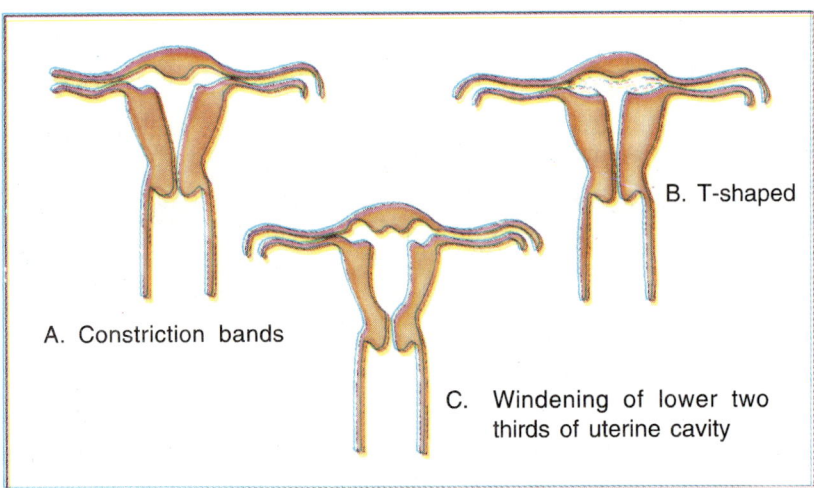

A. Constriction bands

B. T-shaped

C. Windening of lower two thirds of uterine cavity

Fig. 4.8a-c. AFS Class VII–Diethystibesterol related anomalies

malignancies in women exposed in-utero to diethylstilbesterol. 'T' shaped uterus, short uterus and cervix with a small uterine cavity and short and narrow fallopian tubes with absent fimbria are some of the anomalies encountered in women exposed to this drug in-utero.

Imperforate hymen

- Although not being an anomaly of mullerian duct development, deserves special mention due to its clinical importance.

- It is usually detected after the age of puberty.

- *Clinical features*

  - Clinical presentation is by cryptomenorrhoea or 'hidden menstruation' as the menstrual fluid collects above the hymen and gives rise to haematocolpos haematometra and haematosalpinx (Fig. 4.9). There is amenorrhoea and cyclical lower abdominal pain.

  - Patient may present with urinary symptoms like frequency or retention. A full bladder or an enlarged uterus may be palpable per abdomen.

  - On separation of the labia-minora a bluish bulging membrane is visible.

  - Rectal examination reveals a bulge anteriorly. If not treated for long it can lead to haematometra and haematosalpinx.

- *Treatment* is by giving cruciate incisions over the membrane to drain the collected fluid. Quadrants of the hymen are partly excised away from the vaginal mucosa. Vaginal examination should be not done as it may lead to infection.

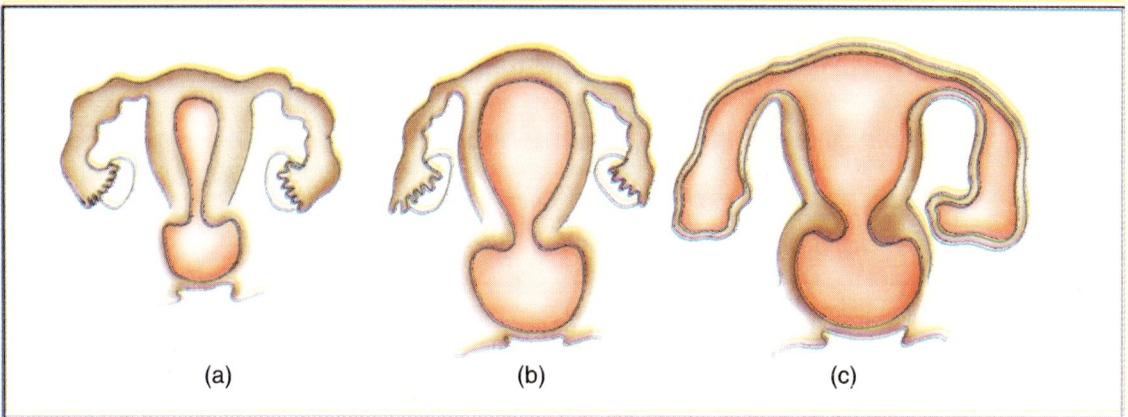

| (a) | (b) | (c) |

Fig. 4.9.   Imperforate hymen with (a) Haematocolpos, (b) Haematocolpos+Haematometra and (c) Haematocolpos+Haematometra+haemato-salpinx

RECURRENT PREGNANCY LOSS AND CONGENITAL UTERINE ANOMALIES

• A woman with three or more spontaneous abortions or premature labour should undergo hysterosalpingography (HSG) to detect if any structural abnormality of uterus is present. In about 10% of such patients an abnormality may be present. In second trimester abortions the incidence of congenital uterine anomalies is higher.

• Complete work-up for recurrent pregnancy loss should be done even if a uterine anomaly is found. Correcting other factors may indeed, correct the problem of reproductive loss without a metroplasty.

5

Sexual Differentiation–
Normal and Abnormal

Sexual differentiation is vital for performing the gender specific role in procreation. Under most circumstances, the assignment of sex in a newborn child is a straightforward issue requiring no specialist consultation. Rarely, infants are born with ambiguous genitalia where a clear-cut sex of rearing cannot be identified and experts have to be called to make a quick diagnosis and assign a sex of rearing.

NORMAL SEXUAL DIFFERENTIATION

Normal sexual differentiation begins with fertilization and culminates in the development of normal internal and external genitalia. Understanding and dealing with these disorders requires application of information in the fields of genetics, embryology, endocrinology and psychiatry.

Knowledge about intersex disorders is essential as–

- There is disfigurement of the genitalia.
- They could be associated with life-threatening emergencies (e.g. CAH with salt-losing crisis) or have a propensity for the development of gonadal tumours when the individual has a Y-bearing cell line.

The orchestrated events that cause normal sexual development are given in Table 5.1.

Table 5.1. Events causing normal sexual development
1.   Establishment of chromosomal (and genetic sex) at fertilization and development of the indifferent gonad
2.   Determination of gonadal sex with differentiation of the indifferent gonad into an ovary or a testis
3.   Sexual differentiation with development of male or female external and internal genitalia

1. **Establishment of chromosomal (and genetic) sex** at fertilization, with XY as male and XX as female. For the first two months of gestation, the two sexes develop in an identical fashion.

2. **Determination of gonadal (primary) sex** by the genetic sex, when the indifferent gonad develops into an ovary or a testis.

3. **Sexual differentiation** with the development of characteristic male or female external and internal genital structures, regulated by the differentiated gonads.

Embryology of sexual differentiation

Establishment of normal genital components involves the development of the internal genital tract and external genitalia.

a) *Internal genital tract* The internal urogenital tracts arise from two sets of ducts, the wolffian and müllerian ducts, present in early embryos of both sexes (Fig. 5.1).

- In females, the müllerian ducts give rise to the fallopian tubes, the uterus, and upper vagina, and the wolffian ducts persist in a vestigial form.

- In males, the wolffian ducts give rise to the epididymis, vasa deferentia, seminal vesicles, and ejaculatory ducts; the müllerian ducts regress.

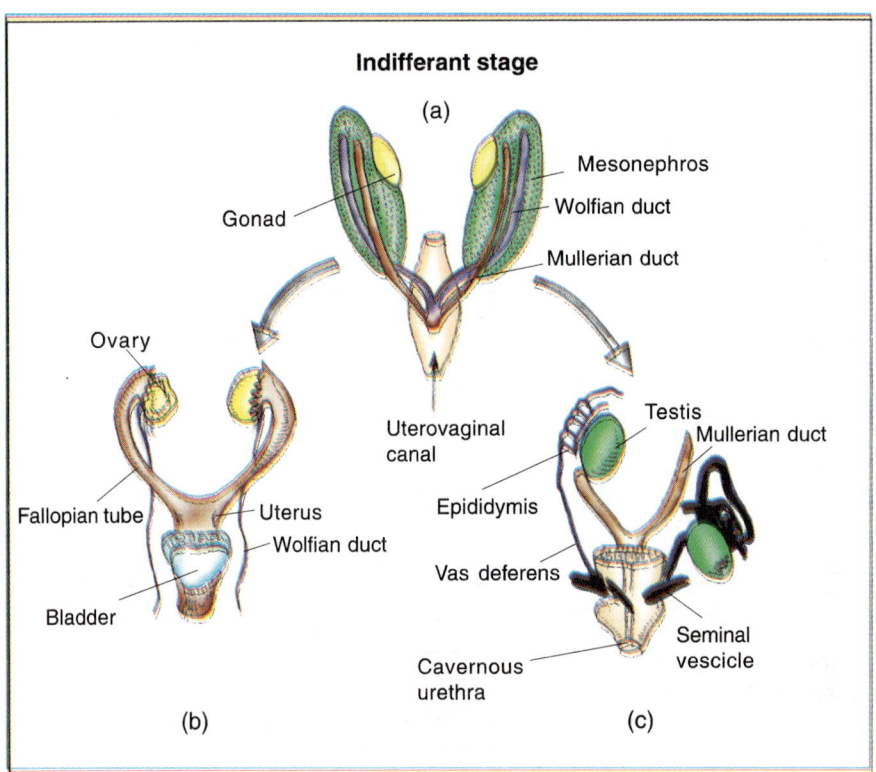

Fig. 5.1.   Differentiation of female and male internal genitalia (a) Indifferant stage (b) Female development (c) Male development

b) *External genitalia* The external genitalia and urethra in the two sexes develop from a common anlagen made up of a cluster of embryonic cells forming the genital tubercle, the genital swellings, and the genital folds (Fig. 5.2).

- In females, the genital tubercle becomes the clitoris, the genital swellings become the labia majora, and the genital folds become the labia minora.

- In males, the genital tubercle becomes the glans penis, the genital swellings fuse to become the scrotum, the genital folds elongate and fuse to form the shaft of the penis and the penile urethra, and the prostate forms in the wall of the urogenital sinus.

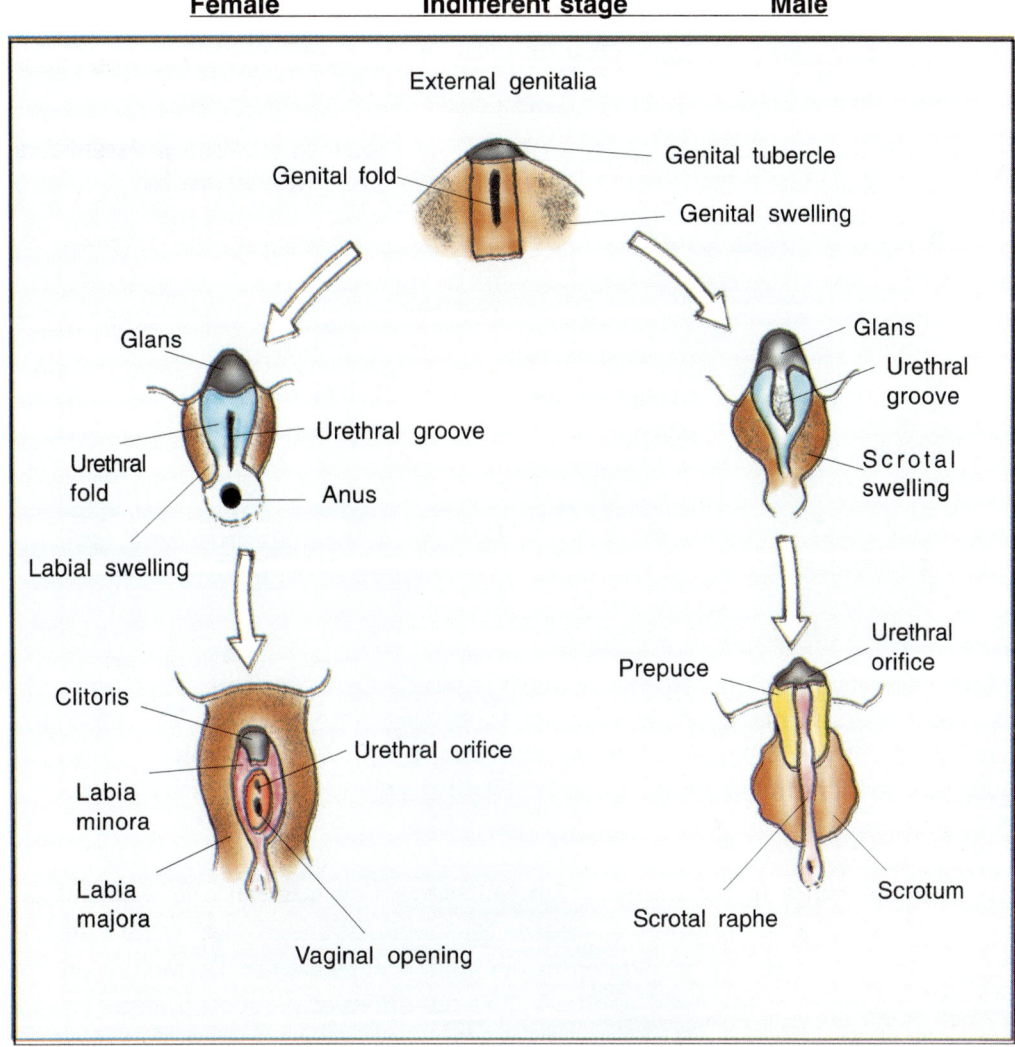

Fig. 5.2. Differentiation of the male and female external genitalia

The differentiation of the male and female external and internal genitalia is summarized in table 5.2.

	Table 5.2. Male and female sexual differentiation	
Female	**Indifferent stage 8 weeks**	**Male**
Gonad		
Granulosa cells, theca cells and interstitial cells ←	Indifferent gonad →	Sertoli cells, leydig cells and rete-testes
Oogonia ⟶ ova ←	Primordial germ cells →	Spermatogonias ⟶ sperms
Genital ducts		
Gartner's ducts ←	Mesonephric ducts →	Epididymis, vas deferens and seminal vesicles
Fallopian tubes uterus and upper vagina ←	Mullerian ducts →	Appendix testis
External genitalia		
Clitoris ←	Genital tubercle →	Glans
Labia majora ←	Genital swellings →	Scrotum
Labia minora ←	Genital/urethral folds →	Shaft of penis and penile urethra
Lower vagina, paraurethral glands and bartholin's glands ←	Urogenital sinus →	Prostate, prostatic utricle and bulbo-urethral glands

Genetic control of gonadal differentiation

The SRY (sex-determining region on the Y) gene located on the short arm of the Y chromosome causes the indifferent gonad to develop into a testis. The mechanism by which SRY promotes differentiation of the testis is not well understood. Translation of gonadal sex into phenotypic sex is the result of hormones secreted by the fetal testes.

Hormonal control of male development

When testicular tissue is not present, the fetus acquires internal and external genitalia of a female. Testicular hormones cause masculinization of the male fetus. Three hormones (testosterone, dihydrotestosterone and anti-mullerian hormone) are responsible for development of the male genitalia. The net effect of these hormones isregression of female internal genital ducts (müllerian) and promotion of male internal (wolffian) and external genitalia as shown in Flow chart 1.

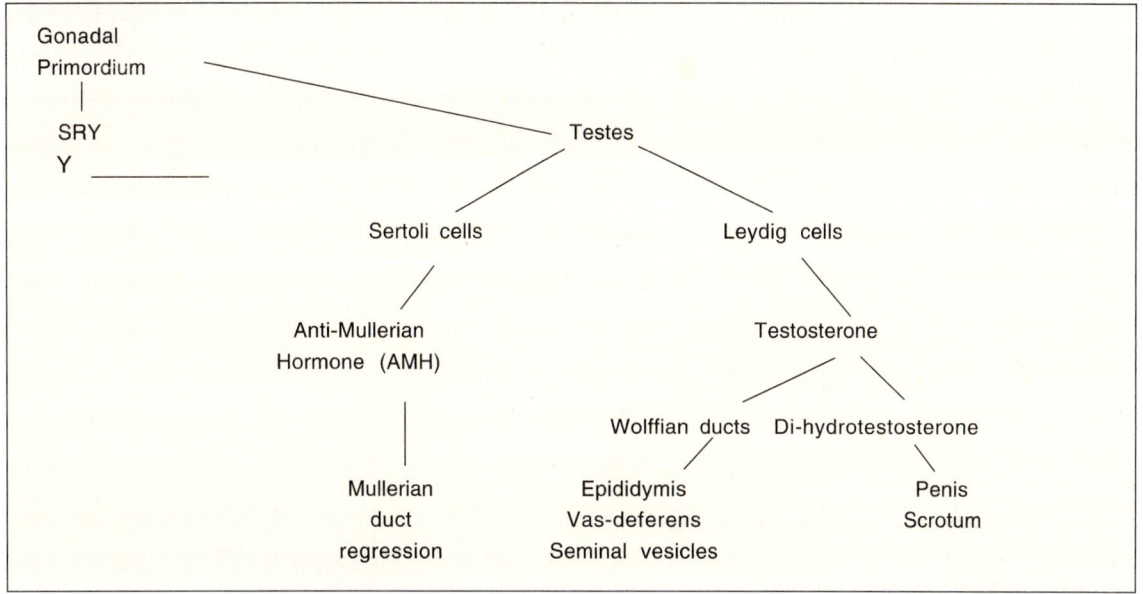

Flow chart 1. A simplified scheme of male sex differentiation

1. *Anti-müllerian hormone (AMH)*, a glycoprotein formed by Sertoli cells of the fetal testis beginning at about six weeks of development, causes regression of the Müllerian ducts, which is completed by about 8 weeks.

2. *Testosterone*, secreted by the fetal testes beginning at about the eighth week of development, directly stimulates Wolffian duct differentiation into epididymis, vas-deferens and seminal vesicles.

3. *Di-hydrotestosterone* formed by peripheral conversion and 5-alpha-reduction of testosterone, causes development of external genitalia (penis, penile urethra) and prostate.

Development of the internal ducts results from a paracrine effect from the ipsilateral gonad.

Timing of sexual differentiation Male sexual differentiation starts from 6th to 7th week of gestation and is completed by 12th week. Female sexual differentiation begins at 11 to 12th week and is completed by 20 weeks.

ANOMALOUS SEXUAL DIFFERENTIATION

Intersex disorders typically are diagnosed at birth as infants with ambiguous genitalia. Disorders associated with minor degrees or no ambiguity may be diagnosed much later. Understanding the diagnosis of intersex states requires an understanding of the steroid biosynthetic pathway Flow chart 2.

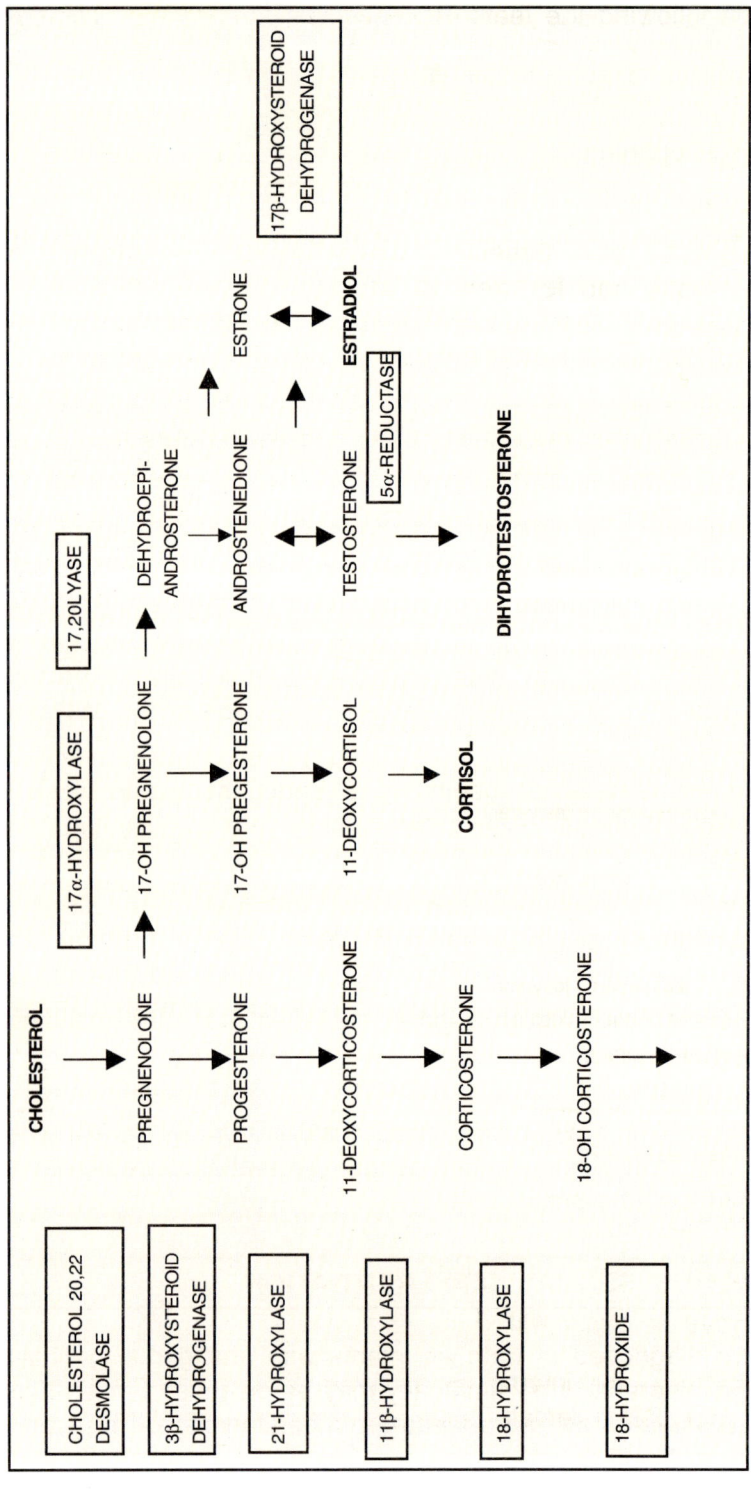

Flow chart 2. Pathway of steroid biosynthesis

Infants with any combination of following the features needs evaluation for an intersex disorder:

1. Small sized phallus

2. An aberrantly located urethral opening

3. At least one impalpable gonad.

The term hermaphroditism originates from Greek mythology wherein the offspring of god Hermes and goddess Sphrodite had features of both–i.e. a true hermaphrodite, whereas a pseudohermaphrodite connotes external genitalia incongruent to internal genitalia. The causes of anomalous sexual differentiation are given below table 5.3.

Table 5.3. Classification of anomalous sexual development

1. Disorders of gonadal differentiation
    • Klinfelter's syndrome
    • Turner's syndrome
    • Complete and incomplete forms of gonadal dysgenesis
    • True hermaphroditism
2. Female Pseudohermaphroditism
    • Congenital adrenal hyperplasia (CAH)
    • Aromatase deficiency
    • Glucocorticoid resistance
    • Iatrogenic maternal ingestion of progesterone or testosterone
    • Virilizing ovarian tumour in the mother
    • Virilizing congenital adrenal hyperplasia in the mother
3. Male Pseudohermaphroditism
    • Enzyme defects affecting both cortisol and testosterone biosynthesis
    • Enzyme defects primarily affecting testosterone biosynthesis in the testis
    • Defective conversion of testosterone (5 alpha-reductase deficiency)
    • Target tissue unresponsiveness to testosterone
4. Unclassified

1. Disorders of gonadal differentiation

- Klinefelter's syndrome
- Turner's syndrome
- Mixed gonadal dysgenesis
- True hermaphroditism–have an ovary with testis or ovotestis.

2. Female pseudo-hermaphroditism–the internal genitalia are female and the external genitalia are virilized. The true sex is female but has the external appearance of a male.

3. **Male pseudo-hermaphroditism**–the internal genitalia are male with poorly virilized external genitalia. The external appearance is of a female when the true sex is male.

4. **Unclassified forms** of abnormal sexual development

1. Disorders of gonadal differentiation

- *Turner's syndrome (45XO)* occurs in 1 in 2500 females and is characterized by X chromosome deletion. There patients have streak ovaries, are short statured and have a characteristic phenotype, including webbing of the neck, widely spaced nipples, increased carrying angle, pigmented naevi and cardiovascular anomalies.

- *Klinefelter's syndrome (47XXY)* occurs in 1 in 700 neonates and is characterized by short statured males with eunuchoid body habitus and gynaecomastia.

- *Mixed gonadal dysgenesis*

  Mosaicism for a Y-bearing cell line, usually the 45X/46XY karyotype, is responsible for most instances of mixed gonadal dysgenesis. Approximately two-thirds have the 45X/46XY karyotype, the remainder have a 46XY karyotype or a variant of mosaicism

  Clinical features: Affected individuals usually have a testis on one side and a streak gonad on the other. The streak gonad, a thin, pale, elongated structure located either in the broad ligament or along the pelvic wall, is composed of ovarian stroma. Both masculinization and mullerian duct regression in utero are incomplete.

  The genital ambiguity include phallic enlargement, a urogenital sinus, and some labioscrotal fusion. The testis may be intra-abdominal, inguinal or scrotal depending on its differentiation. The streak gonad is always intra-abdominal. A uterus, vagina, and at least one fallopian tube are almost invariably present on the side of streak gonad.

  ### Treatment

  - In phenotypic females prophylactic gonadectomy (to prevent gonadoblastoma/seminoma) is followed by oestrogen replacement to induce and maintain feminization.

  - In phenotypic males scrotal testes should be preserved; streak gonads and intra-abdominal testes should be excised (in view of increased risk of gonadal tumours). Reconstructive surgery of the phallus should be performed when appropriate.

  When the diagnosis is established in early infancy and the genitalia are ambiguous, gender assignment is usually female. Resection of the phallus and gonadectomy can be performed in infancy, sometimes in one procedure.

- *True hermaphroditism*

  Clinical features: True hermaphroditism is a condition in which both male and female types of gonadal epithelium are documented histologically in the same individual.

Classification

(1) Bilateral–ovotestes on each side

(2) Unilateral–an ovotestes on one side and an ovary or a testis on the other

(3) Lateral–a testis on one side and an ovary on the other.

A wide spectrum of external genital appearances are seen. The affected individuals are sufficiently masculinized to be reared as males, most have hypospadias and incomplete labioscrotal fusion. The phenotypic females have an enlarged clitoris, and a urogenital sinus. Differentiation of the internal ducts usually corresponds to the adjacent gonad. The ovary is usually in the normal position, but the testis or ovotestis may be found at any level along the route of testicular descent, frequently associated with an inguinal hernia. Variable feminization and virilization ensue at puberty.

Pathophysiology most have a 46XX karyotype, 10% have a 46XY karyotype, the remainder are chimeras or mosaics in whom a Y cell line is present.

Feminization (gynaecomastia and menstruation) is the result of secretion of oestradiol by ovarian tissue. In masculinized patients, secretion of androgen predominates, and some produce sperm.

Treatment Gender assignment depends on the anatomic features. Gonads and internal duct structures that are contradictory to the predominant phenotype (and the gender of rearing) should be removed, and the external genitalia should be modified when appropriate. In true hermaphrodites who carry Y chromosome sequences the possibility of future development of gonadal tumours is to be kept in mind when taking decisions to preserve gonadal tissue.

2. **Female pseudo-hermaphroditism** (Genetic female with external appearance of a male)

As mentioned earlier the causes usually include those that result in androgen exposure in a female fetus.

- Exposure to androgens during the critical period of organogenesis (between 8-12 weeks) results in varying degrees of ambiguity.

- Androgen exposure after 12 weeks gestation results only in varying degrees of clitoromegaly, the labioscrotal folds remaining separated.

The source of androgens could be the fetus itself or transplacental transfer from mother.

A. Fetal source

- Congenital adrenal hyperplasia

- Aromatase deficiency

- Glucocorticoid resistance

B. *Maternal source*
   - Iatrogenic–progesterone or testosterone ingestion
   - Virilizing ovarian or adrenal tumour
   - Virilizing congenital adrenal hyperplasia (CAH) in the mother.

C. *Non-androgen induced disturbances in differentiation of urogenital structures.*

Congenital adrenal hyperplasia (CAH)

Congenital adrenal hyperplasia (CAH) is the commonest cause of genital ambiguity. It results from mutations resulting in loss of function of any of the enzymes involved in cortisol production (Flow chart 2). The ensuing deficiency of cortisol releases pituitary corticotrophs from feedback inhibition, resulting in increased ACTH secretion that drives the adrenal to produce increasing amounts of cortisol precursors which are shunted to form androgens.

Causes of CAH include:

1. 21 hydroxylase deficiency
2. 11-beta hydroxylase deficiency
3. 3-beta hydroxy steroid dehydrogenase deficiency

1) *21 hydroxylase deficiency* This is an autosomal recessive condition and commonest cause of CAH and hence of female pseudohermaphroditism. Depending on the severity of the functional deficiency of the enzyme, a female patient may present with either one of the following:
    - virilization only
    - virilization and salt-losing syndrome classical form
    - non-classical form with neither virilization nor salt loss at birth

    A male child will have normal external genitalia but will have genital pigmentation and fails to thrive. The diagnosis is often missed at birth unless the physician is aware of the condition in the siblings and evaluates the child.

    The condition should also be considered in

    1. Patients with ambiguous genitalia with features of female pseudohermaphroditism
    2. Phenotypic males with bilateral cryptorchidism
    3. Infants who present in shock or severely dehydrated condition–as the salt losing crisis most often occurs in the second week of life, and
    4. Boys and girls who virilize before puberty.

    The family history may reveal a previously affected sibling, an unexpected death in infancy, or a male sibling with sexual precocity. Investigation of the child reveals the following:

- Biochemistry – hyperkalemia, hyponatremia, hypoglycemia and metabolic acidosis.

- Karyotype – 46XX

- Ultrasound pelvis shows presence of mullerian structures

- Hormonal work up reveals increased 17 hydroxy-progesterone (17 OHP).

Prenatal diagnosis is possible by chorion villus biopsy or amniocentesis. The 21-hydroxylase gene is located on the 6th chromosome adjacent to MHC genes.

Treatment of CAH: the treatment of choice is corticosteroid replacement with either hydrocortisone or prednisolone to suppress the raised ACTH levels.

2) *11-beta hydroxylase deficiency* features are similar to CAH due to 21 hydroxylase deficiency but the affected female infants also have hypertension. Salt loss does not occur due to increased aldosterone precursors with mineralocorticoid activity namely de-oxycorticosterone and corticosterone.

3) *3-beta hydroxy steroid dehydrogenase deficiency* results in adrenal insufficiency in addition to virilization in a female.

3. Male pseudohermaphroditism

Ambiguity results in a male fetus if the pathway for production of testosterone is defective, or there is a block in the conversion of testosterone to its active form, or if the target tissues are unresponsive to testosterone. Depending on the severity of involvement, the phenotype of the external genitalia varies, from those of a normal appearing female to those of a male with a micropenis, cryptorchidism and hypoplastic external genitalia.

Causes of male pseudohermaphroditism (MPH)

A. Enzyme defects affecting both cortisol and testosterone (CAH) biosynthesis

B. Enzyme defects primarily affecting testosterone biosynthesis by the testis

C. Defective conversion of testosterone to its active form by peripheral tissues due to 5-alpha reductase deficiency

D. Target tissue unresponsiveness to testosterone (androgen insensitivity)

- Complete androgen insensitivity (testicular feminization) syndrome

- Partial androgen insensitivity syndromes

A) *CAH* They present as phenotypic females or incompletely virilized males with adrenal insufficiency. Absence of mullerian structures and 46XY karyotype identify them as males.

B) *Deficiency of enzymes* affecting testosterone biosynthesis result in male pseudohermaphroditism without adrenal insufficiency.

C) *Defects in conversion of testosterone to its active form by peripheral tissues due to 5-alpha reductase deficiency* These patients have 46XY karyotype, normally differentiated testes, male internal ducts and ambiguous external genitalia; as the development of external genitalia is based on the active form of testosterone (Fig. 5.2). Various degrees of hypospadias and blind vaginal pouch are seen; at puberty, the other signs of masculinization appear. These patients if reared as females in childhood change their gender role behaviour to male at puberty.

D) *Androgen insensitivity syndromes* There is tissue unresponsiveness to testosterone

- Complete androgen insensitivity (*Testicular feminization*) syndrome: Patients with complete androgen resistance have an female phenotype. At birth and in childhood, the diagnosis should be suspected in a female with bilateral inguinal herniae or with gonads palpable in the inguinal region or the labia. They are more commonly brought to medical attention at puberty with primary amenorrhoea. Physical findings include well developed breasts, a blind vaginal pouch and lack of axillary and pubic hair. Ultrasound reveals absence of mullerian structures. Diagnosis is by testosterone levels, LH levels and the karyotype which is 46XY.

- Incomplete forms of androgen resistance: They are a heterogeneous group of 46XY individuals with external genitalia ranging from perineoscrotal hypospadias, blind vaginal pouch with cryptorchidism and micropenis to clitoromegaly with partial labial fusion. Patients with subtle involvement may have a normal male phenotype with a small penis and are fertile. Mullerian structures are absent. Decreased to normal axillary and pubic hair, sparse beard growth and body hair, and gynaecomastia is common at puberty. They have increased testosterone, oestrogen and LH levels and a 46XY karyotype.

EVALUATION OF A NEWBORN WITH AMBIGUOUS GENITALIA

Evaluation of a newborn with ambiguous genitalia requires a team effort (Flow chart 3). The most common intersex condition, CAH, results in virilization of a 46XX female. The clinician's challenge is to distinguish CAH from other less common causes.

History

A detailed family history is essential and should include the following:

- A family history of genital ambiguity, infertility, or unexpected changes at puberty may suggest a genetically transmitted trait.

- Recessive traits (CAH, testosterone biosynthetic defects, 5 α-reductase deficiency and aromatase deficiency) tend to occur in siblings while sparing parents, while X-linked abnormalities (androgen receptor defects) tend to appear in males who are scattered sporadically across the family.

- A history of early death of infants in a family may suggest a previously missed CAH, especially common in male infants with CAH because they have no ambiguity to arouse suspicion.

- A history of maternal drug ingestion is important, particularly during the first trimester, when ambiguity may be produced in a gonadal female exposed to exogenous progesterone (commonly but inappropriately prescribed in patients with previous early pregnancy loss) or androgens (Danazol is the commonly used androgen in patients with endometriosis, patient may continue to take the pill without realizing that she has become pregnant).

- Although extremely rare, a history of maternal virilization may suggest an androgen-producing maternal tumour, or CAH in mother.

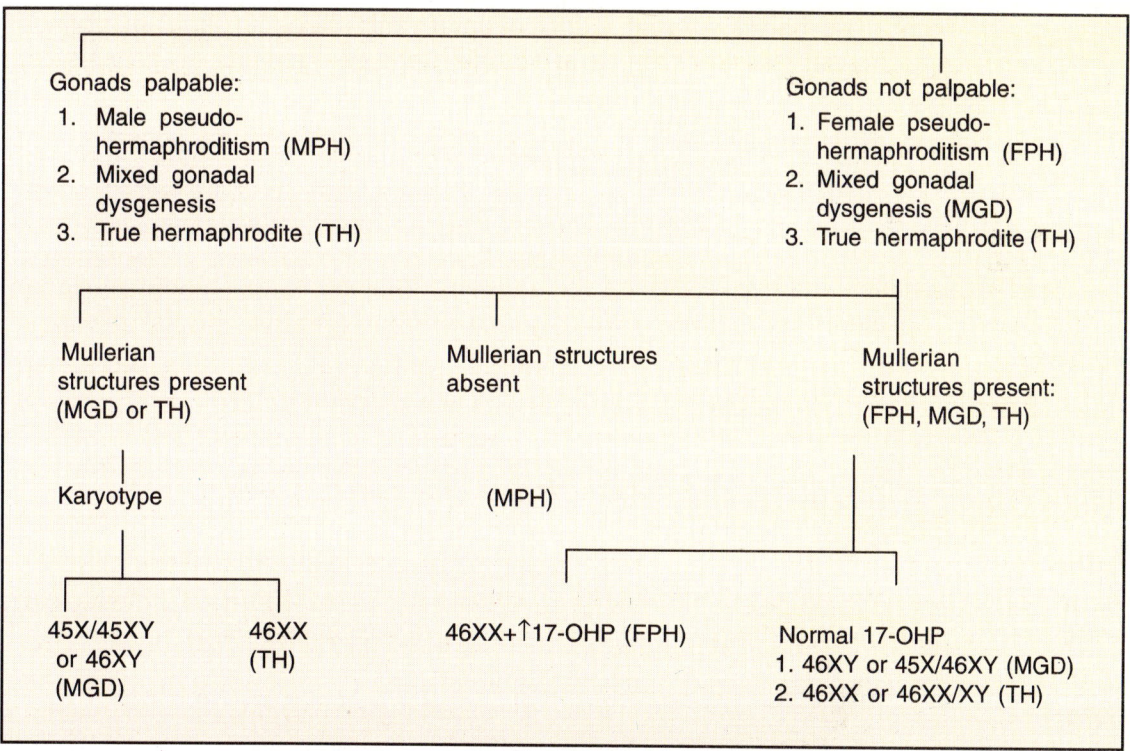

Flow chart 3. Steps in the diagnosis of intersex disorders

Physical examination

Certain physical characteristics may suggest the directions toward which a successful investigation might be pursued, though the diagnosis of intersex is considerably laboratory oriented.

Examination of the external genitalia

- *Phallus* Note the size and degree of differentiation of the phallus, since variations may represent clitoromegaly or hypospadias; besides, the adequacy of phallic length decides the sex of rearing.

- *Position of the urethral meatus* The hypospadias can be coronal, penile, penoscrotal or perineoscrotal depending on where the urethral opening is located.

- *Labioscrotal folds* may be separated or folds may be fused at the midline, giving an appearance of a scrotum. Rugose scrotal or labioscrotal folds with increased pigmentation suggest the possibility of increased corticotropin levels as part of CAH.

Gonadal examination

- Documentation of palpable gonads is important. Although ovotestes have been reported to descend completely to the bottom of the labioscrotal folds, in most patients, only the testicular material descends fully. If examination reveals palpable inguinal gonads; diagnosis of a gonadal female, Turner's syndrome, and pure gonadal dysgenesis can be eliminated.

- Impalpable gonads, in an apparently fully virilized infant, should raise the possibility of a virilized female pseudohermaphrodite with CAH.

Rectal examination

- Rectal examination may reveal a cervix and uterus, confirming internal müllerian structures. The uterus is relatively enlarged in a newborn because of the effects of maternal oestrogen, permitting easy identification.

6

Puberty and Menopause

In this chapter, physiological changes in puberty and menopause are described, and the common problems in both stages are discussed.

PUBERTY

Puberty is defined as the period of transition from childhood to adulthood and involves physical growth, development of sex organs and secondary sexual characters and attainment of menarche culminating in complete physical and psychological maturation.

This period usually takes 8 to 18 yrs.

Changes in the prepubertal period leading to attainment of puberty

1. *Adrenarche*   The growth of pubic and axillary hair due to increased production of adrenal androgens.

   - Starts from 6-7 yrs. to adolescence (13-15 yrs.) and is not under the direct control of gonadotropins or ACTH.

   - Precedes linear growth spurt by 2 yrs.

2. *Decreasing repression of the gonadostat* (hypothalamo-pituitary system controlling secretion of gonadotropins)

   Till 6-7 yrs. of age the gonadostat is highly sensitive to the negative feedback of even the low amounts of circulating oestrogens. From age 8 onwards, the repression of the gonadostat is lifted and there is progressive responsiveness of the anterior pituitary to GnRH and follicle reactivity to FSH and LH.

3. *Increased secretion of gonadotropins*

   There is increase in the amplitude and frequency of the pulsatile GnRH secretion. Following this, FSH rises initially and plateaus in mid-puberty while LH rises more slowly and reaches adult levels in late puberty.

Timing of puberty

The major factor that determines the timing of puberty is genetic. The other factors like geographic location, exposure to light, general health and nutrition and psychological factors influence the time of initiation and rate of progression. The earlier the onset, the longer is the duration. It has been argued that a critical body weight (47.8 kg) or more importantly a greater percentage of body fat (23%) is required to attain menarche.

Pubertal events

The events occur in the following sequence.

1. Physical growth

Growth spurt occurs at about 11-12 years, and doubles in one year. The increase in height is between 6 and 11 cm. The growth peak is attained 2 years after breast budding and 1 year prior to menarche. This is due to increased levels of oestrogen and growth factor I.

2. Changes in genital organs

- *Ovaries* show follicular enlargement and development at various stages. There is stromal cell hyperplasia and the ovaries become bulky and oval in shape.

- *Uterus* shows endometrial and myometrial proliferation. The ratio of uterine body to the cervix changes from 1:2 at birth, to 1:1 at menarche. The uterus further enlarges in the reproductive period and the ratio becomes 2:1 and finally in the postmenopausal period the ratio is 1:1.

- *Vaginal epithelium* becomes stratified squamous non-keratinized, and acquires glycogen due to the effect of oestrogen. It becomes host to a profusion of Doderlein's bacilli that convert glycogen to lactic acid. Thus the vaginal pH changes from alkaline in the prepubertal period to acidic (4-5) in the reproductive period.

- *The vulva* becomes more reactive to steroid hormones.

- *Mons pubis and labia minora* also increase in size.

3. Secondary sexual characters

- *Breast* There is ductal proliferation and fat deposition in response to oestrogens while progesterones lead to glandular development. Tanner described five stages in breast (Fig. 6.1) and pubic hair (Fig. 6.2) development, that relate morphological age to the change expected in secondary sexual characters.

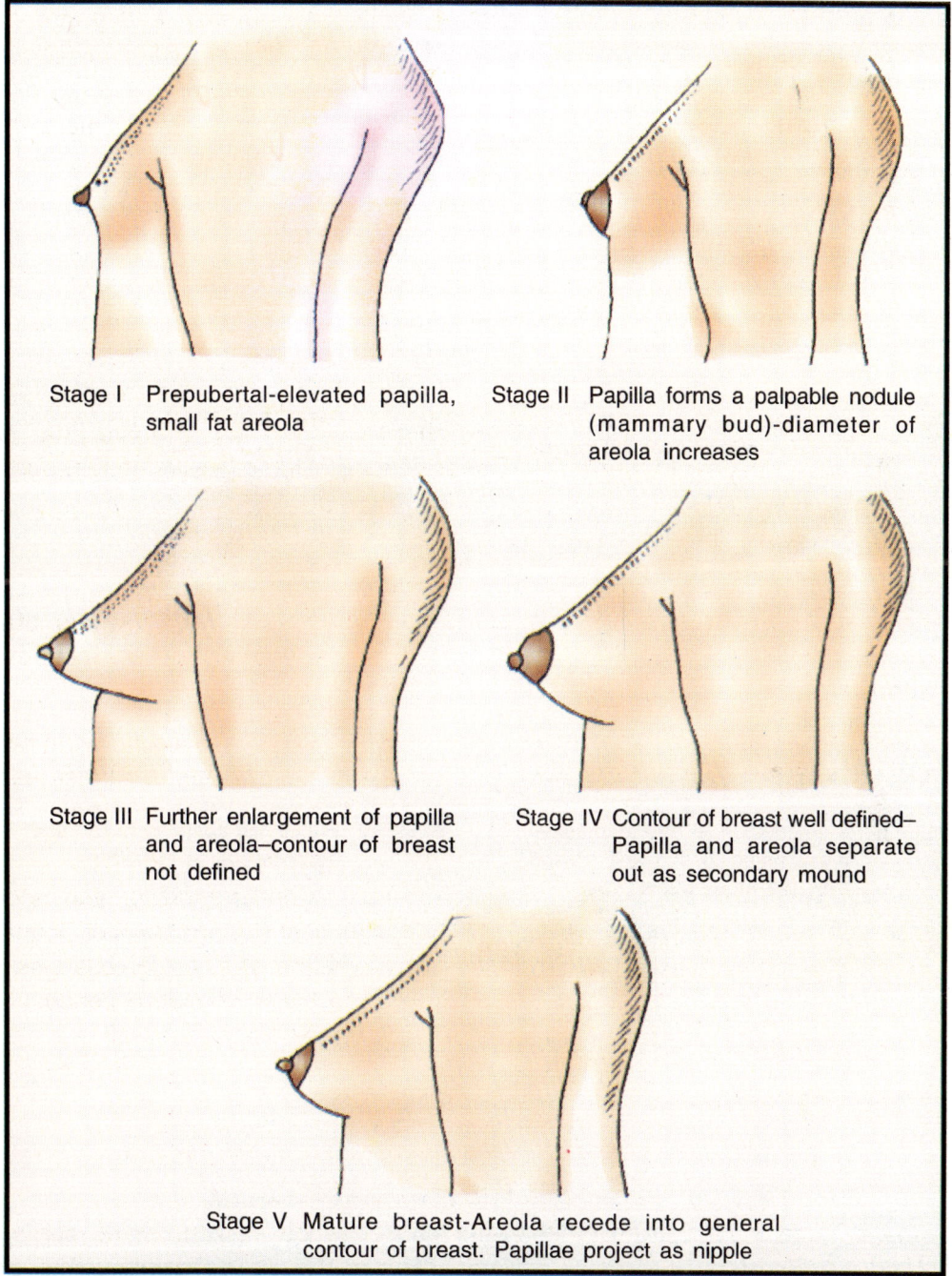

Stage I Prepubertal-elevated papilla, small fat areola

Stage II Papilla forms a palpable nodule (mammary bud)-diameter of areola increases

Stage III Further enlargement of papilla and areola-contour of breast not defined

Stage IV Contour of breast well defined– Papilla and areola separate out as secondary mound

Stage V Mature breast-Areola recede into general contour of breast. Papillae project as nipple

Fig. 6.1a-e. Stages of breast development described by Tanner

- *Pubic and axillary hair* There is increased secretion of adrenal sex steroids from 7 years of age, which are mainly responsible for increased sebum formation, pubic and axillary hair and change in voice.

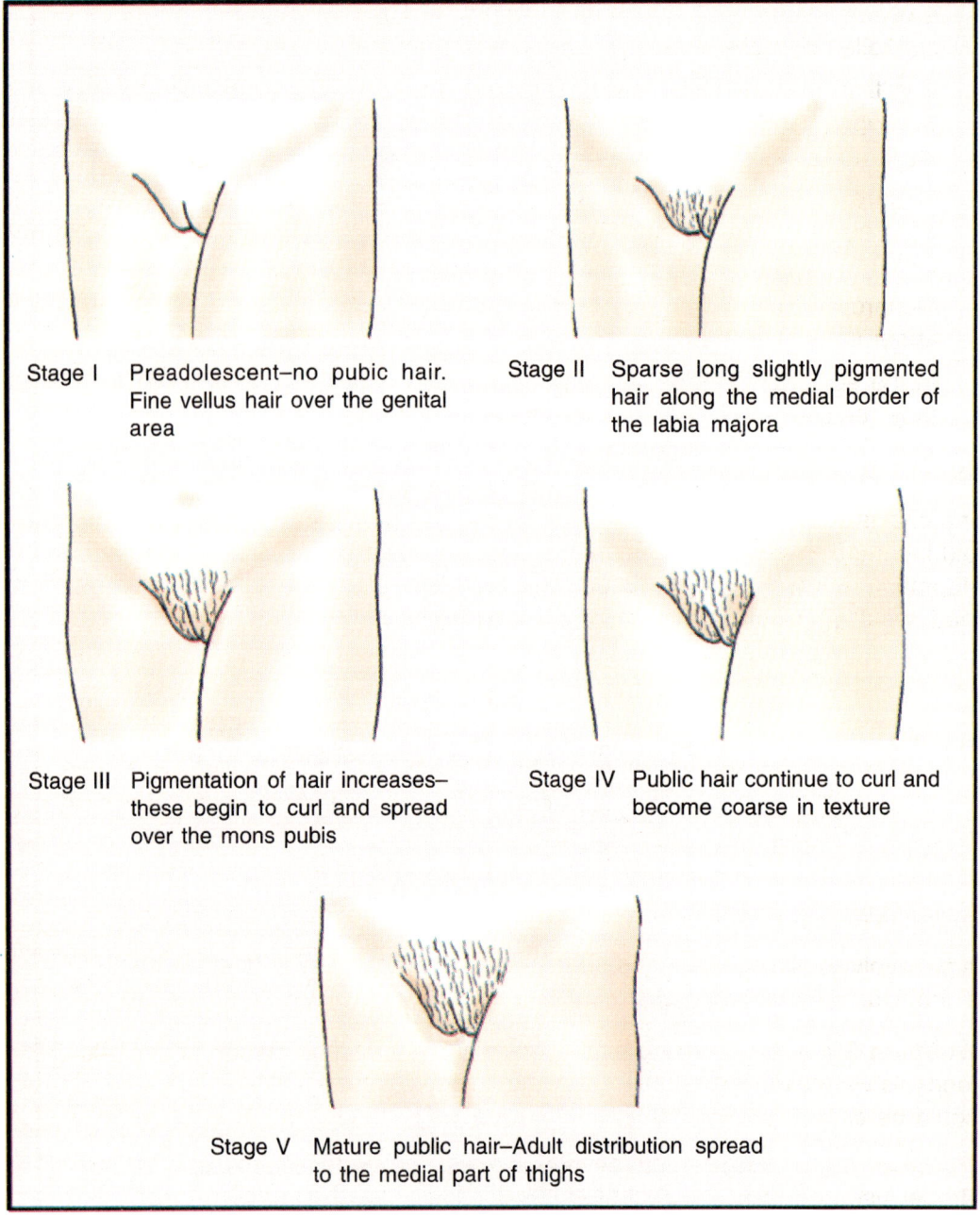

Stage I   Preadolescent–no pubic hair. Fine vellus hair over the genital area

Stage II   Sparse long slightly pigmented hair along the medial border of the labia majora

Stage III   Pigmentation of hair increases– these begin to curl and spread over the mons pubis

Stage IV   Public hair continue to curl and become coarse in texture

Stage V   Mature public hair–Adult distribution spread to the medial part of thighs

Fig. 6.2a-e.   Stages in development of pubic hair described by Tanner

- Female body habitus Oestrogens lead to subcutaneous fat deposition leading to the typical female body habitus.

4. *Menarche* is the first menstruation in life.

- It usually occurs between 9 to 17 yrs. with a median age of 12.8 yrs. It is chiefly controlled by genetic factors when the environment is optimal.

- It is the final endocrine hallmark of puberty and denotes attainment of a positive oestrogen feedback on the HPO axis leading to a mid-cycle surge of LH required for ovulation.

- Menarche also denotes an intact hypothalamo-pituitary axis, functioning ovaries, endometrium responsive to endogenous ovarian steroids and a patent uterovaginal canal.

- Menarche occurs after the peak in growth velocity has passed. Slower growth of about 6 cm is noted after menarche.

- In the earlier stages the menstrual cycles are anovular, but after two to three years they regularize and become ovular.

Sequence of pubertal events

Adrenarche is followed by an increase in gonadal oestrogen (gonadarche) followed by a rapid increase in skeletal growth resulting in a growth spurt. This is followed by breast development, female fat distribution, vaginal and uterine growth. Menarche is finally attained resulting in the culmination of pubertal changes (table 6.1).

Table 6.1. Sequence of pubertal changes
<ul><li>Adrenarche</li><li>Growth spurt</li><li>Thelarche</li><li>Menarche</li></ul>

Management of puberty

Puberty involves radical changes that occur at such a pace that an adolescent mind finds them difficult to comprehend and deal with.

- *Nutrition* Since this is the period of rapid growth, special stress should be given on foods rich in proteins. Anaemia is a common adolescent problem and periodic deworming could be carried out.

- *Personal hygiene* Menarche involves the ability to deal with monthly cyclical bleeding. Proper use and disposal of sanitary napkins and regular baths should be advised.

- *Sex education* With teenage pregnancy acquiring epidemic proportions, adolescents should be educated regarding reproduction, and the various contraceptive methods available.

Abnormal conditions in relation to puberty

Important conditions of clinical interest are precocious puberty, delayed puberty and pubertal menorrhagia

1. Precocious puberty

- Precocious puberty is defined as the development of secondary sex characteristics before the age of 8 years or attainment of menarche before 10 years of age. It can be of two types

   1. GnRH dependent precocious puberty also known as **true precious puberty** due to early activation of the HPO axis.

   2. GnRH independent precocious puberty also known as **precocious pseudo-puberty**. It is due to extra-pituitary secretion of hCG or sex steroid secretion independent of HPO stimulation.

   Precocious puberty may also present as isolated thelarche, pubarche or menarche.

- *Premature thelarche* Refers to isolated development of breast tissue before age 8. It may be unilateral or bilateral.

- *Premature pubarche* Refers to isolated development of pubic or axillary hair before the age of 8 years. It is due to either increased sensitivity of the end organs to circulating hormones or to increased androgen production.

- *Premature menarche* Refers to the isolated event of cyclical vaginal bleeding. It is due to the unusual sensitivity of the endometrium to low levels of oestrogens, an oestrogen producing ovarian tumour, a foreign body in the vagina or injury to the vagina.

Diagnosis of precocious puberty The evaluation of a patient with precocious puberty is shown in Flow chart 1.

1. True precocious puberty

   The commonest cause is constitutional. There is history of early menarche in mother or sisters. Pubertal changes are in an orderly sequence and no detectable cause can be found. Investigations include x-ray of the hand and wrist for bone age as there is acceleration of growth, a pelvic USG to detect an ovarian tumour, skull x-ray and CT head to detect an intracranial lesion.

   Diagnosis of pseudo-puberty involves isolating the underlying pathology.

2. Premature pubarche

   There is usually ovarian enlargement which can be detected by bimanual examination

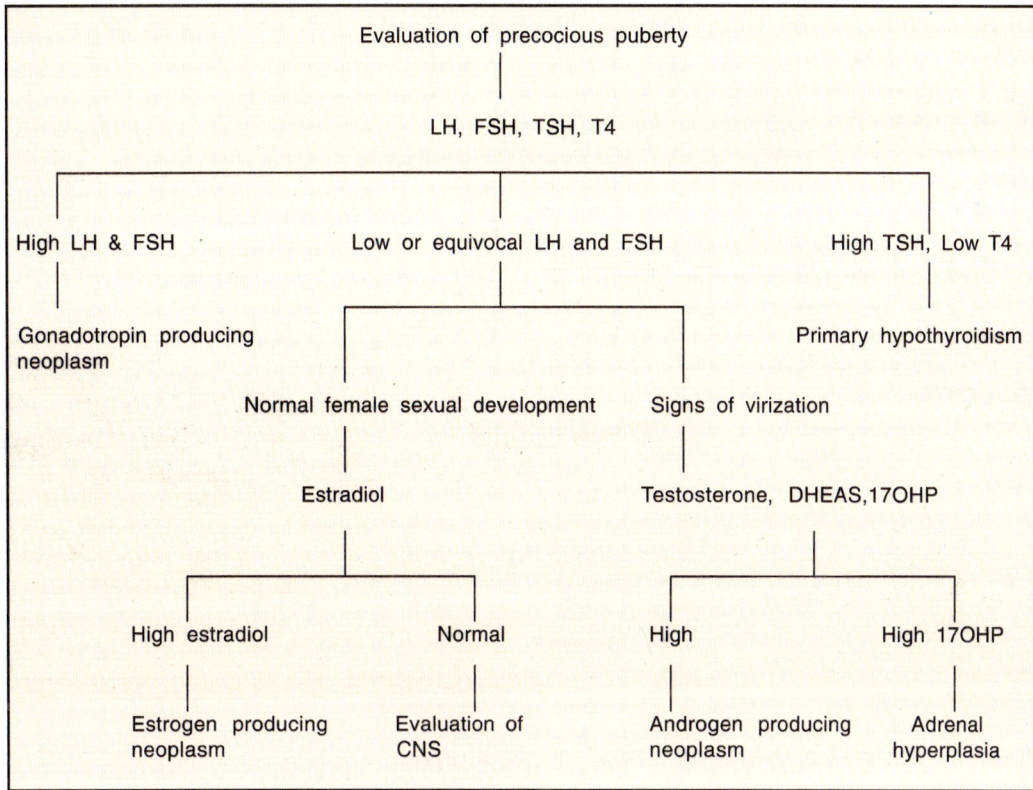

Flow chart 1. Evaluation of precocious puberty

or on USG. Adrenal tumours can be detected by an IVP or CT scan of a abdomen. Adrenal hyperplasia can be diagnosed by measuring levels of 17 hydroxyprogesterone, testosterone and dehydroepiandrosterone (DHEAS).

3. *Premature menarche*

A foreign body or vaginal injury should be ruled out in the first place. Cyclical vaginal bleeding clinches the diagnosis. When no other cause is detected, periodic evaluation is recommended at 6 monthly intervals

Management of precocious puberty

- In true precocious puberty: apart from short stature there is normal menstrual pattern and future fertility is not impaired.

- In idiopathic precocious puberty, most patients only require assurance and counselling.

- In the remaining the goal is to reduce gonadotropin secretion, to reduce or counteract the peripheral action of sex steroids and stabilize the growth rate to normal thereby slowing skeletal maturation. For the others, treatment depends on dealing with the cause.

- Drugs used
  1. Medroxy progesterone acetate: suppresses menstruation and breast development
  2. Cyproterone acetate: Anti-androgen used for treatment of excess androgen production in girls with premature adrenarche
  3. GnRH analogues: Suppress premature activation of the HPO axis by down regulation and slow the process of skeletal maturation
  4. Danazol: Produces amenorrhoea and arrests breast development.

2. Delayed puberty

When breast tissue and/or pubic hair have not appeared by 13-14 yrs. of age or menarche has not set in by 16 yrs., it is known as delayed puberty.

Causes

- Constitutional–there is no cause.
- Secondary to chronic diseases e.g. tuberculosis, chronic liver or renal disease.
- Endocrinal due to true gonadal insufficiency which could be at the hypothalamo-pituitary level or ovarian level.

Diagnosis

Comprises history, physical examination and investigations as mentioned in Flow chart 2.

Treatment

In constitutionally delayed puberty assurance, improvement of general health and treatment of any illness is necessary.

- When hypogonadism is detected, cyclical oestrogens or contraceptive pills can be given.
- In cases of hypergonadotropic hypogonadism, chromosomal studies to exclude intersexuality should be carried out.

3. Pubertal Menorrhagia

The evaluation and management of pubertal menorrhagia is summarized in Flow chart 3.

The initial periods can be heavy and prolonged due to anovulatory cycles. The unopposed action of oestrogen causes endometrial hyperplasia leading to delayed cycles and sometimes excessive blood loss.

Very rarely in patients not responding to medical treatment, a Mirena coil (progesterone

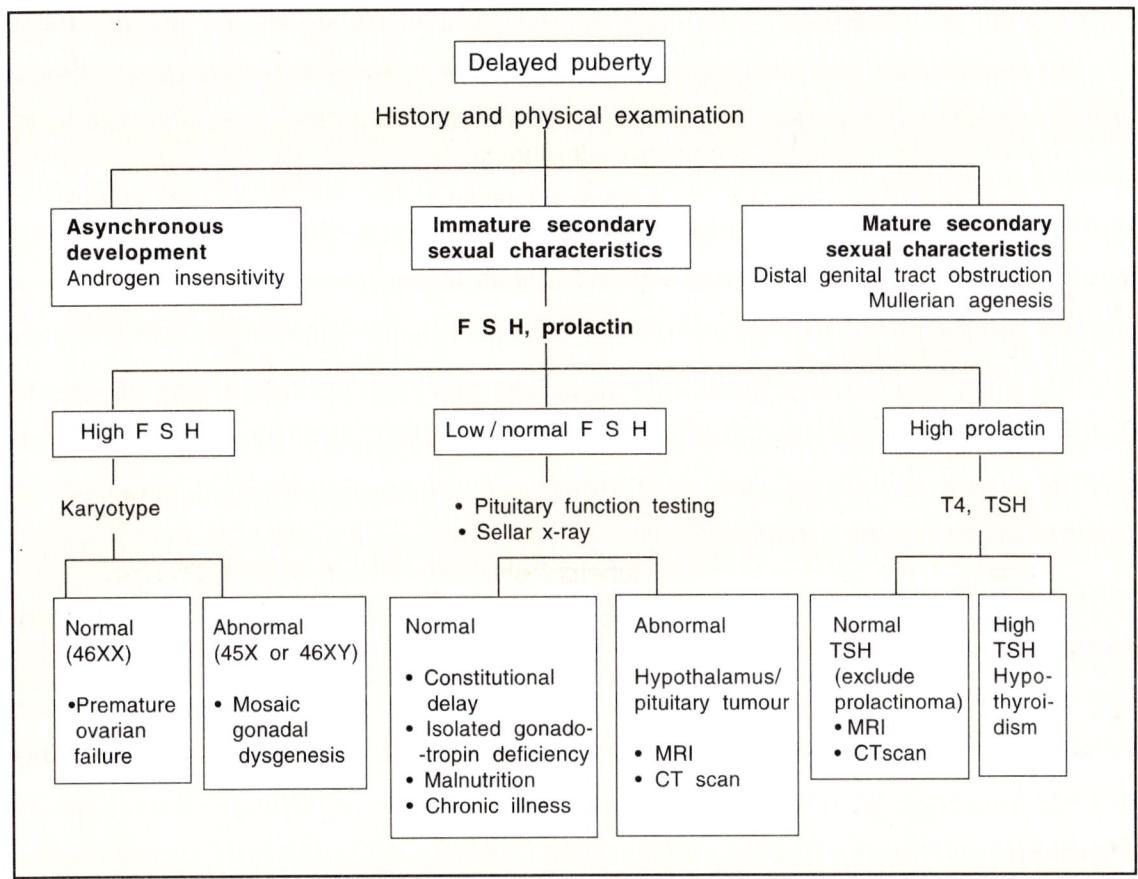

Flow chart 2. Diagnosis of delayed puberty

releasing IUCD) can be inserted in order to avoid surgical intervention and high doses of hormones

MENOPAUSE

Total cessation of menstruation for six consecutive months is known as *menopause*. The period before menopause is called the *premenopause* and that after, is the *postmenopause*. *Perimenopause* refers to the period around menopause (40-55 yrs.) while *climacteric* is the period 10-15 yrs. before and after menopause.

The age of menopause is usually 45-55 yrs. with an average of around 50 yrs. With increasing life expectancy more women are now experiencing menopause for a longer time. The age of menopause is genetically predetermined. Cigarette smoking or severe malnutrition can hasten its onset.

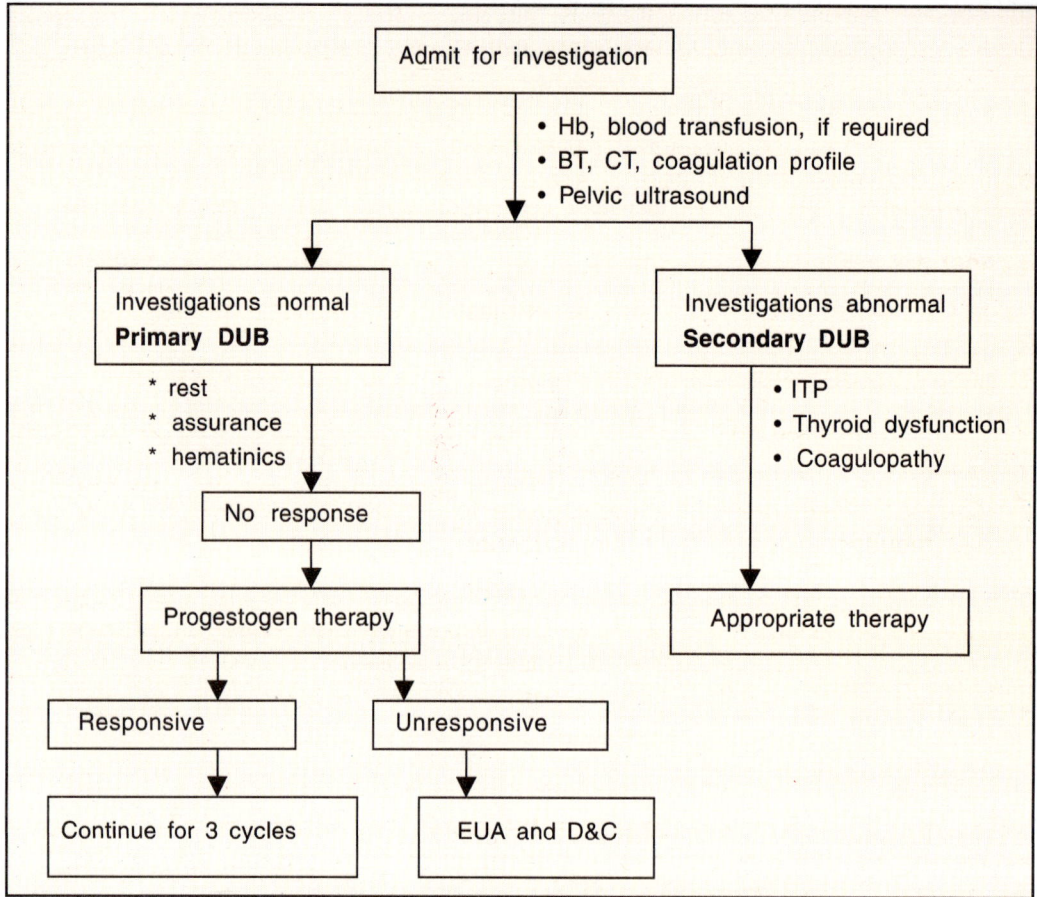

Flow chart 3. Evaluation of pubertal menorrhagia

Menstruation pattern prior to menopause

Any of the following patterns are observed:

1. Sudden cessation of menses
2. Gradual decrease in the amount of blood flow during menses (hypomenorrhoea) or infrequent cycles (oligomenorrhoea)
3. Irregular bleeding.

In case of heavy periods or inter-menstrual bleeding, one should always exclude genital tract malignancy.

Anatomical changes

*   In the **breasts**, fat is resorbed and glands atrophy. The nipples decrease in size and the breasts become progressively flat and pendulous.

- The *ovaries* shrink, and while there is thinning of the cortex, there is an increase in medullary components and an abundance of stromal cells with secretory activity.

- The *fallopian tubes* atrophy.

- The *uterus* becomes smaller and the uterocervical ratio becomes 1:1. The endometrium becomes thin and atrophic and in some women with high endogenous oestrogens (usually obese), the endometrium becomes proliferative or hyperplastic.

- *Cervical secretions* become scanty.

- The *vagina* gets narrower due to loss of elasticity, the epithelium becomes thin, and rugae progressively flatten. There is no glycogen secretion by the vaginal epithelium, Doderlein's bacilli are absent and the vaginal pH becomes alkaline.

- In the *vulva*, the labia flatten, pubic hair are scantier and the introitus is narrowed.

- *Bladder and urethra* undergo similar changes to those of the vulva and vagina. The epithelium becomes thin and is more prone to damage and infection. There may be dysuria, frequency, urge or even stress incontinence.

- *Loss of muscle tone* leads to pelvic relaxation and anatomical changes in the urethra and neck of the bladder. The pelvic cellular tissues become scanty and the ligaments supporting the uterus and vagina lose their tone. As such preexisting weakness gets aggravated and the degree of uterine descent may increase.

Menopausal symptoms

Menopause is a physiological state and in the majority of women, apart from cessation of menstruation, no more symptoms are evident. In some, symptoms appear which may be grouped as follows:

(a) Psychological

(b) Vasomotor

(c) Genital & Urinary

(d) Skeletal

(e) Cardiac

(a) *Psychological* There is increased frequency of anxiety, headache, insomnia, irritability and depression.

(b) *Vasomotor* The characteristic symptom of menopause is the "hot flush". It starts as a wave of heat from the extremities going up, associated with sweating and a feeling of uneasiness. The woman experiences palpitations and the pulse rate may rise by 20 beats per minute. It lasts only for 1-2 minutes. Hot flushes are due to peripheral vascular instability. All the major sex steroids-oestrogen, progesterone and androgen are probably involved in the aetiology. Sleep may be disturbed due to night sweats. It is probably related to a low level of oestrogens and peripheral vasodilatation.

(c) *Genitourinary* The *genital* symptoms include features of atrophic vaginitis and endometritis, most importantly dyspareunia and a feeling of dryness in the vulva and vagina. *Urethral* symptoms are urinary urgency, dysuria, recurrent urinary infection and stress incontinence.

(d) *Skeletal*   Increased osteoclastic activity leads to greater resorption of bone and osteoporosis. There is decline in the collagenous organic matrix. The vertebral body, femoral neck and distal radius are markedly affected resulting in a greater liability to fracture.

(e) *Cardiovascular effects* There is increased risk of coronary heart disease, which may be due to a rise in the lipid levels, both triglycerides and cholesterol. LDL increases more compared to the cardioprotective HDL.

The symptoms of menopause are summarized in table 6.2.

Table 6.2. Menopausal symptoms

Anxiety, headache, insomnia, irritability and depression
Hot flushes
Night sweats
Dryness of the vulva and vagina
Bone pains due to osteoporosis
Chest pain due to ischaemic heart disease

Diagnosis of menopause

The following criteria should be present

1. Cessation of menstruation for six consecutive months during climacteric.
2. Appearance of menopausal symptoms 'hot flushes' and 'night sweats'.
3. Vaginal cytology–showing features of low oestrogen.
4. Serum oestradiol <20pg/ml
5. Serum FSH and LH >30IU/l

Management of menopause

Prophylaxis

A healthy lifestyle which includes moderate exercise and a high calcium intake from early adolescence right through reproductive years will ensure a healthy menopausal transition. Sixty percent of total calcium deposition in bones occurs in the adolescent period itself.

Prevention

Once menopause sets in, adverse changes in coming years can be prevented by reassurance regarding physiology of menopause, a high calcium diet with micronutrient intake, and regular exercise.

Treatment

1. Non-hormonal treatment

- Good nutritious diet
- *Calcium* salts in the dose of 1100-1200mg per day reduce the bone turn over and reduce the risk of vertebral fractures.

  Excercise improves the muscle strength, postural stability, chronic pain and causes an increased sense of well-being.
- *Hypnotics, tranquilisers* and sedatives can allay the psychologic symptoms but cannot relieve the true symptoms or underlying pathology.
- *Clonidine*, an alpha adrenergic agonist may be used sometimes to reduce the severity and duration of hot flushes. It is helpful where oestrogen is contraindicated as in hypertensives.

2. Hormone replacement therapy (HRT)

HRT is indicated in menopausal women to overcome the short-term and long-term consequences of oestrogen deficiency. It is beneficial in symptomatic women when non-hormonal treatment has not been effective. Though it has a beneficial effect on osteoporosis, atherosclerosis, cardiovascular disease, urogenital atrophy and degenerative changes in the skin, the benefits last only until the duration of therapy, hence compliance with therapy is essential. The monitoring prior to and during HRT is given in table 6.3.

Table 6.3. Monitoring prior to and during HRT

A base level parameter of the following and their subsequent check up annually are mandatory.
      Blood pressure recording
      Breast palpation
      Pelvic examination
      Cervical cytology
      Mammography

A special group of women to whom HRT should be routinely prescribed include:

-   Premature ovarian failure
-   Gonadal dysgenesis
-   Surgical or radiation menopause

The contraindications to HRT are given in table 6.4.

Table 6.4. Contraindications to HRT
• Previous history of breast cancer • Family history of breast cancer • Deep vein thrombosis–past or present • Recent history of endometrial cancer • Active liver disease

HRT includes oestrogen alone or in combination with progesterone. If the uterus is present, progestogens must be prescribed in addition to prevent endometrial hyperplasia and subsequent development of endometrial carcinoma.

Modes of oestrogen HRT (table 6.5)

1. *Oral* It may be given continuously or cyclically.

    a) *Continuous combined therapy:* This involves the daily use of oestrogens and progesterones for 21 days. The oestrogen used are natural oestrogen (oestradiol, oestrone, oestriol, conjugated equine oestrogens) as synthetic oestrogens are less suitable because of their greater metabolic impact. The progesterones used are nearly all synthetic, i.e., 17-hydroxyprogesterone derivatives (dydrogesterone, medroxyprogesterone acetate) and 19 nor-testosterone derivatives (norethisterone, norgestrel). The woman will thus have no menstrual bleeding.

    b) *Cyclic:* Oestrogen is given from day 1 to day 25 and progestogen added from day 14 to day 25. These women will have cyclical bleeding.

2. *Vaginal cream* Conjugated vaginal oestrogen cream 1.25mg daily is very effective specially in atrophic vaginitis.

3. *Percutaneous oestrogen cream* 5 gm applicator of cream delivering 3 mg of oestradiol daily is applied on to the skin over the anterior abdominal wall.

4. *Subdermal* 17-ß oestradiol as pellets or implants 25 mg, 50 mg and 100 mg are available and can be kept for 6 months. The method is suitable in patients who have had a hysterectomy.

5. *Transdermal patch* contains 3.2 mg of 17-ß oestradiol, releasing about 50µg of

oestradiol in 24 hours. It should be applied below the waist line and changed twice a week.

Table 6.5. Modes of HRT	
Oestrogens–	Oral-continuous combined/cyclical
	Vaginal cream
	Percutaneous cream
	Subdermal implants
	Transdermal patches
Tibolone	
Bisphosphonates	
Selective Estrogen Receptor Modulators (SERMS)	

* *Risks of oestrogen HRT*

1. Breast cancer–HRT increases the risk by 2.3% per year of use, when started after 50 years of age. The risk is higher in combined HRT users. The magnitude of increase is roughly equivalent to the rise in relative risk associated with each year of menopause after the age fifty.

2. Endometrial cancer–The relative risk is increased with prolonged duration of use. The addition of progesterone for 10 days has a protective effect.

3. Venous thromboembolism–There is an increased risk of venous thromboembolism with an absolute risk of 3 per 10,000 users per year i.e., an excess of 2 cases per 10,000 users per year. The risk is further increased with a previous episode.

Other Options

– **Tibolone** is a synthetic compound having a mixed oestrogenic, progestogenic and androgenic action. It is useful for vasomotor, psychological, libid problems and osteoporosis prevention in the dose of 2.5 mg daily.

– **Bisphosphonates** Etidronate, Alendronate and Risedronate inhibit bone resorption and have a protective effect on osteoporosis.

– **Selective Estrogen Receptor Modulators (SERMS)** These have an oestrogenic effect on the bone and lipids and an antagonist effect on the breast. Raloxifine (the only licensed SERM) reduces vertebral fractures by 40-50%. It is not suitable for women with vasomotor symptoms.

Abnormal menopause

- **Premature menopause** If the menopause occurs before the age of 35 years, it is said to be premature. Often there is familial diathesis and cytogenetic studies reveal no abnormality. Treatment by substitution therapy is of value.

- *Delayed menopause* If the menopause fails to occur even beyond 55 years, it is called delayed. The common causes are constitutional, uterine fibroids, diabetes mellitus and oestrogenic tumours of the ovary. In the absence of palpable pelvic pathology, endometrial aspiration should be done to exclude endometrial malignancy.

- *Artificial menopause* can occur following surgery or radiation.

  1. *Surgical* Menstruating women who have had bilateral oophorectomy and/or hysterectomy, experience sudden menopausal symptoms which may sometimes be more troublesome than natural menopause.

  2. *Radiation* The ovarian function may be suppressed by external gamma radiation in women below the age 40. The castration is not permanent. The menstruation may resume after 2 years and even conception is possible. Intracavitary introduction of radium can cause castration by destroying the endometrium and also by suppressing the ovarian function. The menopausal symptoms are not so intense as found in surgical menopause.

7

Amenorrhoea

Regular menstruation is dependant on a functioning hypothalamo-pituitary ovarian axis. Amenorrhoea or lack of visible evidence of menstruation results due to a weakening or a break in the axis.

Physiological amenorrhoea occurs prior to the onset of puberty, during pregnancy, lactation and after menopause.

Pathological amenorrhoea is defined as failure to menstruate for atleast 6-12 months during the normal reproductive years and is not related to pregnancy or lactation.

Amenorrhoea can be classified as:

1. Primary
2. Secondary

Primary Failure to menstruate at the onset of puberty (i.e., 16 yrs.) in the presence of well developed secondary sex characters and 14 yrs. in the absence of well developed secondary sex characteristics.

Secondary When there has been evidence of prior menstruation, but there is amenorrhoea for atleast 6 months.

Prevalence 1-2% of women in the reproductive age group. Endocrine disturbances are the underlying cause in 99% and anatomical defects in 1%.

PRIMARY AMENORRHOEA

The causes could be due to problems in the hypothalamus, pituitary, ovary, uterus or the outflow tract and are outlined in Flow chart 1.

Evaluation of a patient with primary amenorrhoea

History
- Age at menarche of other siblings (could be familial)

87

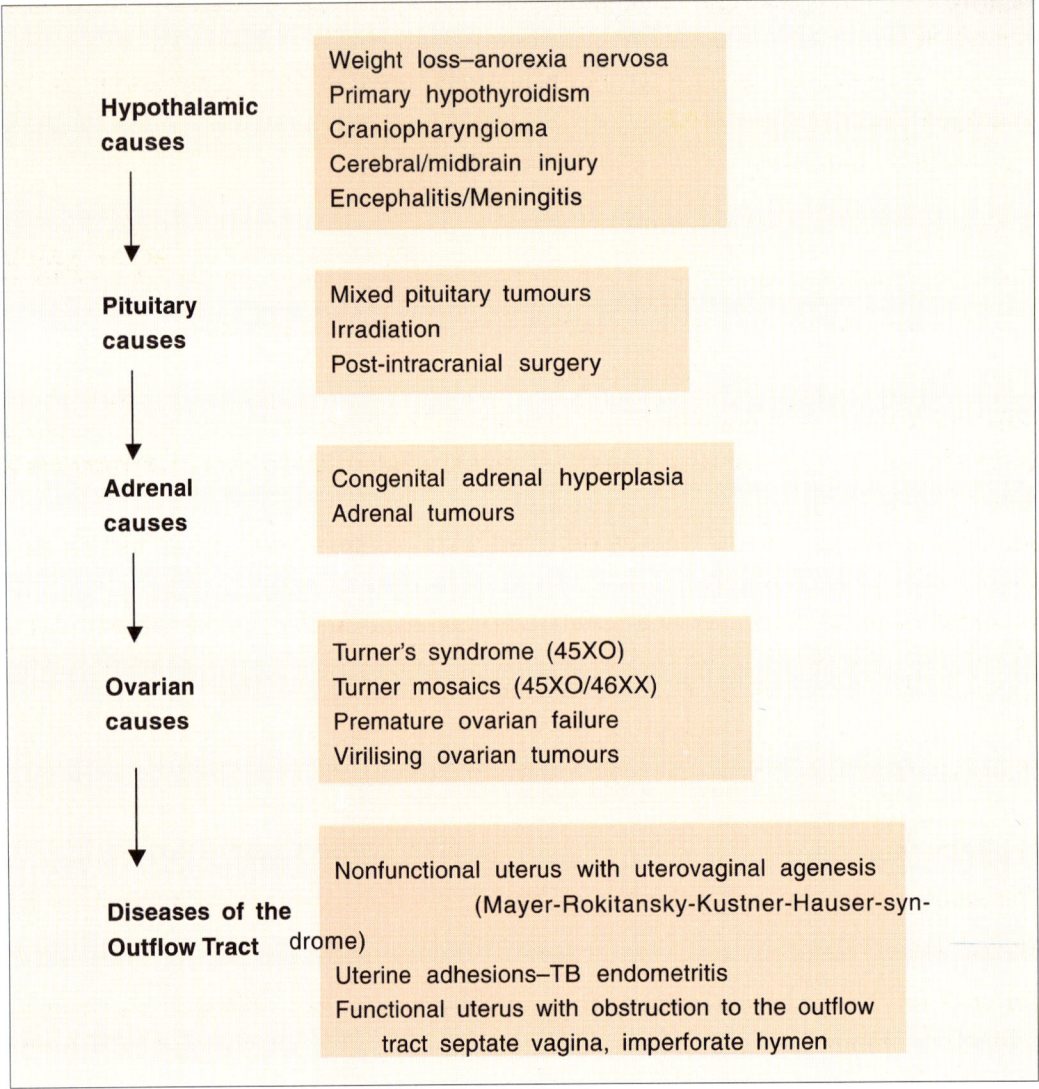

Hypothalamic causes
- Weight loss–anorexia nervosa
- Primary hypothyroidism
- Craniopharyngioma
- Cerebral/midbrain injury
- Encephalitis/Meningitis

Pituitary causes
- Mixed pituitary tumours
- Irradiation
- Post-intracranial surgery

Adrenal causes
- Congenital adrenal hyperplasia
- Adrenal tumours

Ovarian causes
- Turner's syndrome (45XO)
- Turner mosaics (45XO/46XX)
- Premature ovarian failure
- Virilising ovarian tumours

Diseases of the Outflow Tract
- Nonfunctional uterus with uterovaginal agenesis (Mayer-Rokitansky-Kustner-Hauser-syndrome)
- Uterine adhesions–TB endometritis
- Functional uterus with obstruction to the outflow tract septate vagina, imperforate hymen

Flow chart 1. Causes of primary amenorrhoea

- Family history of chromosomal abnormalities
- History of excessive weight loss of 10-15% of body weight by dieting, exercise (seen in *anorexia nervosa*)
- History of cyclical lower abdominal pain-suggests *cryptomenorrhoea* (unseen menstruation) due to obstructive lesions in the outflow tract
- History of anosmia (suggests Kallman's syndrome)
- History of headaches, visual disturbances suggests intracranial tumours

- History of meningitis, tuberculosis (amenorrhoea could be due to hypothalamic involvement)
- History suggestive of virilization, hirsuitism, change in voice (indicate hyper androgenisation as the cause)
- History of radiotherapy to the pelvis or chemotherapy.

Examination

- Build and nutritional status
- Height–short stature is seen hypothyroidism and Turner's syndrome
- Development of secondary sex characters
- Signs of virilization–change in voice, hirsuitism, acne
- Stigmata of Turner's syndrome–webbed neck, pectus-cavum, cubitus-valgus, widely spaced nipples
- Abdomen-abdominal mass may be detected (uterine-cryptomenorrhoea; lumbar-adrenal tumours).
- External genitalia–note if the external genitalia are male/female; a bulging hymenal membrane indicates an imperforate hymen, clitoromegaly (indicates virilization), undescended testes in the groins suggests Testicular Feminization.
- Vagina–note the presence/absence of vaginal canal by one finger examination. If vagina is present note if it is communicating with the cervical canal or not.

Investigations

- Ultrasound abdomen and pelvis to assess the presence/absence of uterus/ovaries.
- Buccal smear–presence of barr body (sex chromatin) indicates normal 46XX-karyotype.
- Serum FSH, LH, prolactin, oestradiol–A low gonadotropin level indicates a hypothalamo-pituitary cause, a high level indicates an ovarian cause (low oestrogen levels lead to absence of negative feed back inhibition).
- Chromosomal analysis (45×O in Turner's syndrome)
- Plain x-ray skull-reveals widening of the sella in pituitary tumours.
- Contrast enhanced CT head (CECT)–may reveal a pituitary tumour or cranio pharyngioma.

Treatment of primary amenorrhoea

Goals of treatment

1. Correct the underlying cause.

2. Correct sexual infantilism and initiate full reproductive potential when possible.

3. Correct short stature.

1. *Correction of underlying cause*

   – Surgical excision of craniopharyngioma and pituitary tumours.

   – XY karyotype–surgical removal of testicular tissue is indicated to prevent the development of gonadoblastoma.

   – Imperforate hymen–Cruciate incisions are given in the hymenal membrane to relieve the collected menstrual blood.

   – Vaginal atresia/septate vagina–vaginoplasty is indicated.

2. *Correction of sexual Infantilism* Exogenous estrogen + progesterone are given for development of breast and uterus.

3. *Correction of short stature* Human growth hormone and exogenous gonadotropins are given to correct short stature.

SECONDARY AMENORRHOEA

The absence of menses in a woman who has previously been menstruating regularly for a period of six months or more is termed as secondary amenorrhoea.

Causes

1. Physiological

   – Pregnancy

   – Lactation

2. Pathological (causes are summarized in table 7.1)

   – Hypothalamo-pituitary causes

   – Ovarian causes

   – Uterine causes

   – Systemic disease

   – Weight loss/anorexia nervosa

Evaluation of a patient with secondary amenorrhoea

History The following points should be noted in the history:

• Date of last menstrual period

• History of lactation

Table 7.1. Causes of secondary amenorrhoea

Hypothalamic causes
- Stress
- Drugs (causing hyperprolactinemia)
- Intracranial tumours
- Craniopharyngioma
- Trauma–head injury or following removal of a large intracranial tumour
- Irradiation

Pituitary
- Postpartum pituitary necrosis–Sheehan's syndrome
- Hyperprolactinaemia–(due to drugs, prolactinemi a, idiopathic)
- Empty-sella syndrome

Ovary
- Premature ovarian failure
- Virilising ovarian tumours

Systemic
- Hypothyroidism
- Chronic renal failure (CRF)
- Chronic liver disease

Uterus
- Asherman's syndrome
- Missed abortion

- History of recent use of oral contraceptive pills (suggests post-pill amenorrhoea)
- History of recent weight loss, diet change, vigorous exercise (suggests anorexia nervosa)
- History of visual disturbances, galactorrhoea (suggests pituitary tumour)
- Family history of premature menopause, suggests idiopatic premature menopause
- History of drug intake-phenothiazines, methyldopa
- History of excessive hair growth over the body and voice change (suggests virilization)
- History of postpartum haemorrhage (suggests Sheehan's syndrome or postpartum pituitary necrosis)
- History of postpartum curettage suggests (Asherman's syndrome–causing intra-uterine synechiae)
- History of tuberculosis (suggests TB endometritis)
- History of thyroid, renal or liver disease as chronic illness could be the cause of secondary amenorrhoea.

Examination   The points to be noted in the examination are:

- Weight and nutritional status
- Sign of virilization–acne, hirsuitism, clitoromegaly
- Signs of Turner's syndrome–webbed neck, widely-spaced nipples, pectus cavum.
- Vaginal examination–rugosity of the vagina, size of the uterus and any adnexal mass are noted.
- Visual fields, fundoscopy are carried out if a pituitary tumour is suspected.

The evaluation and investigations of a patient with amenorrhoea are given in Flow chart 2.

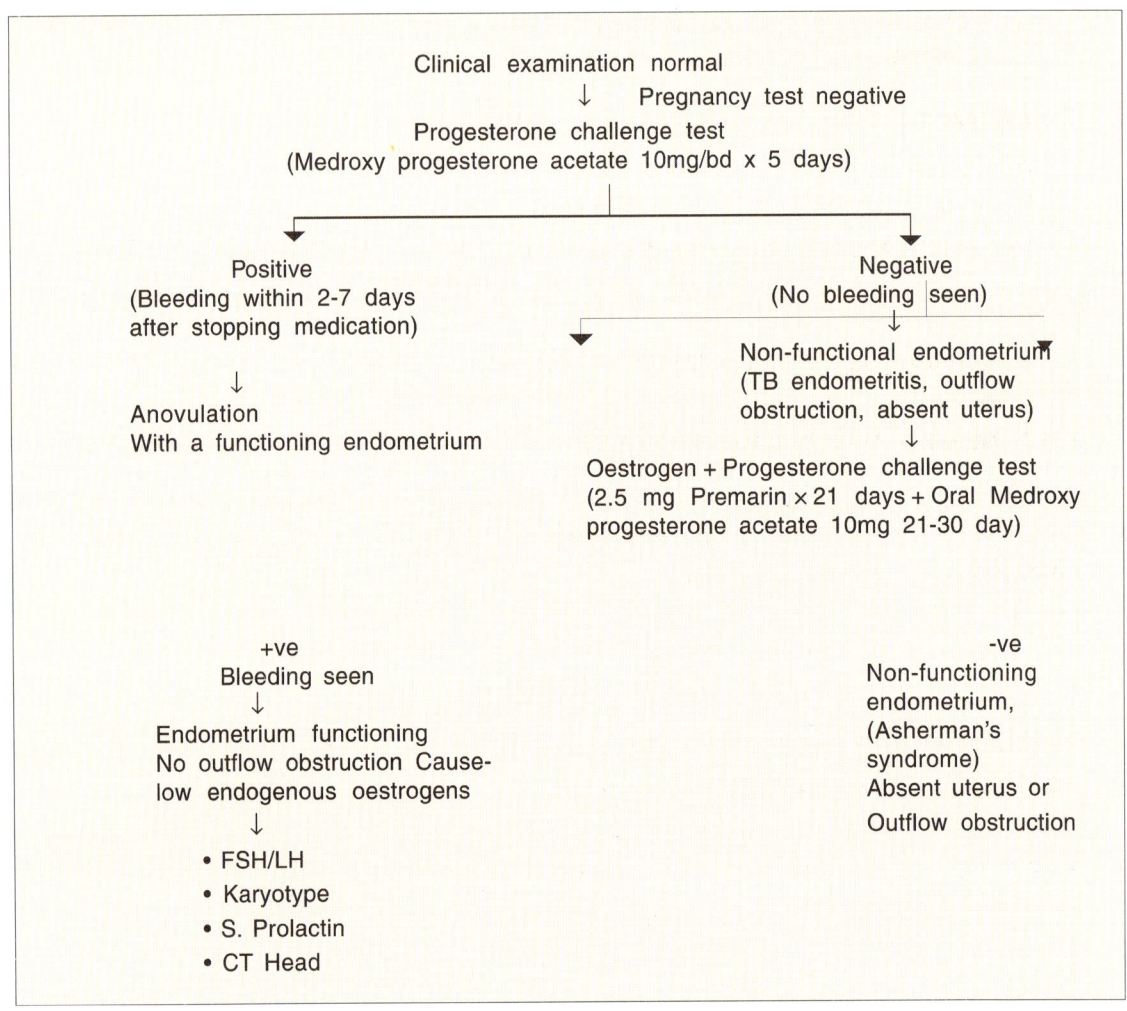

Flow chart 2.   Evaluation of patient with amenorrhoea

Management of secondary amenorrhoea

The management of a patient with secondary amenorrhoea depends on the cause identified.

1. *Hypothalamo-pituitary causes* Identification and elimination of the stressful factors, removal of intracranial tumours may result in return of menses. Patients who have had brain injury (due to surgery or RT) and have low gonadotropin levels need ovulation induction with gonadotropins or pulsatile GnRH therapy to restore fertility.

   • *Hyperprolactinaemia* –

     a) Dopamine agonists (Bromocriptine, Cabergoline) are indicated in small prolactinomas and in idiopathic hyperprolactinaemia.

     b) Surgery is indicated in macro-adenomas and those patients who are unresponsive to drugs.

2. *Ovarian causes*

   • Premature ovarian failure need cyclical oestrogens and progesterones to protect the female skeleton from demineralization.

   • Virilizing ovarian tumours–need excision.

3. *Uterine causes*

   • Hysteroscopic division of intrauterine adhesions with HRT is indicated in Asherman's syndrome.

   • A patient with missed abortion needs dilatation and evacuation under antibiotic cover.

4. *Systemic diseases* need to be managed, menstrual cycles resume when the organ functions are restored.

8

Menstrual Dysfunction

Menstrual dysfunctions commonly encountered are:

- Menorrhagia
- Polymenorrhoea
- Dysmenorrhoea
- Premenstrual syndrome

MENORRHAGIA

- A Greek word *mene*-moon *rheghyme*-to burst forth.
- Regular heavy bleeding every month, 50 to 80 ml per cycle is considered normal, 80 ml being the upper limit.
- Normal menstrual cycle:

    Occurs every 22 to 35 days.

    Normal menstrual flow lasts 3 to 7 days, with most blood loss occurring within the first 3 days.

    The menstrual flow amounts to 35 ml and consists of effluent debris and blood.

    Approximately 16 mg of iron is lost with each menstrual cycle, this will rarely result in anaemia in women with an adequate intake of dietary iron.

- In menorrhagia patients lose more than 80 ml of blood with each menstrual cycle and often develop anaemia. Other common Greek names for menstrual symptoms are–

    Polymenorrhoea – frequent periods

    Polymenorrhagia – frequent heavy periods

    Oligomenorrhoea – infrequent periods

    Oligomenorrhagia – infrequent heavy periods

    Metrorrhagia – irregular acyclical bleeding

Metropathia haemorrhagica – continuous vaginal bleeding for weeks preceded by a period of amenorrhoea

To understand the management, it is important to know something about aetiological factors, pathogenesis of various presentations and proper assessment of the problem.

Aetiology

Menorrhagia could be **Primary** or **Secondary**.

Primary menorrhagia – DUB (see below)

- There is no local or extra genital cause.
- Aetiology is purely hormonal.
- Hyperplasia and hypertrophy of the endometrium is caused by a high titre of endogenous oestrogen.

Secondary menorrhagia – is secondary to systemic, local or iatrogenic causes.

1. *Systemic disease*

    - blood dyscrasias–leukaemia, coagulopathy, thrombocytopenic purpura
    - hypothyroidism

2. *Local causes*

    - Uterine – uterine fibroids, submucosal polyps
    - Ovarian causes – PCOD, feminizing ovarian tumours
    - Tubo-ovarian causes – endometriosis, pelvic inflammatory disease
    - Immediate puerperium and post abortion – due to altered vascularity in the pelvis.

3. *Iatrogenic*

    - IUCD – 10% of cases can be associated with menorrhagia.
    - Post sterilization – 15% of cases seen following PPS, due to altered blood supply to the pelvis.
    - Progestogens – minipill, depo-provera

Dysfunctional uterine bleeding (DUB)

- Dysfunctional uterine bleeding is defined as excessively heavy (> 80 mls per month) or prolonged uterine bleeding in the absence of systemic or genital tract pathology. It is a diagnosis of exclusion.

- It affects 10% of women and is the most common cause of iron deficiency anaemia and gynaecological referrals.

- Although up to 30% of women report symptoms, this is confirmed on objective measurement in less than a third of cases. Dysfunctional uterine bleeding is divided into *ovulatory*, which is associated with regular painful periods, and *anovulatory*, which is more common in the postmenarchal and perimenopausal age groups.

Metropathia Haemorrhagica

- It is a specialized form of dysfunctional uterine haemorrhage.

- *Symptoms* are very typical. The most common complaint is of continuous vaginal bleeding which may last for many weeks. In half the cases the continuous bleeding is preceded by a short period of amenorrhoea, an interval of about eight weeks elapsing between the last period and the onset of the continuous haemorrhage. The bleeding is always painless since it is anovulatory.

- *Physical signs* that are usually obtained are those of a slight symmetrical enlargement of the uterus together with the presence of a cystic ovary.

- *Pathology* There is a mild degree of myohyperplasia of the myometrium, causing a symmetrical enlargement of the uterus. The endometrium is thick, haemorrhagic, and polypoidal, with thin, slender polypi projecting towards the internal os. Microscopy shows the characteristic *cystic glandular hyperplasia* with dilated cystic glands and a hyperplastic stroma (*swiss cheese pattern*).

- *Investigations* planned are determined by the history and clinical examination findings. They include basic haematological investigations followed by ultrasound for endometrial thickness and hysteroscopy with directed biopsies.

- *Treatment* of metropathia

  - Progesterone is the most effective therapy; the dose of orally active progestogen varies according to the age of the patient, the amount of bleeding and the time in the cycle at which treatment commences. Norethynodrel, norethisterone and lynestrenol are the progestogens most commonly used which are usually continued for about 21 days.

  - The use of combined oral oestrogen/progestogen contraceptives leading to anovulation is a useful second line of management and should be continued for 9-12 months if symptoms improve.

  - Clomiphene 50-100 mg daily for five days is indicated in young women who are also infertile with anovulation. Clomiphene acts by inducing ovulation, after which the metropathic syndrome cannot continue.

Evaluation of a patient with menorrhagia

History

A detailed history should be taken regarding

- Age and parity of the patient
- Duration of symptoms
- Duration and amount of bleeding
- Whether the bleeding is cyclical / acyclical
- History suggestive of PID eg. white discharge, abdominal pain associated with bleeding
- History of dysmenorrhoea, dyspareunia suggests endometriosis
- History of IUCD in-situ, or previous tubal ligation
- Any history of amenorrhoea preceding the bleeding episode as it could be an incomplete miscarriage.
- History of recent delivery or abortion should be asked.
- History suggestive of a bleeding disorder eg. easy bruisability, bleeding from wounds should be asked.

Examination

A full general examination to look for anaemia, hypothyroidism, any purpuric spots suggestive of thrombocytopenia, abdominal and pelvic examination to look for fibroids, any adnexal mass suggestive of endometriosis or PID should be looked for.

Investigations

- Haemogram and platelet counts, coagulation profile
- Thyroid function tests
- LH/FSH ratio if the history is suggestive of PCOS.
- Ultrasound to exclude any pelvic pathology.
- Endometrial sampling with a Pipelle or 4mm Karman's cannula is good to assess the endometrial histology but can miss polyps as only 4% of the endometrium is sampled.
- Dilatation and curettage, primarily for biopsy, samples only 50% of the uterine cavity.
- Hysteroscopy is an optimum method of investigation for intermenstrual bleeding (IMB), menorrhagia at any age or postmenopausal bleeding. Hysteroscopy is now the gold standard worldwide for diagnosis as well as treatment.

Below the age of 40 years, the risk of endometrial cancer is very low, endometrial sampling is not normally required for menorrhagia. However, irregular bleeding warrants hysteroscopy and sampling to rule out endometrial pathology.

The RCOG (Royal College of Obstetricians and Gynaecologists) guidelines recommend screening for coagulation disorders and hypothyroidism only in cases where no cause is found.

Medical management of menorrhagia

The treatment of DUB should be with the simplest effective regimen with minimum side effects. First-line therapy is medical and will depend on the patient's need for contraception and on the severity of the problem. Regardless of which therapy is chosen, treatment should be reviewed after 3 months and, if there is no response, the patient should be referred for further investigation. The treatment is tailored based on the need for contraception (table 8.1).

Table 8.1. Medical management of menorrhagia	
Patients not needing contraception	**Patients needing contraception**
– NSAIDs (Mefenamic acid) – Antifibrinolytics (Tranexamic acid) – Progestogens	– Combined oral pill – DMPA – Mirena – GnRH analogues – Danazol

Patients with a regular cycle who do not require contraception

1. *Antifibrinolytics* (*Tranexamic acid*) This is the most effective first-line drug. It acts by inhibiting tissue plasminogen activator (a fibrinolytic enzyme that has raised levels in women with DUB) and reduces menstrual blood loss (MBL) by around 50%. The dose of tranexamic acid is 1g three to four times a day during menstruation. The side effects are mainly minor gastrointestinal with high doses. It is contraindicated where there is a history of thromboembolic disease.

2. *Nonsteroidal anti-inflammatory drugs (NSAIDS)* such as Mefenamic acid are effective, well tested and tolerated. They act by inhibiting cyclooxygenase and decrease the endometrial prostaglandin release. NSAIDs reduce MBL by 25-40%; they are also analgesic drugs, so they are often used as first-line treatment in the presence of dysmenorrhoea. Mefenamic acid is commonly used at a dose of 500 mg three times a day for 5 days during menses. The main side effect is gastrointestinal irritation.

3. *Progestogens* Synthetic progestogens (norethisterone 5mg 8-hourly from day 12-26 or day 5-26) are the most popular drugs prescribed in general practice for the treatment of menorrhagia even though they have minimal or no effect on MBL. Progestogen therapy can be of value in regulating an irregular cycle. The main side effects are weight gain, bloating, and androgenic symptoms such as acne.

Patients with an irregular cycle or who need contraception

1. *Combined oral contraceptive pill (COC)* is commonly used especially in young women. It reduces MBL by 50%, helps to regulate periods, and provides contraception. The mode of action is by inhibition of ovulation, production of an inactive endometrium, possibly by reduction in the endometrial prostaglandin synthesis and fibrinolysis. In the perimenopausal age group sequential combined hormone replacement therapy (HRT) can be used in a similar way to regulate the cycle and reduce the mean blood loss.

2. *Injectables* Depo-Provera used for contraception is also associated with reduced MBL and amenorrhoea in some women.

3. *Levonorgestrel-releasing intrauterine contraceptive device (Mirena)* releases 20µg of levonorgestrel per 24 hours over 5 years. The modes of action of levonorgestrel are a reduction in the endometrial prostaglandin synthesis, the production of an inactive endometrium, and a reduction in the endometrial fibrinolytic activity. It reduces MBL by 86% after 3 months. If a copper intrauterine contraceptive device is already in-situ, treatment should be given with either tranexamic acid or NSAIDS or the IUCD changed to levonorgestrel intrauterine device. Patients should be warned that irregular bleeding is common during the first 3 months after insertion.

Second-line medical treatment

1. *Danazol* (100mg/6-24 hourly) is a synthetic steroid that acts in a number of ways. It inhibits steroid synthesis, blocks the androgen and progesterone receptors, and inhibits pituitary gonadotropins. These actions combine to inhibit endometrial growth. However, its use is limited by the androgenic side-effects (acne, hirsuitism, breast atrophy, weight gain) and the high cost of the drug.

2. *Gonadotropin-releasing hormone analogues (GnRHa)* (*Goserelin, Buserelin, Prostap*) down regulate the pituitary and inhibit follicle-stimulating hormone (FSH) and luteinizing hormone (LH) production. They are highly effective in producing amenorrhoea; treatment cannot given for longer than 6 months because of the risk of osteoporosis on prolonged therapy.

Surgical management of menorrhagia

1. **Curettage** the age old, most commonly used treatment somehow cures 30 to 40% patients. It is recommended in young women if hormone therapy fails, for diagnosis in

the older age group, to exclude atypical hyperplasia, tuberculosis and endometrial carcinoma. Joshi and Deshpande reported the endometrial histology in DUB as given in the table 8.2.

Table 8.2. Endometrial histology in DUB		
Normal endometrium	–	54.0%
Hyperplastic endometrium	–	31.0%
Irregular ripening	–	3.0%
Irregular shedding	–	6.0%
Atrophic endometrium	–	3.0%
Chronic endometritis	–	1.0%
Others	–	2.0%

2. *Hysterectomy* indicated, when the woman wants permanent amenorrhoea or there is uterine pathology. It can be performed transabdominally, transvaginally or assisted by laparoscopy.

3. *Minimally invasive surgical options* are becoming a more attractive alternative to hysterectomy (particularly in the developed world) as they are almost equally effective in reducing the heavy flow, safe in experienced hands, have a short period of recovery and are cost effective.

   The aim is to destroy the endometrial glands. The various procedures used for endometrial ablation are–

   • *Hysteroscopic TCRE (Transcervical Resection of the Endometrium)*–The uterine cavity is distended by 1.5% glycine by using a C-infusor pressure cuffs or irrigation pump. Resection of endometrium is done by a resectoscope under direct vision; myomas and polyps can also be removed at the same time and tissue obtained for histopathology. The main complications are uterine perforation and fluid absorption.

   • *Uterine thermal balloon ablation*–Endometrium is destroyed by heated fluid in a balloon. The disposable balloon is expensive, and is suitable for a uterus of normal size and shape only.

   • *Microwave endometrial ablation (MEA)*–Microwave energy is supplied by microwave generator to a probe placed in the uterine cavity. The probe is moved slowly across the fundus and down through the uterine cavity, destroying the endometrium.

POLYMENORRHOEA

• Frequent regular menstruation eg. every 2-3 wks.

- It is common at the time of menarche and the menopause.

- It occurs due to a disordered hypothalamo-pituitary ovarian axis. It could also be due to ovarian hyperactivity seen with salpingo-oophoritis, chocolate cysts of the ovaries.

- Frequent menstruation is usually associated with increased flow.

- Treatment of polymenorrhoea is the same as outlined in the section of menorrhagia.

DYSMENORRHOEA

Dysmenorrhoea or painful menstruation is when the menstrual periods are accompanied by either a sharp, intermittent or a dull, aching pain, usually in the pelvis or lower abdomen.

Dysmenorrhoea refers to menstrual pain severe enough to limit normal activities or require medication.

There are two types of dysmenorrhoea based on the cause.

- *Primary dysmenorrhoea* refers to menstrual pain that occurs in an otherwise healthy women. This type of pain is not related to any specific problems with the uterus or other pelvic organs. Increased endometrial levels of the hormone prostaglandin, PGF2 alpha, is thought to be a factor in primary dysmenorrhoea.

- *Secondary dysmenorrhoea* is menstrual pain that is attributed to some underlying disease process or structural abnormality either within or outside the uterus.

Aetiology

The causes of dysmenorrhoea are given below:

Primary dysmenorrhoea The pain is due to muscular spasm, sufficiently intense to cause ischaemia. The theories postulated are:

a) *Endocrine causes* Invariably associated with ovulatory cycles. Progesterone stimulates myometrial contraction which further stimulates production of prostaglandin F2 that accentuates pain.

b) *Nerve pathways* Muscle spasm of uterus may be the result of an imbalance of the autonomic nerve supply of the uterus. Surgical division of the presacral nerve at *Cotte's operation* interrupts the sensory pathway of pain and alleviates pain during menstruation.

Secondary dysmenorrhoea The pain occurs due to muscular spasms in a uterus which has a foreign body eg. an IUCD or a mass acting like a foreign body eg. fibroid.

The other common causes are endometriosis and adenomyosis, pelvic inflammatory disease, fibroids, cervical stenosis, unicornuate or bicornuate uterus.

Investigations

Investigations are planned based on the history and clinical examination findings. They are carried out primarily to exclude any pelvic pathology.

- Ultrasound pelvis
- Dilatation and curettage of the cervix may be diagnostic and therapeutic.
- Laparoscopy to diagnose endometriosis, PID, uterine anomalies
- Hysteroscopy–to diagnose a submucosal fibroid
- High vaginal swab cultures are taken to exclude PID.

Treatment

- If no cause is found a combined oral estrogen/progestogen contraceptive is given leading to an anovulatory cycle. They are useful as a therapeutic test and should be continued for 9-12 months if symptoms improve.
- For pain caused by an IUCD, removal of the IUD and alternative birth control methods may be needed.
- Antibiotics are necessary for pelvic inflammatory disease (see chapter on PID).

Membranous dysmenorrhoea It is a familial condition characterized by passage of membranes which take the form of casts. The cause is deficiency of a tryptic ferment secreted by the endometrium in normal menstruation. Treatment is same as spasmodic dysmenorrhoea.

PREMENSTRUAL SYNDROME

Premenstrual syndrome (PMS) involves symptoms that occur in relation to the menstrual cycle and interfere with the woman's life. The symptoms usually begin 5 to 11 days before the start of menstruation and usually stop when menstruation begins, or shortly thereafter.

An exact cause of PMS has not been identified. However, it may be related to social, cultural, biological and psychological factors. PMS can occur with apparently normal ovarian function (regular ovulatory cycles).

Symptoms

The most common symptoms include:

- Headache
- Swelling of ankles, feet and hands

- Backache
- Abdominal cramps or heaviness
- Abdominal pain
- Abdominal fullness, a feeling of gaseous distension
- Breast tenderness
- Weight gain
- Acne flare-ups
- Nausea
- Bloating
- Constipation or diarrhoea
- Food cravings
- Decreased tolerance for noises and lights
- Painful menstruation

It important that a complete history, physical examination (including pelvic exam), and in some instances a psychiatric evaluation be conducted to rule out other causes or symptoms that may be attributed to PMS. Physical examination is usually negative.

Treatment

There is no specific treatment. The following could be tried:

- Self-care, methods, exercise and dietary measures.
- Nutritional supplements–vitamin B6, calcium, and magnesium.
- Prostaglandin inhibitors (aspirin, ibuprofen, other NSAIDS) may be prescribed for women with significant pain, including headache, backache, menstrual cramps and breast tenderness.
- Diuretics may be prescribed for women found to have significant weight gain due to fluid retention.
- Psychiatric medications may be used for women who exhibit a moderate to severe degree of anxiety, irritability, or depression.
- Hormonal therapy may include a trial of oral contraceptives, which may either decrease or increase PMS symptoms. The use of progesterone vaginal suppositories during the second half of the menstrual cycle is controversial.

9

Bleeding in Early Pregnancy

First trimester bleeding is any bleeding noted during the first 12 weeks of pregnancy, and it is one of the most common symptoms reported by pregnant women. Until a non-threatening cause is identified, all first trimester bleeding is labelled as "threatened miscarriage". The common causes of bleeding in early pregnancy are–

1. Miscarriage
2. Ectopic pregnancy
3. Hydatidiform mole

MISCARRIAGE

The incidence of first trimester bleeding is 25-30%, miscarriage occurs in 50% of patients with bleeding mostly in the first 12 weeks. Even if pregnancy continues post-bleed, there is a higher risk of complications.

Definitions

- **Spontaneous miscarriage** is pregnancy loss before 20 wks of gestation, the weight of the conceptus being less than 500 grams. It is considered early if it occurs before 12 weeks.

- **Threatened miscarriage** is uterine bleeding with the cervix closed, with no evidence of fetal demise (Fig. 9.1a).

- **Inevitable miscarriage** is bleeding and rupture of the gestational sac at <20 wks. of gestation with a dilated cervix accompanied by menstrual-type of cramping. The products of conception have not been expelled yet (Fig. 9.1b).

- **Incomplete miscarriage** is incomplete evacuation of the products of conception.

- **Complete miscarriage** signifies complete evacuation of the products of conception. It is may difficult to differentiate from incomplete abortion if the amount of retained products are minimal and may require an ultrasound or a check curettage for diagnosis.

- **Missed miscarriage** (fetal demise) is a retained non-viable pregnancy (Fig. 9.1c).

- **Blighted ovum** (embryonic resorption) is a type of missed miscarriage when a gestational sac and placenta can be identified on ultrasound but the embryo fails to develop.

- **Sporadic miscarriage** is miscarriage which has occurred for the first time.

- **Recurrent miscarriage** is defined as three or more consecutive miscarriages; occurs in 0.5-20% of women.

- **Septic abortion** is an induced abortion which is complete or incomplete with secondary infection. This results in endometritis, parametritis or peritonitis.

- **Induced abortion** can be elective or therapeutic, and is discussed in the chapter on Medical Termination of Pregnancy.

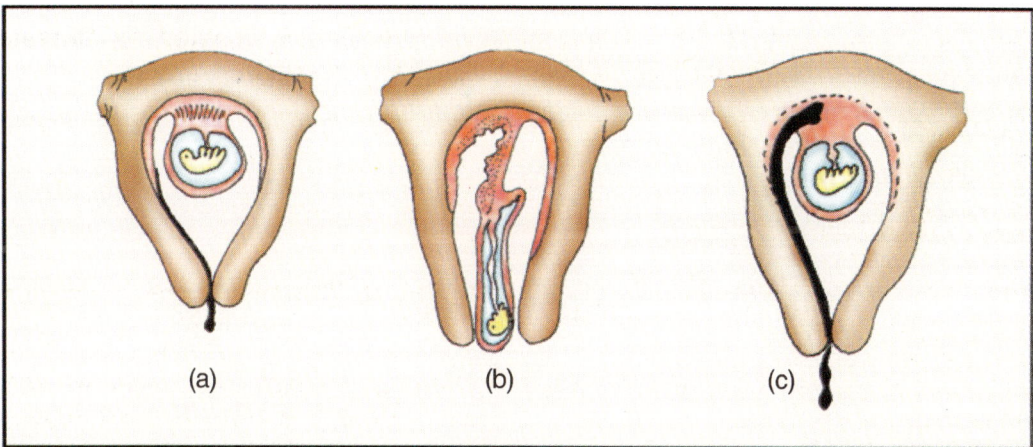

Fig. 9.1a-c. Types of miscarriage (a) Threatened miscarriage (b) Inevitable miscarriage and (c) Missed miscarriage (with a dead fetus)

Causes of miscarriage

The causes of sporadic first trimester pregnancy loss are different from those that are recurrent.

Causes of sporadic miscarriage

1. *Chromosomal anomalies* account for 50% of all cases

   - Autosomal trisomy is the most common and is seen in 30% of cases.

   - Chromosomal triploidy or monosomy seen in 20%.

2. *Infection* Several organisms are associated with early miscarriage eg. rubella, listeria,

toxoplasmosis, herpes, varicella zoster and malaria. Syphilis and parvo-virus B19 are commonly associated with late miscarriage. Group B streptococcal infection and bacterial vaginosis have been implicated in late second trimester miscarriage and preterm labour. High grade fever associated with any infection can also cause a miscarriage.

3. *Placental abnormalities* Abnormal placental villus development has been reported in 30-40% of miscarriages.

4. *Multiple pregnancy, maternal age and parity* The risk of early pregnancy loss with multiple pregnancies is twice that of singleton pregnancies. The rate of late pregnancy loss in monochorionic twin pregnancies is also increased. The risk of miscarriage rises with parity and also after 39 years of age.

5. *Maternal health* Poorly controlled diabetes, severe medical diseases, cigarette smoking, cocaine abuse, alcohol abuse have been associated with an increased risk. Chemical agents including lead, ethylene oxide, solvents, pesticides, anaesthetic gases have some association with fetal loss. Radiotherapy and chemotherapeutic agents are accepted causes of miscarriage and fetal abnormality; a dose of >25 rads is associated with a 0.1% risk of abnormality.

Causes of recurrent miscarriage

1. *Genetic factors* Parental chromosomal abnormalities (balanced or reciprocal translocations) are the most important genetic anomalies currently detectable amongst couples with recurrent miscarriage. Molecular mutations or single gene defects could also be a cause of recurrent miscarriage.

2. *Anatomical factors* Uterine anomalies, submucosal fibroids are associated with an increased risk of first and second trimester miscarriage possibly due to decreased vascularity of the placenta. Cervical incompetence is usually associated with early second trimester miscarriage. It usually presents as silent dilatation of the cervix with bulging of membranes, which eventually rupture spontaneously.

3. *Infections* Syphilis is a cause of recurrent late second trimester miscarriages and stillbirths. Malaria in endemic areas is also associated with recurrent miscarriages. Bacterial vaginosis is associated with recurrent late second-trimester miscarriage and preterm labour.

4. *Endocrine causes*

   – Uncontrolled diabetes has a higher risk of both fetal malformations and miscarriages.

   – Luteal phase defects–Corpus-luteum is essential for the implantation and maintenance of pregnancy; disorders have been reported to occur in 20-60% of women with recurrent miscarriage.

5. *Autoimmune and thrombophilic factors*

   – Autoimmune disease–Sporadic and recurrent miscarriage rates are increased in women with systemic lupus erythematosus (SLE).

   – Antiphospholipid syndrome–The antiphospholipid syndrome (APS) refers to a syndrome associaed with antiphospholipid antibodies (APL), anticardiolipin antibodies (ACC), recurrent miscarriage and thrombosis. Pregnancy loss with APS is attributed entirely to defective embryonic implantation and later to thrombosis of the uteroplacental vasculature and placental infarction.

6. *Other thrombophilias* Thrombophilias are inherited conditions causing a thrombotic tendency. Activated protein C resistance, hyperhomocystinaemia, protein S, protein C deficiency, antithrombin III deficiency are all associated with recurrent miscarriage as well as a risk of thromboembolism during pregnancy.

Evaluation of a patient with miscarriage

This includes a detailed history and examination.

History

A complete history with special emphasis on the following should be taken.

1. Quantity and rate of blood loss / passage of products of conception.

2. Pelvic pain or cramping

3. History of amenorrhoea

4. Symptoms of pregnancy eg. nausea, vomiting.

5. Any pregnancy confirmation test-urine pregnancy test, previous record of pelvic examination, USG.

6. History of fever, rash etc.

Physical examination

A thorough general physical and systemic examination should be carried out, including–

1. Temperature, pulse and blood pressure–a patient who has lost a significant amount of blood may have pallor, hypotension and tachycardia. In septic abortion, the patient may be febrile and tachycardic.

2. General physical examination should note any pallor, icterus, thyromegaly, pedal oedema.

3. Abdominal examination to note

   – any organomegaly

– signs of peritoneal irritation or haemoperitoneum which suggest a ruptured ectopic pregnancy e.g. rebound tenderness, abdominal distention.

4. Local examination

a) Per-speculum examination to note

– Bleeding through the os if present.

– Any cervical erosion, polyp etc. which may also be a cause of bleeding.

b) Per-vaginum examination to note

– Any cervical excitation to rule out ectopic

– Cervical dilatation–note if the os is open or closed. The os is open in cases of inevitable or incomplete miscarriage.

– Bimanual examination for size of the uterus, any adnexal mass or tenderness.

Differential diagnosis

The other causes of bleeding in the first trimester should be excluded.

- *Ectopic pregnancy* is associated with lower abdominal pain, giddiness, cervical excitation and adnexal tenderness on pelvic examination.

- *Twin loss* loss of one fetus of a twin pregnancy.

- *Hydatidiform mole* there may be a history of passage of vesicles, ultrasound and hCG are diagnostic.

- *Cervical ectopy* (commonly known as cervical erosion) is caused by the normal hormonal changes of pregnancy and can be cause of bleeding.

- *Subchorionic haemorrhage* represents a small clot that causes bleeding and then dissolves away harmlessly. Rarely, the clot dissects between the placenta and the decidua and causes a miscarriage.

- *Implantation bleeding* In the past it has been thought that an egg eroding into the uterine lining would cause bleeding because of a burrowing effect. It is usually considered the aetiology when no cause is identified and in which the pregnancy goes on successfully to term.

Investigations

Once a diagnosis of threatened abortion has been made, the following tests help to confirm viability and establish a diagnosis

1. **Urine pregnancy test**

2. **Ultrasound** (transabdominal or transvaginal if required) An intrauterine pregnancy is confirmed if a gestational sac is seen within the uterus. The presence of cardiac activity indicates it is viable. *Snow-storm appearance* is seen in cases of a vesicular mole.

Adnexal mass or a gestational sac in the adnexa with free fluid in the peritoneal cavity are suggestive of an ectopic pregnancy.

3. *Quantitative β HCG* If the beta hCG doubles in 48 hrs., it indicates a viable intrauterine pregnancy. If it fails to double in 48 hrs., it indicates a possible ectopic pregnancy.

4. *Examination of the expelled products of conception* any tissue passed should be evaluated and sent to pathology for a complete examination. Findings that confirm an intrauterine pregnancy are:

   - Chorionic villi–Rinse and put it in saline, if it floats, it indicates the tissue as chorionic villi, if it sinks down it could be decidua. This examination can be done even before sending the tissue to the laboratory.

   - Finding an intact embryo

   - Intact gestational sac

   - Histopathology indicates chorionic villi. A decidual cast is shed in an ectopic pregnancy

5. *Blood grouping and Rh typing* should be done and patients who are rhesus negative given anti-D.

Management

The management is summarized below:

- *Missed miscarriage* Dilatation and evacuation after using agents for cervical ripening (prostaglandin analogues) to reduce the risks of cervical trauma.

- *Threatened miscarriage*

  - Abstinence and bed rest–although there is paucity of clinical evidence to support this, many continue to advise it.

  - Maintain hydration and nutrition

  - Folic acid 1mg/day as prophylaxis against neural tube defects.

  - Progesterone supplementation (oral/vaginal)–there is limited evidence to support its use.

  - Give Anti-D prophylaxis if the mother is Rh negative and father is Rh positive.

- *Inevitable, incomplete or complete miscarriage*

  - Intravenous fluids are given if the patient is hypotensive or has lost a considerable amount of blood.

  - Anti-D prophylaxis if mother is Rh negative.

  - Expectant management of incomplete miscarriage–In women with minimal retained products (15-50ml), expectant management has been associated with complete miscarriage in 80%.

– Dilatation and evacuation with suction or ovum forceps is carried out followed by inj. ergometrine to contract the uterus and minimize bleeding.

- ***Recurrent miscarriage***

    The investigations which need to be carried out in recurrent first trimester miscarriage are given in table 9.1. Testing for thyroid function, random blood glucose, auto-antibody screen and TORCH titres has not been shown to be of any benefit.

Table 9.1. Investigations for recurrent miscarriage
• Male and female chromosome analysis • Anticardiolipin antibody (ACL) • Antiphospholipid antibody (APL) • Clotting studies • Activated protein C resistance • Testing for factor V Leiden mutation • Pelvic ultrasound scan • Hysterosalpingogram • Hysteroscopy • Laparoscopy

Treatment of recurrent first trimester miscarriage

- The only proven treatment is in antiphospholipid syndrome. The use of subcutaneous heparin and low-dose aspirin until 34 wks of gestation has been shown to be currently the most effective treatment

- Reassurance and psychological support have a 75% chance of a live birth in unexplained recurrent miscarriage.

ECTOPIC PREGNANCY

When the implantation of the fertilized ovum occurs anywhere outside the normal uterine cavity, the gestation is said to be ectopic. The most common site of implantation is the fallopian tubes (95%) when it is called a tubal pregnancy. The other sites of implantation are shown in table 9.2.

Table 9.2. Classification of ectopic pregnancy according to the site of implantation

• Tubal: This can be further divided as–
    Ampullary 80%
    Isthmic 12%
    Fimbrial 5%
    Interstitial 2%
• Ovarian 0.2%
• Abdominal 1.4%
• Cervical 0.2%

Pathophysiology

Natural course of a tubal pregnancy There is local enlargement of the tube resulting in either **tubal rupture** due to uncontrolled invasion of the trophoblast with destruction of the tubal wall or **tubal abortion** when the conceptus is excluded via the fimbrial end into the peritoneal cavity. This could either cause intraperitoneal bleeding from the site of implantation; or the expelled embryo may be absorbed and the symptoms resolve spontaneously. Recurrent choriodecidual haemorrhage around a dead conceptus results in the formation of a blood mole or ***carneous mole.*** A pregnancy in the cornual and isthmic end of the fallopian tube ruptures earlier than one at the ampullary end, as there is less space for expansion at the former sites.

Changes in the uterus The uterus becomes soft and slightly enlarged. The endometrial glands undergo hyperplasia and are closely packed with irregular hyperchromatic nuclei and evidence of hypersecretion; this change being known as the ***Arias-Stella reaction***. The stroma gets decidualized in response to the hormones and may be expelled as a ***decidual cast***.

High risk factors

- ***Pelvic inflammatory disease (PID)*** Infection of the tubal epithelium results in damage to the ciliated epithelium and formation of intraluminal adhesions and pockets.

- ***IUCD*** users are at an increased risk as an IUCD can prevent an intrauterine but not an ectopic pregnancy. Progesterone containing IUCD also affects the tubal motility, thus increasing the risk of implantation in the tube. Women who conceive with an IUCD have seven times increased risk of having an ectopic pregnancy.

- ***Previous history of ectopic pregnancy*** increases the risk and there is a 10-20% chance of having an ectopic in the subsequent pregnancy.

- ***Tubal reconstructive procedures*** interfere with tubal motility and are associated with an increased risk of an ectopic pregnancy.

- ***Tubal ligation*** increases the risk with a 20% chance of a pregnancy after sterilization being an ectopic.

- ***Assisted reproductive techniques (ART)***

- ***Smoking***-one study has found an increased risk possibly due to interference with tubal motility.

Diagnosis This is based on a detailed history and examination

History The clinical picture depends on whether the ectopic pregnancy is ruptured or not.

- A ruptured ectopic pregnancy is an acute emergency and presents classically with fainting attacks and collapse, associated with intra-abdominal haemorrhage.

- History of amenorrhoea of short duration (6-8 wks.) as tubal rupture occurs early. However, patients with interstitial or abdominal pregnancy can have amenorrhoea of longer duration.
- Abdominal pain due to tubal rupture and intraperitoneal collection of blood. The pain radiates to the shoulder due to diaphragmatic irritation.
- Vaginal bleeding is usually scanty but persistent.

General examination

- In ruptured ectopic with massive intraperitoneal haemorrhage, the patient is ill-looking with pallor, tachycardia and other features of shock.
- There may be abdominal distension in case of massive intraperitoneal haemorrhage.
- In tubal abortion, the presentation is sub-acute, the patient is symptomatic, but clinically stable.

Per-vaginal examination reveals

- Tenderness on cervical excitation.
- Uterus is usually normal sized or bulky.
- Palpable adnexal mass on the site of the ectopic due to the dilated tube, adherent omentum and bowel.
- Fullness in the pouch of douglas may be noted due to collection of blood in the cul-de-sac.
- The pelvic examination may be completely normal in an unruptured ectopic or a tubal rupture.

Investigations

- *Urine pregnancy test* is usually positive.
- *Quantitative serum beta hCG levels* In an intrauterine pregnancy, the hCG levels usually double in 48 hrs. In an ectopic pregnancy, there is sub-optimal rise in the beta hCG and does not double in 48 hrs.
- *Ultrasonography* Trans-vaginal sonography shows an empty uterus with an adnexal mass or increased vascularity at the site of the ectopic with free fluid in the pouch of douglas. A pseudo-gestational sac may be seen in the uterus due to the decidual cast.
- *Culdocentesis* (needle aspiration in the posterior fornix) reveals altered blood. It is not indicated routinely and should be performed in the OT, if laparoscopy is not available and the diagnosis is doubtful.
- *Abdominal paracentesis* may reveal blood in case of a ruptured ectopic with haemoperitoneum.

- **Laparoscopy** remains the gold standard for diagnosis; the tube appears distended and bluish with presence of free blood in the peritoneal cavity.

Management

The management depends on the general condition of the patient, the duration of symptoms and the desire for future fertility.

- Acute ruptured ectopic in shock demands immediate resuscitation followed by laparotomy and salpingectomy.
- Sub-acute onset, when the general condition is stable, laparoscopic or open surgery can be used depending on the facilities available and the skill of the surgeon. There is no statistically significant difference in the reproductive outcome with either laparotomy or by laparoscopic technique. However, laparoscopic approach provides a shorter duration of hospitalization and has a lower risk of developing intra-abdominal adhesions in the post-op period.

Surgical options

The types of surgery which can be performed are:

1. **Salpingectomy** involves removal of the fallopian tube and is indicated in
   - Ruptured tubal pregnancy
   - Recurrent ectopic pregnancy in a tube already treated conservatively
   - Previous sterilization and reversal of sterilization
   - Previous tubal surgery for infertility
   - Pre-existing tubal damage as a consequence of a frozen pelvis.

2. **Conservative surgery** is indicated in patients who wish to preserve their fertility. The types of surgeries which can be performed are:
   - Linear salpingotomy—An incision is given over the tube and the products of conception removed.
   - Segmental resection is carried out when the ectopic is located in the isthmic region of the fallopian tube.
   - Fimbrial evacuation is indicated when the pregnancy lies at the fimbrial end. It involves gentle and progressive compression of the tube starting first proximal to the site of pregnancy towards the fimbrial end to achieve a tubal abortion.

Medical management

Methotrexate is given in a patient with an unruptured tubal pregnancy who is asymptomatic and haemodynamically stable. It is indicated when

- Initial pre-treatment beta hCG is <10,000 iu/l.

- Tubal diameter is <2 cm as defined by direct visualization or by ultrasound.

- Fetal heart beat is absent on ultrasound scan.

It is given in a single dose of 50mg/m^2 of body surface area and the beta hCG levels are monitored for two weeks.

Non-tubal ectopic pregnancy

1. ***Cervical pregnancy*** is one that implants within the cervical canal. It causes profuse vaginal bleeding with crampy abdominal pain. On examination, the uterus surrounding the distended cervix feels smaller and curettage reveals no evidence of trophoblastic tissue. On ultrasound scan, there is ballooning of the cervical canal, the gestational sac is in the endocervix and the internal os is closed.

2. ***Ovarian pregnancy*** is the most common non-tubal type of ectopic pregnancy. The diagnosis is usually made on laparoscopy or laparotomy. Spielberg (1878) defined certain criteria for the diagnosis of ovarian pregnancy.

   - the gestational sac must occupy a portion of the ovary.

   - the gestational sac must be connected to the uterus by the ovarian ligament.

   - ovarian tissue must be identified in the wall of the sac.

   - the fallopian tube on the affected side should be normal.

3. ***Abdominal pregnancy*** could be of two types

   i)   Primary abdominal pregnancy due to primary peritoneal implantation of the blastocyst.

   ii) Secondary due to peritoneal implantation of the conceptus following tubal abortion, or rupture. This is more common than primary.

   The treatment of both is by an immediate laparotomy with removal of the fetus and placenta if technically feasible, as the placenta may be implanted on the bowel etc.

4. ***Intra-ligamentous pregnancy*** due to penetration of the tubal wall with advancement into the broad ligament by the trophoblastic tissue. The diagnosis is usually made on laparotomy.

5. ***Heterotopic pregnancy*** is a combination of an intrauterine and extrauterine pregnancy. It is more common in IVF pregnancies.

HYDATIDIFORM MOLE

It is an abnormal development of the placenta (abnormal trophoblastic proliferation) resulting in the formation of grape like vesicles, as the fetal part of the pregnancy fails to develop. It could be *complete* or *partial*.

Complete mole–the entire fetus and placenta are replaced by grape like vesicles.

Partial mole–if only part of the placenta and/or the fetus are converted to molar tissue.

Risk factors

- Age – <20 and > 35 yrs.
- Low socioeconomic status
- Race/ethnic origin-more common in women of south-east asia, however recent studies have shown that the incidence has decreased possibly due to altered dietary habits.
- Dietary deficiency of high quality protein, folic acid and iron
- Parity–increasing parity increases the risk
- Previous molar pregnancy–also increases the risk.

Genetics   A complete mole contains only paternal DNA due to fertilization of a haploid sperm (23X) with an empty ovum which then duplicates to form 46XX, of which both the x-chromosomes are from the male partner (***androgenisation***). A partial mole has a triploid set of chromosomes with two paternal and one maternal set (Fig. 9.2).

Pathology

- A *complete mole* grossly resembles a bundle of grapes due to hydropic degeneration and swelling of all the chorionic villi. The embryo is not developed.

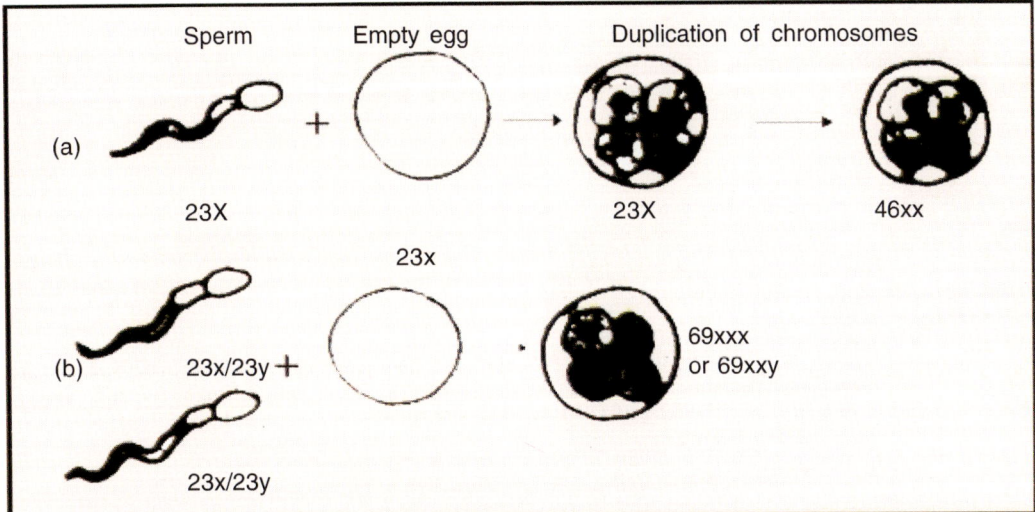

Fig. 9.2.   Genetics of molar pregnancy (a) Complete mole–one sperm fertilizes an empty egg followed by duplication and (b) Partial mole–fertilization of one egg with 23x chromosomes with two sperms giving a triploid set of chromosomes

- In a *partial mole*, villus swelling affects only some villi and the embryo is also present.
- In an *invasive mole*, the molar tissue invades the myometrium and surrounding pelvic structures and can present with intraperitoneal haemorrhage.
- *Choriocarcinoma* grossly appears as a soft, purple, largely haemorrhagic mass. Microscopically, it has cores of cytotrophoblast surrounded by multinucleated syncytiotrophoblast with the absence of chorionic villi, and extensive areas of haemorrhage and necrosis. It can arise from a normal pregnancy, a complete or a partial mole.

Clinical features

History The following symptoms are characteristic, however all of them may or may not be present.

- Amenorrhoea
- Vaginal bleeding-intermittent or continuous
- History of passage of grapelike vesicles
- Abdominal pain
- Hyperemesis (30%)
- Severe pre-ecclampsia and thyrotoxicosis (due to cross-reactivity between hCG and TSH at the TSH receptor site).
- Invasive mole can present with persistent abdominal pain or intraperitoneal bleeding from an invading mole.
- Choriocarcinoma usually presents as irregular bleeding and an enlarged uterus following an abortion or term pregnancy. One third of them present with symptoms due to distant metastases in the lungs, brain or liver.

Examination

- Pallor which is disproportionate to the amount of bleeding described by the patient.
- Tachycardia and hypertension may be seen with associated thyrotoxicosis and pre-ecclampsia.
- Size of the uterus may be normal or more than the period of amenorrhoea.
- Uterus has a doughy consistency due to the absence of fetal parts and amniotic fluid.
- Cervix is soft as in a normal pregnancy.
- Grapelike products of conception may be seen on per-vaginum examination.

Investigations

1. **Ultrasound** scan is usually diagnostic.

- Complete mole–no fetal parts are seen, **snow storm appearance** is seen due to multiple vesicles and areas of haemorrhage.
- Partial mole–fetal parts are seen with multiple cystic spaces in places.
- Theca-lutein cysts may be seen in the ovaries.
- Metastases to the liver or kidneys can be identified.

2. **Complete haemogram** is carried out to assess the degree of anaemia and blood arranged.
3. **Serum beta hCG** (prior to evacuation and every weekly)–to know the risk of persistent disease.
4. **X-ray chest** to look for lung metastases.
5. **Thyroid function tests**

Management

- **Suction evacuation** is the method of choice for complete mole, as it enables a rapid and complete evacuation of the uterus. It is carried out after arranging adequate amount of blood. All the curettings are to be sent for histopathological examination. A repeat curettage is not recommended routinely due to the risk of perforation and metastases.
- **Follow-up** is done by weekly beta hCG levels till they become negative (usually within 8 weeks). Subsequently the patient is called every three monthly for the first year and six monthly for two years.
- **Contraception** is advised for one year as the risk of recurrence is maximum in this period. Barrier contraceptive is the method of choice. Combined oral contraceptives can interfere with the beta hCG levels and are not recommended.
- **Chemotherapy** indications for chemotherapy are given in table 9.3.

Table 9.3. Indications of chemotherapy
• Histological evidence of choriocarcinoma or invasive mole
• Heavy vaginal bleeding or evidence of gastrointestinal or intraperitoneal haemorrhage
• Evidence of metastases in the brain, liver or gastrointestinal tract; or radiological opacities of >2 cm on the chest x-ray
• Pulmonary, vulval or vaginal metastases
• Rising hCG after evacuation
• Serum hCG of 20,000 iu/l more than 4 weeks after evacuation
• High hCG levels 6 months after evacuation

Prognostic scoring Patients with gestational trophoblastic neoplasia (invasive mole and choriocarcinoma) are assessed regarding their risk of persistent disease. A unified WHO and FIGO scoring system is given in table 9.4. Each variable carries a score, which when added together for an individual patient, correlates with the risk of the tumour being resistant to single-agent therapy.

Table 9.4. Prognostic scoring of gestational trophoblastic neoplasia

Prognostic factor	Score			
	0	1	2	4
Age in years	<39	>39		
Antecedant pregnancy	Mole	Abortion	Term	
Interval from last pregnancy in months	<4	4-6	7-12	>12
Largest tumour (cm)	3-5	>5		
Site of metastases		Spleen, kidney	GI tract	Brain, liver
hCG levels iu/l	<1000	1,000-10,000	10,000–100,000	>100,000
Number of metastases identified	1-4	1-4	5-8	>8
Prior failed chemotherapy			Single drug	>2 drugs

The scoring system is used to subdivide patients into three groups. Low, medium or high risk depending on their overall score and chemotherapy given accordingly as shown in the table 9.5.

Table 9.5. Chemotherapy regimes in gestational trophoblastic neoplasia

Low and medium risk patients–single agent chemotherapy
- Methotrexate 50 mg/m^2 IM repeated every 48 hourly for four doses,
- Folinic acid 15 mg IM given alternating with methotrexate

The course is repeated 2 weekly till two consecutive beta hCG levels come negative.

High risk patients–combination chemotherapy with EMACO regime comprising Etoposide, Methotrexate, Actinomycin D, Vincristine (Onconovin) and Cyclophosphamide

Sexually transmitted diseases in Women

Sexually transmitted diseases (STD) are important causes of morbidity in women.

The sequelae of some of these infections cause salpingitis, and pelvic inflammatory disease, which may result in tubal blockage causing infertility or ectopic pregnancy. Some of these infections could be even life threatening to the fetus or neonate if present during pregnancy and may cause serious deformities or permanent stigmata.

The common STDs that occur in women can be classified into three major groups: bacterial, viral and others as shown in the table 10.1.

SYPHILIS

Syphilis is an STD caused by *Treponema pallidum.*

The incubation period is variable (9-90 days, usually 3-6 weeks).

Untreated, syphilis has a natural course having three stages: primary, secondary and tertiary.

Clinical features

Primary syphilis

- Classical lesion is the *chancre* which is a painless genital ulcer commonly on the cervix. It is classically indurated, firm, non-tender, round to oval with minimal or no discharge, and does not bleed on palpation.

- The other sites are the labia, fourchette, urethra, and perineum

- Extragenital sites include the anus, mouth, oropharynx and breast.

- *'Kissing lesions'* may occur in areas of skin-to-skin contact as on the vulva.

- The regional lymph nodes are often involved as discrete, non-tender nodes having a rubbery consistency.

Table 10.1. Common sexually transmitted diseases in women and their causative organism	
Disease	**Causative organism**
Bacterial STDs	
Syphilis	*Treponema pallidum* (a spirochaete)
Chancroid	*Haemophilus ducreyi* (a gram negative bacillus)
Donovanosis	*Calymmatobacterium granulomatis* (a gram negative bacillus)
LGV	*Chlamydia trachomatis* (L1-3 serovars)
Bacterial vaginosis	*Gardnerella vaginalis* (an anaerobic bacterium) and *Mycoplasma hominis*
Gonorrhoea	*Neisseria gonorrhoeae* (a gram negative diplococcus)
Non-gonococcal urethritis	*Chlamydia trachomatis, Mycoplasma genitalium, Ureaplasma urealyticum* and rarely other organisms
Viral STDs	
Genital herpes	*Herpes simplex virus-1 (HSV1), Herpes simplex virus-2 (HSV2)*
Anogenital warts	*Human papilloma virus (HPV)* (various subtypes)
Molluscum contagiosum	*Poxvirus (Molluscum contagiosum-1 and 2)*
Hepatitis	*Hepatitis virus A, B, C and E*
Infectious mononucleosis	*Cytomegalovirus (CMV)*
Others	
Trichomoniasis	*Trichomonas vaginalis* (a protozoan)
Candidial vulvovaginitis	*Candida albicans* and other species of *Candida*
Scabies	*Sarcoptes scabies* (itch mite)

Secondary syphilis

- Develops as the chancre disappears or up to 6 months later in two-thirds of untreated patients.

- Two types of lesions are seen:

  1) *Rash* which is an asymptomatic erythematous to coppery-red hyperpigmented rash affecting the trunk, palms and soles and mucous membranes.

  2) *Condylomata lata* moist papules and plaques occurring over the vaginal and perianal region and are highly infectious.

- Secondary syphilis may be asymptomatic and may be detected in women with a history of recurrent spontaneous abortions.

Latent syphilis

- A majority of patients with untreated secondary syphilis enter the latent phase.

- The patients are asymptomatic with positive serological tests for syphilis, detected during routine antenatal investigations. If the latent period is less than two years after the primary infection, it is called *early latent syphilis* and, if more than two years have elapsed from the primary infection it is called *late latent syphilis*.

- One-third of patients with latent syphilis develop tertiary syphilis.

Tertiary syphilis

- Tertiary syphilis is rarely seen nowadays due to prompt treatment of the primary lesion.

- There is involvement of the neurological and cardiovascular system.

Effect on pregnancy

Syphilis is a systemic infection from the onset and has multi-systemic manifestations.

- The effect on pregnancy depends upon the duration of the disease stage i.e., longer the duration of untreated maternal syphilis, lesser is the effect on the fetus (*Kassowitz' law*).

- With primary and secondary syphilis, there is a 50% chance of preterm labour, still birth, neonatal death or congenital syphilis in the neonate.

- With latent syphilis 9% go into preterm labour, 11% are stillborn, and only 10% are born with congenital syphilis.

- However a patient who has previously had several miscarriages, stillbirths and children with congenital syphilis may later give birth to a healthy non-infected child.

- A positive serology at birth does not necessarily indicate the presence of neonatal infection. Rising titres in serial tests or failure of the test to become negative after a few weeks indicates active infection. Usually the last infant has fewer signs and symptoms of the disease.

Significance of routine antenatal screening

Routine antenatal serological screening with VDRL or rapid plasma regain (RPR), a card test, for all pregnant mothers should be undertaken even in a low prevalence areas as early diagnosis and treatment can prevent congenital syphilis. A possibility of biological false positive (BFP) reaction during healthy pregnancy should be kept in mind, which can occur at a titre of 1:8 or less. If the VDRL test is positive, specific tests for syphilis (TPHA, FTA-ABS test) are indicated.

Diagnosis

1. Screening tests–VDRL & RPR (Rapid plasma reagin tests)

2. Specific Tests–TPHA (Treponemal pallidum haemagglutination assay) FTA–ABS (Fluorescent Treponemal Antibody Absorption Test), Treponema pallidum particle agglutination tests are specific T. pallidum antigens (see Fig. 10.1)

3. Dark ground illumination (DGI) microscopy demonstrating the presence of *T. pallidum* from ulcers, moist lesions and mucous membranes.

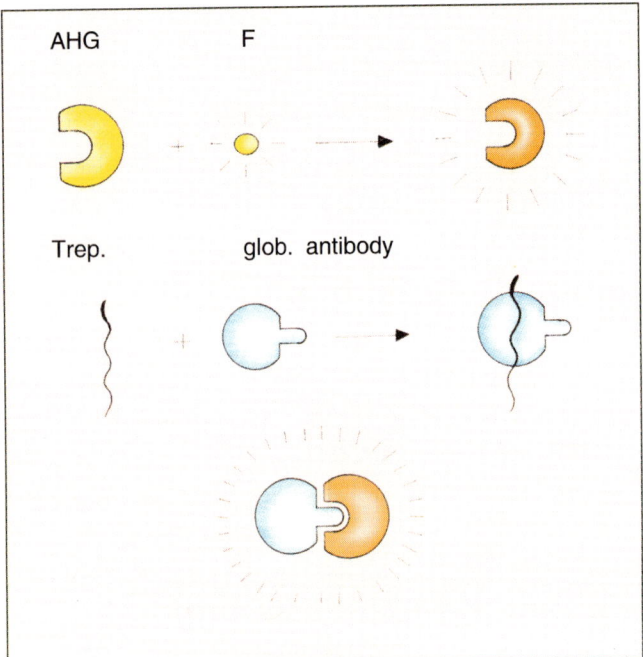

AHG   F

Trep.   glob. antibody

a) Anti-human globulin is combined with fluorescein

b) Dead trepronema is com-bined with test serum. If subject is infected, the treponema acquires a coating of globulain antibody

c) 1& 2 are combined and the treponeme becomes flourescent

Fig. 10.1. Principle of flurorescent treponemal antibody test

Treatment

The recommended regimens for adults are as follows:

- *Primary, secondary, or early latent stage* benzathine penicillin G, 2.4 million units intramuscularly as a single dose (half in each buttock).

- *Late latent syphilis or syphilis of unknown duration* benzathine penicillin G, 2.4 million units intramuscularly once a week for 3 consecutive weeks.

- *Neurosyphilis* Crystalline penicillin G, 3 to 4 million units intravenously every 4 hours or 18 to 24 million units daily as continuous infusion for 10 to 14 days.

- *Treatment of pregnant women* The appropriate penicillin regimen should be given depending upon the stage of syphilis. Women who are allergic to penicillin should be given erythromycin 500 mg 4 times daily for 14 days. While on treatment the pregnant women with early syphilis may experience a *Jarisch-Herxheimer reaction.* There is a risk of premature labour or fetal distress if this reaction takes place after 20 weeks of gestation.

- *Treatment of the family* The sexual partner should be examined, in all patients who test positive; serological testing carried out and treatment given accordingly. If the exact duration of the disease is not known, the patient's other children should also be investigated to rule out latent syphilis and treated. Testing for HIV status is mandatory after appropriate counselling.

CHANCROID

Chancroid, also called as soft sore, is caused by the Gram-negative bacillus *Haemophilus ducreyi*. The organism is inoculated through micro-trauma or abrasion during sexual intercourse.

Clinical Features

Symptoms

Most female patients report pain on micturition or defecation, vaginal discharge, dyspareunia as the usual symptoms as the women are unaware of their lesions.

Signs

- Multiple ulcers are diagnostic, the common sites of involvement are the fourchette, vestibule, labia, clitoris, vagina and the perianal area.
- Extragenital lesions on the breasts, finger, thighs and in the oral cavity have been described.
- Painful and tender inguinal lymphadenopathy (*bubo*) usually starting on one side and then appearing bilaterally is common, though less than in male patients.

Diagnosis

Often made on clinical examination and has an accuracy rate of only 30-50%.

A probable diagnosis of chancroid can be made if following are present:

- One or more painful genital ulcers
- Regional lymphadenopathy
- Dark ground examination (DGI) of ulcer exudates is negative for *T. pallidum*. (However it must be borne in mind that more than one STD often occur simultaneously).
- The serological test for syphilis performed at least 7 days after the onset of ulcers is non-reactive.

- The test for herpes simplex virus (HSV) is negative.

- *Isolation of H. ducreyi from the genital ulcer or bubo*–Smears are taken with cotton swabs from beneath the undermined edges of ulcers and stained with gram or Wright stain. Pleomorphic gram negative coccobacilli arranged in parallel chains of twos or fours with a *"school of fish"* or *"rail track"* appearance when present, are diagnostic.

- *Culture*–A definitive diagnosis of H. ducreyi infection requires growth of the organism on culture.

- *Multiplex PCR* combining PCR for *H. ducreyi, T. pallidum* and HSV has been developed and may be a useful tool in the future.

Treatment

Several antibiotic regimens are effective, but the sensitivity may vary from time to time and between populations. Any one of the following drugs can be given.

- Azithromycin 1 g orally, as a single dose, or

- Ceftriaxone 250 mg intramuscularly, as a single dose,

- Ciprofloxacin 500 mg orally, twice a day for 3 days,

- Erythromycin base 500 mg orally, four times a day for 7 days.

Ceftriaxone or erythromycin are preferred in pregnant and lactating women.

DONOVANOSIS/GRANULOMA INGUINALE

It is a progressively destructive ulcerative disease of the genital area which is caused by a gram negative bacillus *Calymmatobacterium granulomatis* or *Klebsiella granulomatis*. It is more prevalent in certain geographical areas, particularly in the southern states of India.

Clinical features

In women the usual sites of infection are the labia and the fourchette.

- It presents as a mildly painful, usually single, fleshy ulcer, usually raised from the surface due to granulation tissue, giving it a beefy red, velvety look.

- Sclerotic lesions cause stenosis of the urethra, vulva or anal orifice.

- Elephantiasis of the vulva, rectovaginal fistula and carcinoma are rare complications.

Diagnosis

The identification of predominantly intracellular *Donovan bodies* is the gold standard for making a diagnosis. It is demonstrated by direct microscopy of the crushed tissue smear stained with Giemsa stain, the organisms classically have a *'safety pin'* appearance, with darker staining at either end.

Treatment

The recommended antibiotics are

- Doxycycline 100 mg, twice a day, or
- Cotrimoazole (800mg/160mg) 2 tablets twice a day, or
- Erythromycin 500 mg orally, four times a day (preferred for the treatment of pregnant patients)

They are to be taken for at least 3 weeks or until all the lesions have healed completely.

LYMPHOGRANULOMA VENEREUM

Lymphogranuloma venereum (LGV) affects primarily the lymphatic system, and is caused by *Chlamydia trachomatis serovars L1-L3*. The disease is characterized by regional suppurative lymphadenopathy following a transient papule or an ulcer.

Clinical features

The incubation period is 3-12 days. Based on the evolution and sequelae of the disease the clinical features can be divided into primary, secondary (inguinal) and tertiary stages.

Primary stage is characterized by an ulcer on the posterior vaginal wall, fourchette, vulva and posterior lip of cervix.

Secondary stage

One third of the patients have inguinal lymphadenopathy and one third have abdominal or back pain due to involvement of the deep pelvic or para-aortic lumbar lymph nodes. The superomedial groups of inguinal lymph nodes are enlarged, which later become fluctuant due to suppuration. They either rupture leading to discharging sinuses or heal with contracted scars

Tertiary stage

There is anorectal involvement known as the *genito-anorectal syndrome*, characterised by protocolitis, hyperplasia of the lymphatic tissue (lymphorrhoids), abscess formation, fistulae, stricture formation, chronic ulceration and scarring. The commonly affected sites are the rectum and the vagina.

Anorectal involvement can occur following penoanal intercourse or due to direct spread from vaginal secretions or by lymphatic dissemination from the cervix or posterior vaginal wall. Perianal oedema is associated with diffuse oedema of the anorectal mucosa is causing a pebbled feel on rectal examination. It may present as pruritus ani, tenesmus and blood stained rectal discharge due to ulceration of the rectal mucosa.

After 3-6 months, the anorectal mucosa becomes rigid with narrowing of the lumen leading to a rectal stricture involving all the layers of the bowel. The stricture may be annular, tubular or funnel-like.

Complications

- Chronic oedema leads to elephantiasis of the vulva often referred to as 'esthiomene'. This presents as swelling of a labium to giant lobulated masses hanging and obstructing the vaginal introitus.
- Rectovaginal and urethrovaginal fistulae.

Diagnosis

Mainly clinical as laboratory investigations are not easily available. Polymerase chain reaction techniques recently have been used to identify the organism.

Treatment

Treatment of lymphogranuloma venereum is with

- Doxycycline 100 mg twice a day, for 21 days.
- An alternative regime is Erythromycin, 500 mg orally, four times a day for 21 days.
- In conjunction with antibiotic therapy, aspiration of nodes (only in fluctuant stage), through adjacent healthy skin should be performed to prevent sinus tract formation.
- Complications need surgical corrections following antibiotic therapy.

GONORRHOEA

Gonorrhoea is caused by *Neisseria gonorrhoeae*, a gram-negative diplococcus. The organisms are present intracellularly in the polymorphonuclear leucocytes.

In contrast to the male, the female urethra often escapes infection owing to its lining with stratified squamous epithelium with only a limited area of columnar epithelium.

Clinical features

- The commonest manifestation of gonorrhoea in women is cervicitis.
- Endometritis, salpingitis, and rarely perihepatitis occur as complications.

- Urethritis is uncommon and when present, manifests as moderate burning micturition, frequency and urgency.
- Conjunctivitis, tonsillitis and proctitis can also occur.
- Chronic asymptomatic infection is also common.
- Gonococcal infection during pregnancy is usually asymptomatic. In the neonate, passage of the fetus through the birth canal can give rise to ophthalmia neonatorum, pharyngitis, proctitis and also meningitis.

Complications

1. *Salpingitis*

- Acute salpingitis or pelvic inflammatory disease (PID) is the most common complication of gonorrhoea in women. It presents as lower abdominal pain, dyspareunia and menstrual abnormalities.
- Chronic infection leads to hydro or pyosalpinx.

2. *Bartholin's gland abscess*
Inflammation is commonly unilateral and remains confined to the ducts and the periglandular tissues. The erythematous orifice exudes pus on pressure. It may present as a small indurated swelling, or a large abscess or as a cystic swelling of the duct or gland due to recurrent infection.

3. *Disseminated infection*
is the most common systemic complication of acute gonorrhoea, characterized by acute arthritis and dermatitis. Other systemic complications are gonococcal arthritis and meningitis.

Laboratory diagnosis

- The diagnosis of gonorrhoea includes microscopy and culture.
- The specimen is taken commonly from the endocervix; the urethra, rectum or oropharynx are also sampled if symptoms arise from there areas.
- The organisms are visualized on gram staining with oil immersion as intracellular gram-negative diplococci.
- The specific media for culture are modified Thayer-Martin, and Chacko-Nayar medium.

Treatment

The recommended treatment regimens for uncomplicated gonorrhoeal infection of the cervix or urethra include third-generation cephalosporins and quinolones.

- Cefixime 400 mg orally in a single dose, or
- Ceftriaxone 125 mg intramuscularly, in a single dose, or
- Ciprofloxacin 500 mg orally, or ofloxacin 400 mg orally or levofloxacin 250 mg orally, in a single dose.

Approximately 10% to 30% of women with genital gonorrhoea are also infected with *Chlamydia*. Therefore, the treatment regimen should always include

Azithromycin, 1g orally, or

Doxycycline, 100mg orally, twice a day for 7 days.

For disseminated gonococcal infection

- Ceftriaxone, 1g IM or IV once daily for 7 days (2 weeks for meningitis), or
- Cefixime, 400 mg twice daily orally for 7 days.

CHLAMYDIAL INFECTIONS

- Chlamydial infections in women are caused by *Chlamydia trachomatis serovars D to K.*
- **Clinical features** It is usually asymptomatic; only about one third of those infected have signs on gynaecological examination. The clinical syndromes due to chlamydia trachomatis are summarized in table 10.2.
- The most common presentations are a mucopurulent discharge and an area of hypertrophy on ectocervix, which is edematous, congested, and bleeds easily.

Table 10.2. Diagnosis of C. Trachomatis infections in women

Clinical Syndrome	Clinical criteria	Laboratory criteria Presumptive	Diagnostic
Mucopurulent cervicitis (MPC)	Mucopurulent cervical discharge, cervical erosion and oedema, spontaneous or easily induced cervical bleeding	Cervical GS* with > 30 PMNL/HPF (x1000)	Positive culture or antigen detection by ELISA
Acute urethral syndrome	Dysuria-frequency syndrome in young sexually active women, recent new sex partner, often > 7 days of symptoms	Pyuria, no bacteria	As above
PID	Lower abdominal pain; adnexal tenderness on pelvic exam; evidence of cervicitis often present	cervical GS positive for gonococcus.	Positive culture from (cervix, FVU, endometrium, tube)
Perihepatitis	Right upper quadrant pain, nausea, vomiting, fever in young sexually active women; evidence of PID	As for MPC and PID	High titre IgM or IgG antibody to C. trachomatis

*GS-Gram stain
PMNL-Polymorpho leucocytes

- Clinical recognition depends on a high index of suspicion and a careful cervical examination as the symptoms are not specific.

- *Urethritis* is usually associated with cervicitis and presents as dysuria, frequency and pyuria.

- *Bartholinitis* an exudative infection of the Bartholin's ducts with purulent discharge may occur, as in gonococcal infection.

- *Endometritis* is present in about 50% of patients with chlamydial cervicitis and may be associated with abnormal vaginal bleeding, menorrhagia and metrorrhagia.

- *Salpingitis* is usually asymptomatic but causes progressive tubal scarring, resulting in ectopic pregnancy and infertility ("*silent salpingitis*").

- *Perihepatitis* (*Fitz-Hugh-Curtis Syndrome*) is a rare complication and should by suspected in young, sexually active women who develop right upper quadrant pain, fever, nausea or vomitings.

- *Infection in pregnancy* can cause spontaneous abortion, low birth weight, prematurity and preterm delivery. Infection during delivery can cause neonatal conjunctivitis, ophthalmia neonatorum, pneumonia, chronic lung and eye disease.

Diagnosis

Many diagnostic tests for *C. trachomatis* have become available over the past decade, from antigen detection by monoclonal or polyclonal antibodies to molecular biologic methods.

- Gram stain of the endocervical discharge usually shows more than 30 polymorphonuclear leucocytes per high power field, presents of intracellular chlamydia in endocervical cells (Fig. 10.2), absence of gonococci and other bacteria.

- Anti-chlamydia antibodies, can be assessed by a micro-immunofluorescence assay.

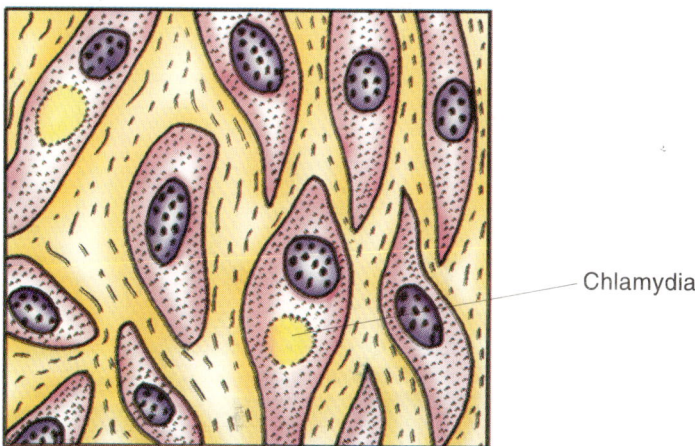

Chlamydia

Fig. 10.2. Intracellular chlamydia seen in endocervical cells

Treatment

Uncomplicated non-gonococcal associated infections (urethral, endocervical and rectal) can be treated with:

- Doxycycline 100 mg bid x 7 days, or
- Tetracycline 500 mg qid x 7 days, or
- Erythromycin stearate 500 mg qid x 7 days, or
- Sulfisoxasole 100 mg qid x 10 days.

BACTERIAL VAGINOSIS

Bacterial vaginosis is a syndrome caused by replacement of the normal vaginal flora with overgrowth of anaerobic microorganisms (including *Prevotella* sp and *Mobiluncus* sp), along with *Gardnerella vaginalis* and *Mycoplasma hominis*.

Bacterial vaginosis is the most common infection of the lower genital tract in women of reproductive age.

Clinical features

- The condition has been increasingly found to be associated with intrauterine infection, preterm birth, postpartum endometritis and post-hysterectomy infections. The pathogenesis of the syndrome is incompletely understood.

Diagnosis

Bacterial vaginosis can be diagnosed clinically using **Amsel's criteria** (three of the following four signs):

- Homogeneous, white discharge that uniformly coats the vaginal walls.
- Presence of clue cells on microscopic exam (Fig. 10.3).

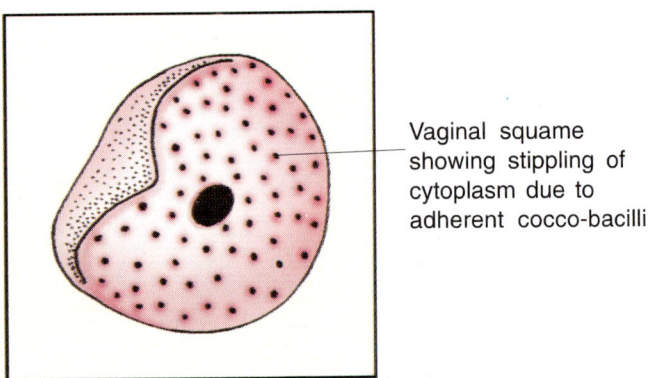

Vaginal squame showing stippling of cytoplasm due to adherent cocco-bacilli

Fig. 10.3. The 'Clue cell' in bacterial vaginosis

- pH of vaginal fluid > 4.5
- Fishy odor after the addition of 10% KOH to the vaginal discharge.

Alternatively, Gram's stain can be used for diagnosis showing the typical 'clue cells'.

Treatment

All women who have symptomatic disease should be treated. Recommended *regimens for treatment* include

- Metronidazole 500 mg orally, twice a day for 7 days
- Metronidazole gel 0.75%, one full applicator (5g) intravaginally, once a day for 5 days
  Clindamycin cream 2%, one full applicator (5g) intravaginally, at bed time for 7 days
- Routine treatment of sex partners is not recommended.

Bacterial vaginosis has been associated with an increase in adverse pregnancy. *Recommended regimens in pregnancy* include

- Metronidazole 250 mg orally, three times a day for 7 days, or
- Clindamycin 300 mg orally, twice a day for 7 days.

GENITAL HERPES

Genital herpes is caused by herpes simplex virus (HSV) serotypes 2 and 1, with HSV 2 being much more frequent.

- *Clinical features* of herpes infection can be broadly divided into:
  (a) primary when the infection is acquired
  (b) recurrent due to reactivation of HSV
    a) *Primary herpes genitalis* is characterized by multiple vesicles on the vulva, vagina, and periurethral area which rupture to form painful erosions causing pain, dysuria and dyspareunia with associated systemic symptoms.
      - Involvement of the sacral nerves leads to retention of urine.
      - Primary pharyngeal and rectal infection is seen following oral or anal intercourse.
      - A primary episode during pregnancy may be more severe. Its importance in pregnancy is mainly due to the devastating obstetric complications and neonatal infection. The risk of transmission to the neonate is especially high (30-50%) if the woman acquires genital herpes at vaginal delivery.
    b) *Recurrent herpes infection* on the other hand, is milder, may be asymptomatic and frequently affects the perineum rather than the cervix.

Laboratory Tests

The diagnosis is usually clinical, but laboratory tests are also available, including tzanck smear, histopathology, viral culture and serology (ELISA & Western Blot).

Treatment

There is no cure for HSV infection, the use of antiviral medications has been shown to reduce the frequency and duration of recurrences, the frequency of asymptomatic shedding, and transmission.

- *First clinical episode* Acyclovir, 400 mg orally, three times a day or 200 mg 5 times a day for 7-10 days

- *For recurrences*, treatment may be:

    (a) *Episodic* at first sign of a recurrence – acyclovir as above, for 5 days, or

    (b) *Suppressive*, to reduce recurrences (if > 6 recurrences/year) – acyclovir, 400 mg orally, twice a day for 6 months. Famciclovir and valacyclovir are also effective.

- *Severe primary or disseminated infection* The recommended treatment is intravenous acyclovir, 5-10mg/kg every 8 hours for 2-7 days or until clinical improvement occurs, followed by oral antiviral therapy till a total of at least 10 days.

- *Herpes infection in pregnancy* has a high risk of neonatal morbidity and mortality.

    - Acyclovir is given orally for the first-episode of genital herpes or severe recurrent herpes; and intravenously to pregnant women with severe HSV infection.

    - The risk of neonatal transmission is influenced by the maternal antibody status and the timing of maternal infection. The risk of vertical transmission to the neonate when a primary out break occurs at the time of delivery is approximately 30% to 50%.

    - At the onset of labour, all women should be questioned carefully about symptoms of genital herpes, and examined carefully for herpetic lesions. In the absence of lesions or prodromal symptoms, vaginal delivery can be allowed. Patients with symptomatic or active lesions in labour should undergo a caesarean delivery, regardless of the duration of membrane rupture.

CONDYLOMA ACUMINATA

Condyloma acuminata or genital warts are caused by human papilloma virus (HPV). Currently, more than 80 sub types of HPV have been identified, approximately 30 of which are associated with genital infection. Subtypes 6 and 11 are most frequently associated with external genital warts, where as HPV types 16, 18, 31, 33, 35, and 39 are more frequently associated with genital cancer.

Clinical features

- Clinically, genital warts present as asymptomatic verrucous papules on the genitalia.
- Diagnosis is most often made by visualization of the lesions. If doubt exists, a biopsy should be performed.

Treatment

- Approximately 10% to 20% of patients have spontaneous resolution of the lesions.
- Any associated infections should be eradicated before treating the warts.
- It is important to counsel patients that although the warts may be eradicated, the virus may persist, commonly resulting in recurrences of warts.
- Several treatments are currently available, which the patient can apply herself.

    1. A *purified podophyllin resin* (*podofilox*) is available as a solution or gel and may be applied twice daily for 3 consecutive days per week for up to 4 weeks.

    2. *Imiquimod 5% cream* can be used topically by a patient three times a week for upto 8 weeks. It should be applied at bedtime and washed off in 6 to 10 hours. It is not recommended in pregnancy.

    3. *Podophyllin (10-25% solution)* applied for 1-4 hrs. is effective in lesions smaller than 2 cm. It is a cytotoxic agent, hence contraindicated in pregnancy. If the warts fail to regress after four applications, an alternative therapy may be needed.

    4. *Bi- or trichloracetic acid* in upto 85% solution in alcohol applied weekly for 6-8 hrs. for up to 4 weeks is an effective treatment for small lesions. It has fewer side effects than with podophyllin, and may be used safely in pregnancy. However, neither compound seems to be effective in treating vaginal or cervical warts.

    5. *Topical 5-fluorouracil* may also be used, but can cause erythema, edema, and shallow ulcerations on the skin, however, it is contraindicated in pregnant women.

    6. *Interferon injection* is effective and useful for recurrent or resistant genital warts, but is very expensive.

    7. *Cryotherapy* is useful for multiple cervical lesions. Burning and ulceration may follow therapy, which usually resolves in 7 to 10 days with little or no scarring.

    8. *Surgical excision* (electrosurgery, scalpel or scissor or punch excision, CO_2 laser) is useful for large perianal lesions.

The risk of laryngeal papillomatosis in the neonate is low and does not indicate a caesarean section to prevent transmission.

MOLLUSCUM CONTAGIOSUM

- Caused by a poxvirus

- Presents as multiple slow growing dome shaped lesions with central umbilication on the vulva from which a whitish core can sometimes be expressed.
- Diagnosis of this lesion is primarily made by gross appearance; skin biopsy is usually only performed when the diagnosis is in question.
- Infection is self-limiting and lasts usually for 6 to 9 months.

Treatment

Effective treatment can be achieved with skin curettage, cryotherapy, expression of the umbilicated core, or excision (causes scarring, hence not routinely recommended). Podophyllin and trichloracetic acid also are effective.

SCABIES

Scabies is a highly contagious infection caused by *Sarcoptes scabiei*, also known as the itch mite, an obligate parasite which resides in human skin.

It is transmitted by intimate contact through sexual intercourse or via fomites.

Clinical features

Patients complain of intense pruritus that is worse at night. On examination, there are erythematous papules, vesicles and excoriations in the body clefts eg. interdigital spaces, wrists, axillary folds, periumbilical and pelvic areas.

Diagnosis

Mainly clinical formal diagnosis is made by microscopically examining the skin scrapings of suspected sites for the organism, eggs or fecal pellets.

Treatment

Scabicidal drugs

1. The drug of choice for treatment of scabies is *permethrin 5% cream*, applied to all areas of the body from the neck down and washed off after 8 to 14 hours. It is safe in pregnancy.
2. *Lindane* (1%), has a lower cure rate, and is applied in a thin layer to all areas of the body from the neck down and thoroughly washed off after 8 hours. Lindane is not recommended during pregnancy.
3. *Oral ivermectin* (200 µg/kg, repeated after 2 weeks) is an alternative treatment for scabies.

General measures

- All household contacts should be treated.

- All clothes should be washed with hot soapy water. Fingernails should be clipped.

- Patients should be counselled that the itching may persist for up to 2 weeks after therapy.

TRICHOMONIASIS

Trichomoniasis is caused by the protozoan *Trichomonas vaginalis*. The most common symptoms are a diffuse, yellow-green vaginal discharge, vaginal malodor, and vulval irritation, though some women may be asymptomatic.

Diagnosis

The diagnosis is commonly made by visualization of the motile organisms using light microscopy (Fig 10.4). Culture of the organism is currently considered the gold standard for diagnosis. A DNA probe with high sensitivity is also used where available.

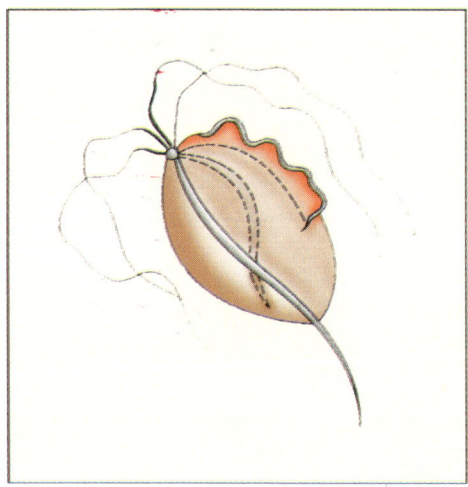

Fig. 10.4. Trichomonas vaginalis

Treatment

The recommended therapeutic agent is metronidazole, 2g orally in a single dose. An alternative regimen is metronidazole, 500 mg orally, twice a day for 7 days. Sexual partners should also be treated.

VULVOVAGINAL CANDIDIASIS

The etiologic agent of vulvovaginal candidiasis (VVC) is typically *Candida albicans*, but infections with other *Candida* species can occur.

The disease is common – an estimated 75% of women will have at least one episode. The predisposing factors are given in table 10.3.

Symptoms of VVC include local pruritus and burning, vaginal discharge, vaginal soreness, dyspareunia, and dysuria.

Recurrent vulvovaginal candidiasis is usually defined as four or more episodes of symptomatic VVC each year. Women with recurrent VVC should have vaginal cultures performed to confirm the diagnosis and identify the unusual species.

'Uncomplicated' VVC indicates episodes which are to (1) sporadic or infrequent, (2) mild-to-moderate, (3) likely to be due to *C. albicans*, and (4) those occurring in non-immunocompromised women

Complicated' VVC includes (1) recurrent VVC, (2) severe VVC, (3) non-albicans candidiasis and (4) uncontrolled diabetes, debilitation, immunosuppression or pregnancy.

Table 10.3. Factors predisposing to vaginal candidiasis
• Immunosuppression due to HIV or immunosuppresive therapy • Diabetes mellitus • Vaginal douching • Conditions causing increased oestrogens eg. pregnancy or combined contraceptive pill • Broad-spectrum antibiotic therapy

Diagnosis

The diagnosis of VVC is often made clinically by the presence of the typical symptoms and signs. Confirmation is by microscopy of the vaginal discharge using 10% potassium hydroxide or by gram stain (Fig. 10.5).

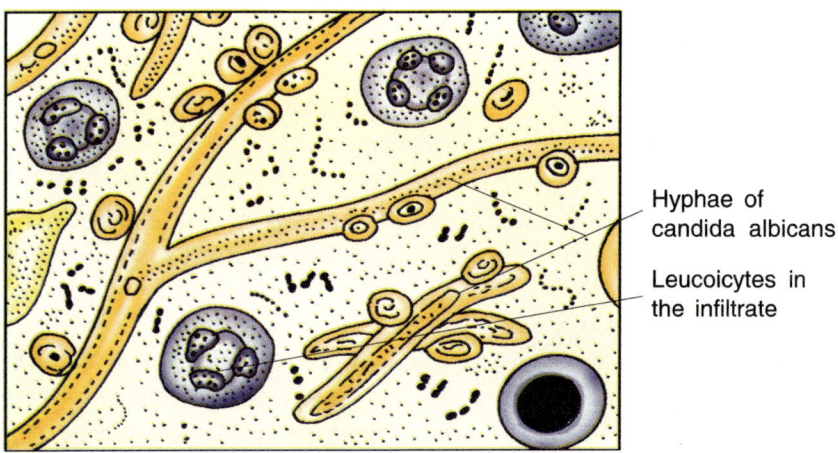

Hyphae of candida albicans

Leucoicytes in the infiltrate

Fig. 10.5.   Microscopy of vaginal discharge in candidaris

Treatment

Asymptomatic colonization can occur in 10-20% of women, so treatment should be reserved for women with symptoms.

Uncomplicated VVC are effectively treated with short-course topical or oral preparations.

- *Topical azole drugs* are more effective than oral nystatin.

    Some of the ***intravaginal agents*** that may be used are:

    - Clotrimazole 1% cream intravaginally for 7 to 14 days, or
    - Clotrimazole vaginal tablet (100 mg for 7 days, 200 mg for 3 days or 500 mg once) or
    - Miconazole 2% cream intravaginally for 7 days, or
    - Miconazole vaginal suppository (100 mg for 7 days or 200 mg for 3 days) or
    - Nystatin 100,000-U vaginal tablet, one tablet for 14 days.

        (Butoconazole, triconazole and terconazole are other topical azoles which have been used).

- *Oral agent:* Fluconazole 150 mg, one tablet as a single dose.

Complicated VVC need longer courses (7-14 days) of conventional therapy. In cases of recurrent VVC, maintenance therapy with weekly clotrimazole suppositories or oral fluconazole may be used every two weekly for 3-6 months.

Treatment of VVC in pregnancy, only the topical azoles are recommended.

APPROACHES TO MANAGEMENT OF SEXUALLY TRANSMITTED DISEASES (STDS)

Patients with STDs may be managed in one of the three ways:

1. **Clinical approach** Here, the health care provider using his or her clinical experience arrives at a specific diagnosis based on the symptoms reported by the patient and the signs found on physical examination. This is the least reliable of the three approaches as even highly experienced specialists may make a wrong diagnosis in a significant proportion of cases. Additionally, STDs commonly occur together and concurrent infections can be missed.

2. **Aetiological approach** The diagnosis is based on laboratory tests to identify the infectious agent, so that the treatment is more specific. However, it is often not practicable as an equipped laboratory may not be available and the patient may have to make a second visit to collect the test results and receive the treatment.

3. **Syndromic approach** is often the best approach in low-resource settings, is based on

the identification of syndromes, which are a combinations of the symptoms the patient reports and the signs the health care provider observes. It differs from the clinical approach in that many STDs can cause a particular syndrome, and treatments simultaneously target all those STDs.

The syndromic approach

The syndromic approach has been recommended since 1990 by the World Health Organization (WHO) and consists of the following elements:

1. *Syndrome identification:* A syndrome is identified based on the patient's symptoms and signs. This can be undertaken without laboratory support.

2. *Use of algorithms:* A flowchart is used to determine the most appropriate treatment for a given set of symptoms and signs. Ideally, these flowcharts are based on the local prevalence of STDs, their associated risk factors, and antibiotic sensitivities.

3. *Treatment:* Treatment that covers all the pathogens with the potential to cause a given syndrome is administered.

4. *Counselling:* Counselling is directed towards promoting safe sexual practices, including promotion of condom use.

5. *Treatment of sexual partners:* All sexual partners are encouraged to be treated for the same syndrome, whether the partner has symptoms or not.

Advantages of the syndromic approach

1. *Immediate treatment:* A major advantage is that treatment is given at the point of first contact with patients, who otherwise may not return for test results and medication.

2. *Effectiveness:* Patients are treated for a potentially mixed infection, reducing the chances of treatment failure.

3. *Ease of use:* It is easy to teach, learn and use the syndromic approach, so that all levels of health care providers and facilities can use it.

4. *Cost effective:* There are cost savings as expensive laboratory tests are not used.

Syndromic management of vaginal discharge

Algorithms

Vaginal discharge is one of the STD syndromes in women managed by the syndromic approach. Three algorithms have been formulated for syndromic management of vaginal discharge, to be used in three different settings with different facilities and levels of expertise:

1. Where vaginal speculum, bimanual pelvic examination and microscopy are not available (Flow chart 1a).

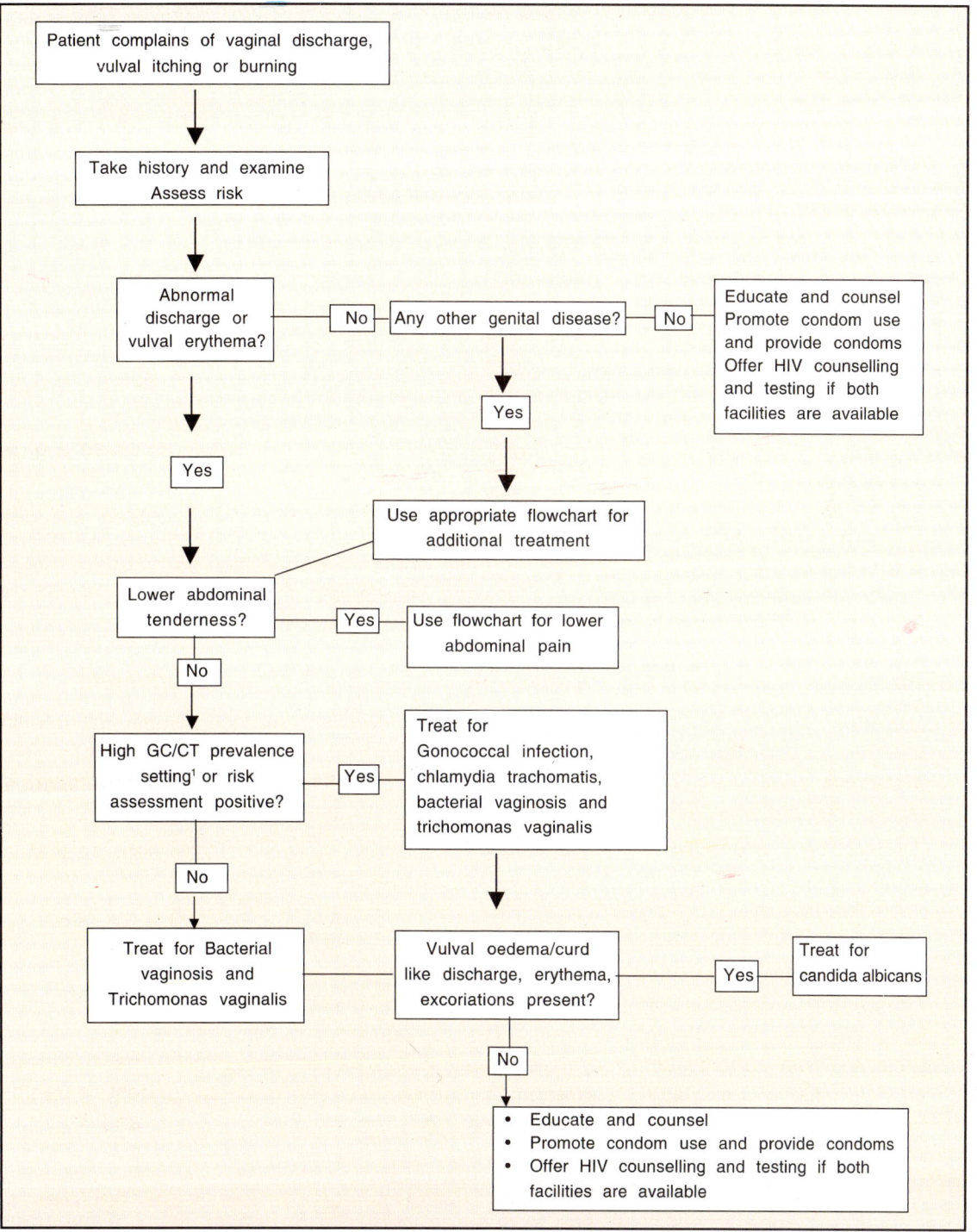

Flow chart 1a. Vaginal discharge

2. Where speculum and bimanual pelvic examination are available (Flow chart 1b).

3. Where speculum/bimanual examinations as well as microscopy are available (Flow chart 1c).

Speculum examination may not be feasible due to lack of a vaginal speculum, private space, gloves, or if the patient refuses it.

Risk assessment

It is difficult to distinguish between vaginal discharge due to vaginal infections (bacterial vaginosis, trichomoniasis, and candidiasis) and the more serious cervical infections (gonococcal and chlamydial). This differentiation is often critical as the cervical infections if left untreated can lead to major complications due to ascent of infection. Risk assessment is based on the principle that vaginal discharge in women at high risk for STDs is more likely to be associated with cervical infection. It is therefore used along with the vaginal discharge algorithms to determine the appropriate treatment and improve the effectiveness of syndromic management. Questions about risk should focus on various factors such as age, marital status, current or past STD symptoms, number of sexual partners, the possibility of partners having other sexual partners, and current symptoms in partners. Local, social, behavioural and epidemiological information must also be incorporated. For example, according to the WHO protocol, symptomatic women are classified as high risk if they are under 21, are single, have more than one sexual partner, or have a new sexual partner.

Limitations of the syndromic approach in vaginal discharge management

Though many of the general advantages of the syndromic approach remain, its use in vaginal discharge poses some problems:

1. *Ineffective against asymptomatic infections:* A major disadvantage of this approach is that it does not cover women with STDs who have no symptoms, as a large proportion of women with cervical infections are known to remain asymptomatic.

2. *Overdiagnosis of STDs:* The vaginal discharge might not be related to an STD, result in overtreatment, or an important non-STD cause of vaginal discharge may be overlooked. Women having non-STD vaginal discharge being told to bring their partners for treatment may lead to relationship problems.

3. *Potential for overtreatment:* Patients are treated for multiple infections, although some will have only one infection, or none. Risk assessment in high-risk populations can result in most patients being labelled as risk-positive, with unnecessary treatment for cervical infections in many. Overtreatment leads to wastage of drugs, and the potential for development of antimicrobial resistance.

Management of other STD syndromes

The syndromic approach is also used to manage women with genital ulcers (Flow chart 2) or lower abdominal pain (Flow chart 3).

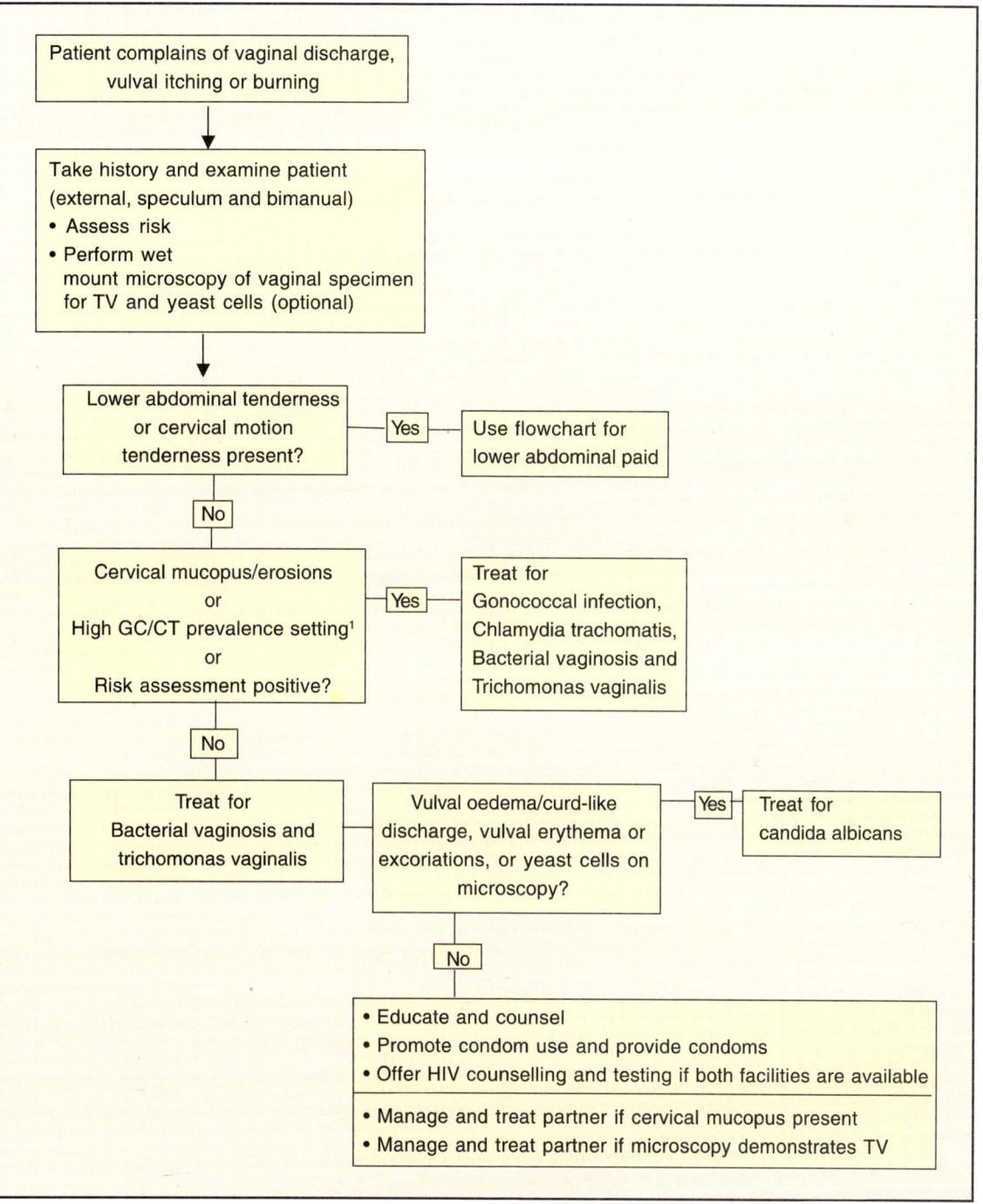

Flow chart 1b. Vaginal discharge: Bimanual & speculum, with or without microscope

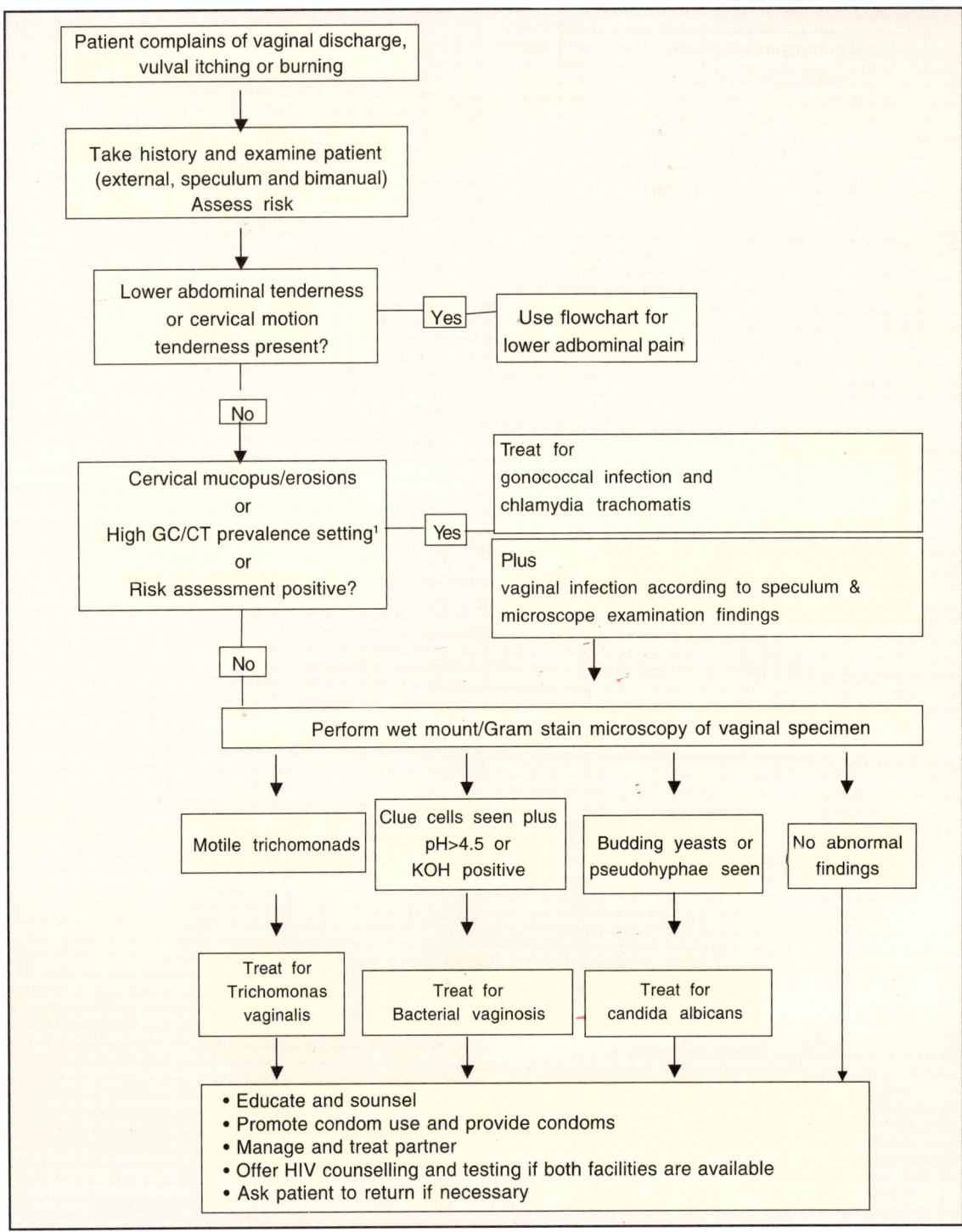

Flow chart 1c.   Vaginal discharge: Bimanual, speculum & microscope

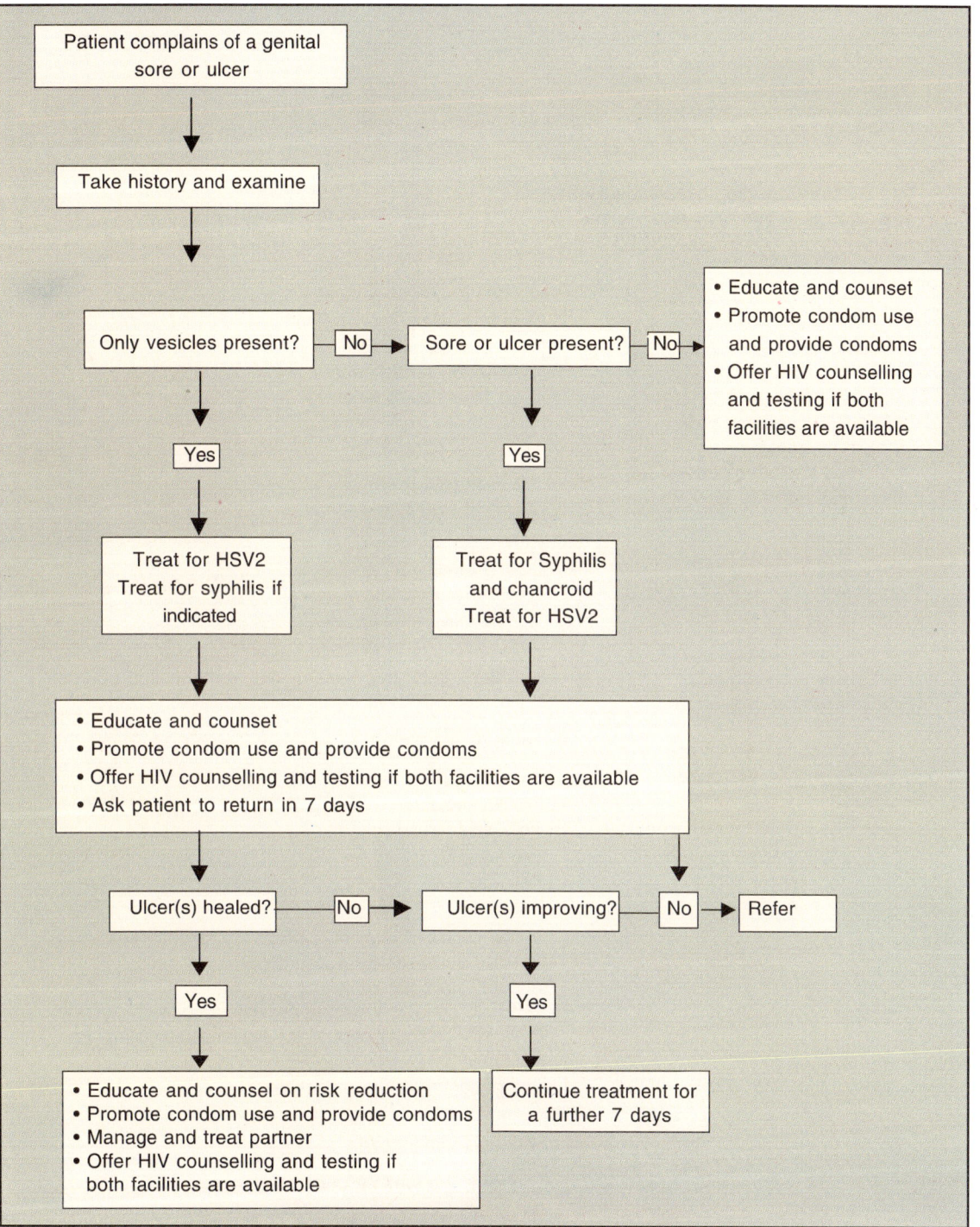

Flow chart 2. Genital ulcers

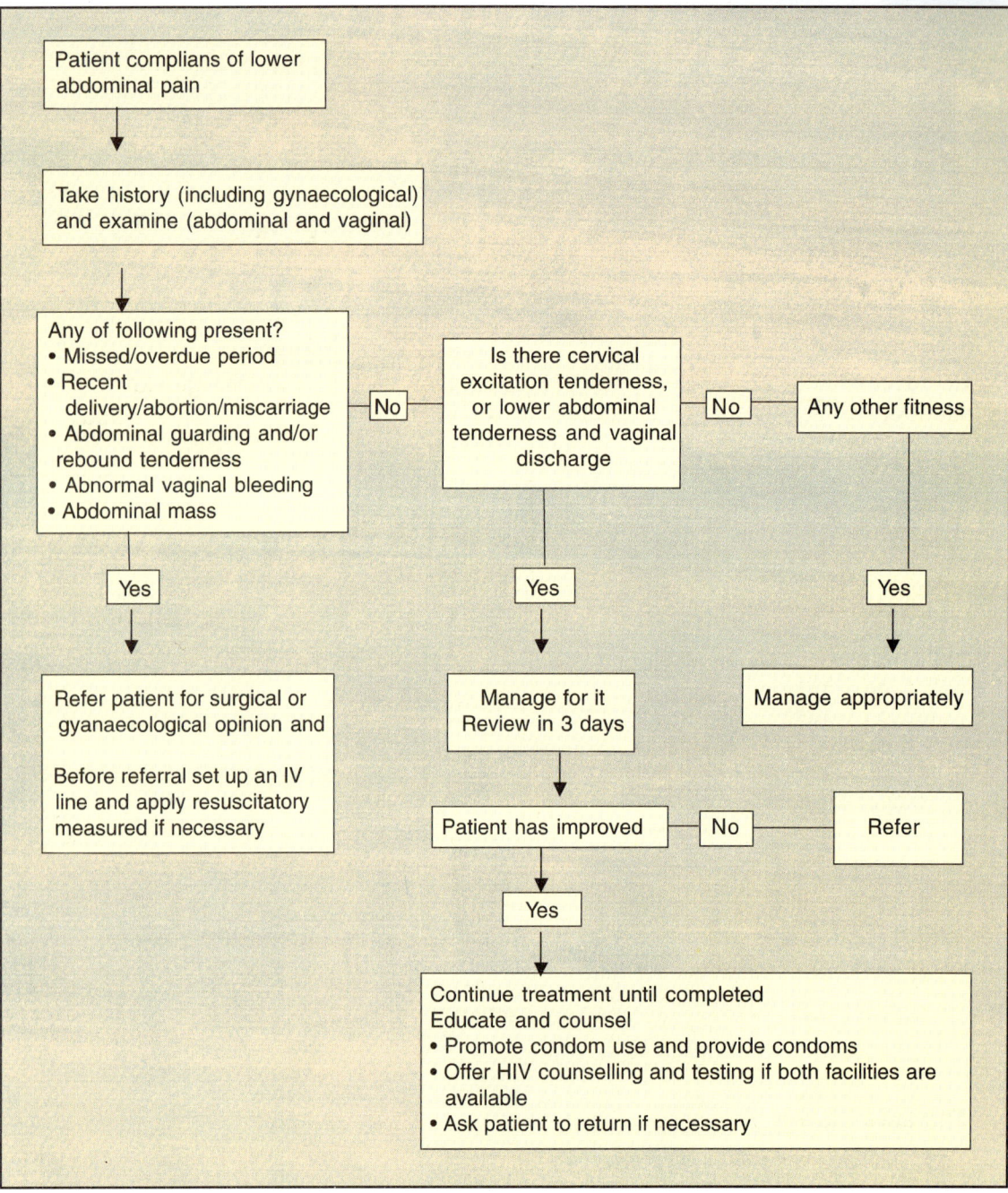

Flow chart 3.   Lower Abdominal pain

Pelvic Inflammatory Disease (PID)

11

Pelvic Inflammatory Disease is infection and inflammation of upper genital tract. The terminology varies as follows according to the part of the genital tract affected.

Uterine cavity–*endometritis*

Tubes and ovaries–*salpingo-ophoritis*

Pelvic peritoneum–*pelvic peritonitis*

Pelvic cellular tissue (endopelvic fascia)–*parametritis*

Prevalence It is an ascending infection and the most common serious infection in the female. It is responsible for

- 30% of patients with infertility
- 50% of patients with ectopic pregnancy, chronic pelvic pain, adhesions and tubal block.

DEFENCE MECHANISMS OF GENITAL TRACT

Female genital tract is open, however not much susceptible to infections, because of the following defence mechanisms:

The **intact hymen** prevents ascent of infection in a virgin.

In the **vulva**

- The labia majora are opposed.
- Vascularity is very high.
- Secretions of bartholin's gland have an anti-fungal and bacteriostatic action.

In the **vagina**

- There is natural apposition of the anterior and posterior vaginal walls.

- Direction of vagina–which is downwards and forwards from the uterus, prevents direct ascending infection
- Lining epithelium–stratified squamous (non-keratinized)
  - Most resistant epithelium
  - Richly stored with glycogen
  - Natural habitat of Doderlien's bacilli, which break down glycogen and maintain a low vaginal pH which prevents the growth of organisms.

In the **cervix**

- The cervix is directed towards the posterior fornix.
- Has complex racemose glands.
- Endometrial glands produce mucus plugs.
- Cervical canal has a relatively small lumen which is normally filled with a plug of alkaline mucus.
- Ciliary movement in the cervix is directed downwards preventing the spread of non-motile organisms upwards.

In the **endometrium**

- Cyclical Loss: Before menstruation there is leucocytic infiltration into the endometrium which protects the raw area which is formed after menstruation.

In the **tubes**

- Tubes ostia are slit like openings.
- Endosalpinx is lined by ciliated epithelium with ciliary movement towards the uterine cavity to prevent the upward spread of non-motile organisms.

Decreased natural resistance

Natural protection mechanism is deficient.

1. *After menses*
   - Cervical canal becomes dilated
   - Raw surfaces are left in the uterus
   - Vaginal pH is increased

2. *After delivery* home deliveries conducted by untrained dais are associated with an increased risk of infection.
   - External os remains patulous throughout

- Internal os closes by 1 week

3. **After MTP**

- Intrauterine manipulations like curettage and suction evacuation in abortion.

4. **After IUCD** The chances of infection are maximum in the first 21 days.

- Vaginal acidity is very high in upper vagina, however organisms can get access via the IUCD threads (length of the IUCD thread is 12 cm).

5. **Menopause**

- Oestrogen deficiency makes the vaginal epithelium bald with an increased risk of infection.

- Decreased glycogen content, with absence of Doderlein's bacilli result in an alkaline pH, increasing the risk of infection.

6. **STD** Gonococcal and Chlamydial infections are the cause of PID in two-thirds of patients. Change in sexual partner within the last 30 days results in introduction of infection.

MICROBIOLOGY AND PATHOGENESIS

The majority of cases of acute PID occur as a result of ascending canalicular spread of microorganisms from the lower genital tract causing infection of the endocervix, endometrium, fallopian tubes and peritoneal cavity. It is predominantly a disease of sexually active women, 75% of cases are seen in women <25 yrs.

Pathology

Mild PID

- Pelvic organs are not much affected.
- Serosal surface of the tubes are hyperaemic.
- Fallopian tubes are edematous but mobile and patent.
- A sticky purulent exudate may be present on the serosal surface.

Moderately severe disease

- Increased inflammation and edema of the tubes.
- There are flimsy adhesions between pelvic and abdominal viscera.
- Tubes may be blocked resulting in pyosalpinx.
- Pelvic organs become adherent forming a complex inflammatory mass.

Microbiology

The aetiology is multifactorial, but three broad types of organisms are responsible.

1. *STD producing*

   These are organisms transmitted by sexual contact and are responsible for 60-75% of cases.

   • Gonococcus seen in 1/3 rd of cases. Gonoccocal inflammation is not seen in females with an azoospermic husband as the bacteria travel up the genital tract along with the sperms.

   • Chlamydia seen in 1/3 rd–the infection is mostly asymptomatic, but tubal damage is more devastating and causes tubal block.

   • Mycoplasma hominis, ureaplasma urealyticum and bacterial vaginosis–their role in the aetiology is unknown.

2. *Pyogenic organisms*

   These are responsible for 15-20% of cases. The organisms responsible are E. coli, bacteroids, anaerobic cocci i.e., peptostreptococci.

3. *Mycobacterium tuberculosis*

   Responsible for 5% of cases of PID and 9% of cases of infertility. The organism spread]s by the blood stream and can cause infection even in a virginal girl.

Iatrogenic causes of PID

1. IUD insertion: The risk of infection is maximum within 20 days of insertion, the organisms are usually of the STD group. Prophylactic Doxycycline 200 mg/orallyx5 days is indicated following IUD insertion. Rarely, pelvic actinomycosis can result if the IUCD is left in the uterine cavity for longer than the specified period.

2. MTP and miscarriage: The incidence is 1-10% and is the major cause of PID in India. Causative organisms are mostly pyogenic bacteria, E. coli, proteus, pseudomonas and bacteroids. Treatment is by broad spectrum antibiotics as the infection is usually polymicrobial.

3. Tubal ligation: The incidence is 0.5 per 1000 following mini-laparotomy and none following laparoscopic tubal ligations.

CLINICAL FEATURES

• The patient is usually young and in the reproductive age group (75% are young and <25 yrs. of age).

- History of exposure (from husband or partner) may be present.

- History of recent MTP/ D&C/ delivery may be given.

- History of an immuno-compromised state may be present.

- History of TB in the husband—TB epididymo-orchitis could cause infection of his wife by ascending infection.

Clinical types

1. Acute PID
2. Chronic PID

Acute PID

Symptoms

- General symptoms like fever, weakness, lassitude, vomiting, malaise, headache etc.

- Discharge: purulent or foul smelling vaginal discharge.

- Lower abdominal pain: The most common symptom is bilateral pain which spreads upwards if general peritonitis follows.

- Bladder and bowel symptoms: frequency, dysuria, diarrhoea due to passage of small quantities of loose stools can occur due to rectal irritation in pelvic abscess.

- Symptoms of complications: Symptoms of acute peritonitis can occur if an ovarian abscess bursts into the peritoneal cavity.

Signs

- Cx and upper vagina may be congested.

- Discharge pouting or pouring may be seen on speculum examination.

- Cervical movements are extremely painful.

- There is tenderness in the fornices.

- Ovary/tube may be palpable and extremely tender.

Per abdomen

- Tenderness and gaurding in the lower abdomen.

- A tender, fixed mass (to mass) may be palpable arising from the pelvis.

- Signs of dehydration may be present.
- Tachycardia and coated tongue may be seen.

Diagnosis of PID

The criteria required for the clinical diagnosis of PID according to CDC-2001 are given in Table 11.1.

Table 11.1. Criteria for diagnosis of PID

Minimum criteria
   • Lower abdominal tenderness
   • Bilateral adnexal tenderness
   • Cervical motion tenderness
 Additional criteria
   • Oral temperature of >38°C
   • Abnormal cervical or vaginal discharge
   • Elevated ESR and C-reactive protein
   • Laboratory documentation of cervical infection with Neisseria or Chlamydia
 Definitive criteria
   • Histopathological evidence of endometritis on endometrial biopsy
   • Tubo-ovarian abscess on sonography or other radiologic tests
   • Laparoscopic abnormalities consistent with PID

Antibiotic therapy should be started if the above criteria are present.

Chronic PID results from relapses of acute PID (Fig. 11.1)

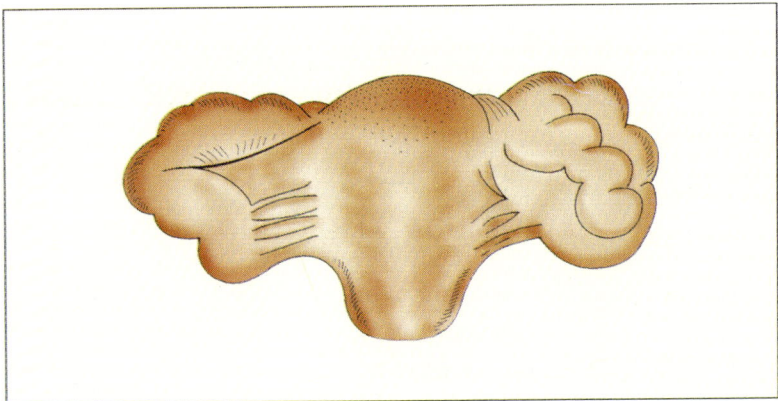

Fig. 11.1. Chronically damaged tubes in chronic PID

Symptoms

- Low backache
- Aggravation of pain during menstruation (dysmenorrhoea)
- Dyspareunia
- Disordered menses–menorrhagia and polymenorrhoea due to ovarian congestion
- Infertility due to tubal or peritubal damage

Signs

- Discharge in the vagina (due to chronic cervicitis).
- Retroverted fixed uterus (due to adhesions) much bigger than normal (due to inflammatory infiltrations in the myometrium).
- Bilateral tenderness in fornices-bilateral adnexal thickenings/swelling/mass.

MANAGEMENT

Investigations

The aim of investigations is two fold:

1. To prove general infection: CBP, TLC, DLC, ESR.
2. To prove local infection: Swabs should be taken after milking the urethra, from the endocervix, high vagina, from the rectum and bladder and after squeezing the bartholin's glands. Both aerobic and anaerobic cultures are to be done. Chlamydia requires special tissue cultures.

Treatment of PID

Principles of treatment

Both partners should be treated. The antibiotics specific for the organisms are–

- Chlamydia–tetracyclines, erythromycin and azithromycin
- Gonococcus and gram negative organisms-co-amoxiclav, ciprofloxacin, ofloxacin and spectinomycin
- Anaerobes–metronidazole and tinidazole

PID with no systemic symptoms antibiotics should be started based on the clinical findings alone:

- Regime A:
  - ofloxacin 400 mg bid for 14 days
  - metronidazole 400 mg/tds for 14 days

- Regime B:
    - IIIrd generation cephalosporin+doxycycline 100mg bd+metronidazole for 14 days

Acute PID with severe systemic symptoms needs hospital admission and iv antibiotics

- Cefotaxime/ Cefoxitin 1 g iv 8 hrly
- Metronidazole 500 mg iv 8 hrly for 3-4 days followed by oral doxycycline and metronidazole for one week
- Symptomatic treatment with analgesics and antipyretics

Surgical treatment The surgical options are:

1. *Laparoscopy* is indicated
    - if the patient is not responding to antibiotic therapy
    - to grade the severity of disease and provide guidance for antibiotic therapy
    - to exclude ectopic pregnancy and appendicitis.
2. *Aspiration of TO mass/pelvic abscess* indicated if there is no response to antibiotic therapy; aspiration can be performed under laparoscopic guidance or transvaginally.
3. *Chronic PID with persistent symptoms*

    Elderly female–TAH + BSO

    Young female–Conservative surgery–(salpingectomy or salpingo-ophorectomy)

Criteria for hospital admission

- When surgical emergencies such as appendicitis cannot be ruled out.
- No response clinically to oral therapy
- Patient unable to tolerate oral regime
- Severe illness
- TO abscess, peritonitis
- HIV with low CD4 counts, immunosuppressive therapy
- Patient in the adolescent age group

SEQUALAE OF PID

1. **Infertility** Due to blockage of the fallopian tubes. The risk after one episode is–8%; following two episodes–19.5% and after 3 episodes the risk is 40%.

2. **Ectopic pregnancy** Due to tubal block or disturbed tubal motility, the fertilized ovum gets lodged in the fallopian tubes.

3. ***Chronic pelvic pain and menstrual irregularities*** If a pyosalpinx or tubo-ovarian abscess responds to antibiotics, the pus contained in it becomes sterile within 6 weeks. But the damage to the tube remains as *chronic pyosalpinx* or *hydrosalpinx*. It is retort shaped due to abnormal dilatation of the ampullary region of the tube filled with clear fluid and may be as large as 15cm. The fimbrial end of the fallopian tube is closed, fimbriae are drawn inwards and the outer surface is smooth and rounded.

Prevention of PID

- 1° prevention–avoid sexual intercourse at an early age.

- 2° prevention–to detect early changes and treatment of all patient partners.

- CDC screening–CDC 1998 advocates universal screening of adolescents or young adults < 24 yrs. undergoing pelvic examination and annual screening of all sexually active females.

DIFFERENTIAL DIAGNOSIS OF ACUTE PELVIC PAIN

The causes of acute pelvic pain are given in the table 11.2.

Table 11.2. Causes of acute pelvic pain	
Gynaecological	**Non-gynaecological**
• Pelvic Inflammatory Disease • Ectopic Pregnancy • Miscarriage • Accidents to ovarian cysts (torsion/rupture) • Mid-cycle ovulation pain (mittelschmerz) • Cervical stenosis with haematometra • Fibroids with degeneration or necrosis	• Ureteric colic • Acute appendicitis • Ileocaecal tuberculosis • Meckel's diverticulitis • Hernias-Inguinal/femoral • Viral mesenteric adenitis • Ischaemic abdominal pain (due to ischaemia of mesenteric vessels)

Evaluation of a patient with acute pelvic pain

History

The points to be noted are–

- Characteristics of the pain-location, mode of onset, constant versus colicky, radiation and relation to the menstrual cycle.

- Menstrual history–date of the last menstrual period, regularity of cycles.

- Contraception used.
- Associated symptoms–vaginal discharge, fever, GI symptoms (vomiting, heartburn, diarrhoea).
- Urinary symptoms (dysuria, haematuria, frequency).
- Past history–history of tuberculosis, previous surgeries, journeys abroad.
- Family history of similar symptoms.

Physical examination

- General appearance–toxic and ill looking or well.
- Vital signs–PR, BP and temperature, fever and shock can cause an increase in PR.
- Abdominal examination to note the site of tenderness, any gaurding or rigidity, abdominal/pelvic mass, hepatosplenomegaly.
- Hernial sites–should be inspected for presence of a cough impulse or swelling.
- Auscultation for bowel sounds.
- Vaginal examination–to look for vaginal discharge, bleeding or expulsion of products of conception (incomplete miscarriage could be the cause).
- Bimanual examination for any evidence of enlarged ovaries, cysts, tubal pregnancy.

Investigations

- Urine for pregnancy test
- High vaginal and endocervical swabs for chlamydia (if there is vaginal dis-charge).
- Mid-stream urine specimen–presence of UTI or any urinary calculus.
- Blood samples–haemoglobin, white cell count and CRP. The CRP is raised in any systemic infection and is a non-specific marker.
- Ultrasound abdomen and pelvis–can diagnose an ovarian cyst, ectopic pregnancy, fibroid causing degeneration, lymphadenopathy in tuberculosis.
- Plain x-ray abdomen–gas under the diaphragm indicates an appendicular or bowel perforation.

TUBERCULOSIS OF THE GENITAL TRACT

Epidemiology

Tuberculosis of the female genital tract has been an important cause of infertility in the developing world. Genital TB is most commonly diagnosed in women of childbearing age from developing countries who have never been pregnant. It is estimated that upto 5 to 10% of infertility in women can be attributed to tuberculosis and in certain regions of India 19% of infertile women have been found to have pelvic TB.

Pathogenesis

Majority of women with pelvic TB have not had a previous diagnosis of pulmonary TB. When there is a history of pulmonary TB, the diagnosis has been made years earlier. The lung disease may be active, quiescent, or healed without radiographic residue. When the primary infection occurs close to the time of menarche, the chance of genital tuberculosis increases. The primary focus is most often situated in the lungs (50%), lymph nodes (40%), urinary tract (5%), and the bones and joints (5%).

Mode of spread

Haematogenous

- Most commonly, infection of the genital tract occurs via haematogenous spread from a primary pulmonary site, although the urinary tract or the abdominal cavity may also be the initial site of infection. Almost all patients have fallopian tube infection and both tubes are usually involved. The cause of the predilection of M. tuberculosis for the fallopian tubes is unknown. The infectious process within the tubes may remain dormant for years and then reactivate years later. From the tubes secondary spread can cause peritonitis (45%) of ovarian disease (10-30%); can involve the endometrium (50-80%) or less commonly the cervix (<5%) or vagina (<1%).

Direct

- About 5% of case of pelvic TB are thought to occur secondary to direct spread. Extension of TB from the bladder, rectum or intestine along the peritoneal surface to the pelvis occurs occasionally.

Sexual contact

- Cervical, vulvar and vaginal TB may result from direct sexual contact with a partner with tuberculous infection of the genito-urinary tract.

Pathology

Fallopian tube

Both the tubes are usually involved, although not to the same degree. The initial site of infection is in the submucosal layer of the ampullary part of the tube (interstitial salpingitis).

- The infection may spread medially along the wall causing destruction of the muscles which are replaced by fibrous tissue. The walls get thickened, become calcified or even ossified. The infection may spread inwards; the mucosa gets swollen and destroyed. The fimbria are everted and the abdominal ostium usually remains patent. The elongated and distended distal tube with the patent abdominal ostium gives the appearance of "*tobacco-pouch*". Occlusion of the ostium may, however occur due to adhesions. The tubercles burst pouring the caseous material inside the lumen producing a tubercular pyosalpix, which may adhere to the ovaries and the surrounding structures. If the infection spreads outwards, it produces *peri-salpingitis* with exudation, causing dense adhesions with the surrounding structures–and a tubercular *tubo-ovarian mass* (Fig. 11.2). Rarely, miliary, tubercles may be found on the serosal surface of the tubes, uterus, peritoneum or intestines, and are often associated with *tubercular peritoniti*s.

The fallopian tubes may look absolutely normal or nodules may be present at the isthmus near the uterine corner, constituting *salpingitis isthmica nodosa*. There is thickening of the tube due to proliferation of tubal epithelium within the hypertrophied muscle layer. It is diagnosed radiologically as a small diverticulum. The microscopic appearance of the fallopian tubes is not distinctive until later stages when the tubal peritoneum is studded with tubercles. Generally pelvic TB mimics chronic non-tuberculous salpingitis.

Uterus The uterus is involved in 50-80% of cases. The infection spreads from the tubes either by lymphatic or direct spread, the cornual ends are commonly affected due to their dual blood supply and anatomical proximity to tubes. Uterine involvement is usually limited to the endometrium. The endometrium may not exhibit tubercles, as the monthly

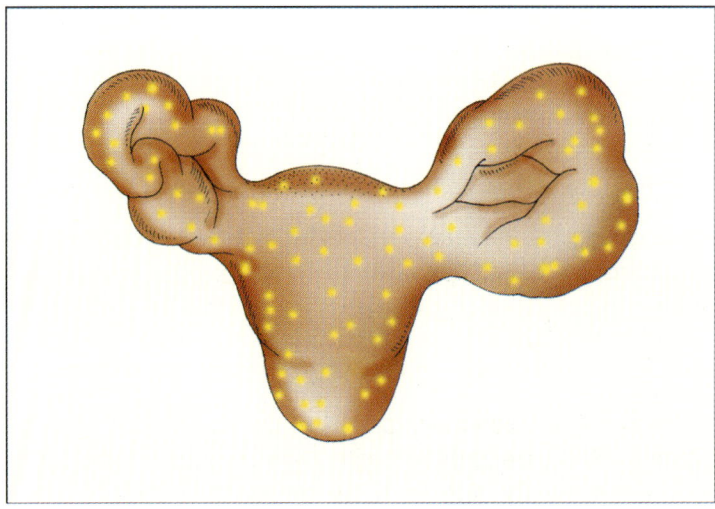

Fig. 11.2. Tuberculosis of the fallopian tubes

sloughing of the endometrium does not allow adequate time for tuberculosis and caseating granulomas to form. Biopsy of the endometrium, will reveal epitheloid and giant cell; AFB are rarely seen. In more advanced cases, caseating material collects in the uterine cavity to form a pyometra. This is more commonly noted in post-menopausal women who have a stenosed cervix. The adhesions within the uterine cavity lead to formation of intrauterine synaechiae and *Asherman's syndrome* and the patient develops secondary amenorrhoea.

Cervix The cervix is involved due to descending infection from the fallopian tube through the uterine cavity; rarely, it could be an ascending infection. The lesion may appears as an ulcer or as a red papillary erosion which bleeds easily on touch. Biopsy is essential to recognize the lesion and exclude malignancy.

Vulva and vagina Tuberculosis of the vulva and vagina usually appears in the form of a painful shallow ulcer with undermined edges, rarely in a hypertrophic form resembling elephantiasis vulva.

Pelvic peritoneum Pelvic peritonitis is present in about 40-50% of cases. Tuberculous peritonitis may be *wet* (exudative type) or *dry* (adhesive type).

In the *wet* variety there is ascites with straw coloured fluid in the peritoneal cavity. The parietal and visceral peritoneum are covered with numerous small tubercles.

In the *dry* variety there are dense adhesions with bowel loops due to fibrosis when the *wet* lesions heal.

Microscopy Granulomas are the characteristic feature consisting of infiltration of multinucleated giant cells (langhans), chronic inflammatory cells and epitheloid cells, surrounding a central area of caseation necrosis. Caseation may not be a constant feature.

Clinical features

Age Infection commonly occurs in women between 20-40 years of age.

Family history A family history of contact may be available.

History There may be past history of tubercular affection of the lungs or lymph nodes. Genital tuberculosis occurs in 10-20 percent of patients who have pulmonary tuberculosis in adolescence.

Symptoms

- *Infertility* may be primary or secondary and is reported in 85% of patients with genital tuberculosis in India. Of all the patients with infertility, 10% have genital tuberculosis. The causes are predominantly due to tubal blockage, adhesions in the endometrial cavity (uterine synaechiae) or associated ovulatory dysfunction.

- *Pelvic pain* is present in about 20-30% cases, is not localized and aggravated by coitus, menses and can be precipitated by tubal patency tests.

- *Menstrual abnormality*   is seen in about 50%. Menorrhagia or irregular bleeding is probably due to ovarian involvement, pelvic congestion or endometrial proliferation and is an early manifestation. These patients fail to respond to hormone therapy. Endometrial tuberculosis is a rare cause of pubertal menorrhagia and post-menopausal bleeding.

- *Amenorrhoea or oligomenorrhoea*   Secondary amenorrhoea is more common due to suppression of the ovarian function by tubercular toxin with compensatory overactivity of the anterior pituitary. It may be also be due to endometrial destruction with uterine synaechiae.

- *Vaginal discharge*   Cervical or vaginal tuberculosis may be associated with post-coital bleeding or blood stained vaginal discharge.

- *Constitutional symptoms*   Loss of weight, malaise, anorexia, pyrexia and anaemia are present in the acute phase of the disease.

Signs   General condition of the patient is generally good. Fever may be absent.

Abdominal examination Abdominal findings may be negative or rarely there may be an irregular tender mass in the lower abdomen arising out of the pelvis due to encysted ascites, matted intestines, pyometra or a tubo-ovarian mass. Abdomen may feel doughy due to the matted intestines. A tubercular encysted cyst may appear as an ovarian cyst, which is usually immobile, often tympanic on percussion due to intestinal adhesions.

Vaginal examination   Pelvic examination may be normal in 50% cases. There may be thickening of the tubes which are felt through the fornix. There may be pelvic masses of varying sizes, which are usually small and fixed. At times the pelvic masses are all matted together and fixed to the uterus–a condition called the *frozen pelvis*. These masses are usually not tender or are less tender than other inflammatory masses unless they are secondarily infected.

Investigations

- *Blood*–The leucocyte count and ESR values may be raised.

- *Montoux tests*–Two days after injection of purified protein derivative of tuberculosis (PPD) to the forearm an induration of 10mm or more is considered positive. A negative test excludes tuberculosis but a positive one is not indicative of location of the disease or its activity.

- Investigations to look for the primary focus–chest X-Ray, sputum for AFB, urine c/s, x-ray of bones

- *Dilatation and curettage*–should be carried out in the late premenstrual phase as the tubercles are present in the superficial layers and are sloughed during menstruation. In the proliferative phase, the tissue is inadequate and fresh tubercles might not have been formed in sufficient numbers for an accurate diagnosis. The first day menstrual fluid is not as satisfactory as the pre-menstrual tissue.

The endometrial tissue is divided into two portions, one for histopathological examination and the other for guinea pig inoculation and tissue culture. This is an OPD procedure. Optimal results are obtained from the endometrial samples curetted from the cornu of the uterus, as the cornual end is the first part of the uterine cavity to be affected. Negative endometrial biopsy may be due to the fact that the endometrium is involved in only 60-70% cases, due to wrong timing of the sample and extensive endometrial destruction due to the disease itself. Other causes of endometrial granulomas are actinomycosis, sarcoidosis, schistosomiasis and foreign body reaction.

- *Hysterosalpingogram* should not be performed until pelvic tuberculosis is excluded by endometrial sampling. Typical hysterosalpingographic findings in pelvic tuberculosis are:

    A rigid non-peristalitic pipe like tube, called *lead pipe appearance.*

    Beading and variation in filling density

    Calcification of the tube

    Cornual block

    A jagged fluffiness of the tubal outline

    Vascular or lymphatic intravasation of the dye

    Shrivelled and obliterated uterine cavity in Asherman's syndrome

    Non-specific changes such as salpingitis isthmica nodosa (SIN)–nodular outpouchings, diverticula and inflammation.

- *Ultrasound*–can reveal a pelvic mass due to encysted ascites or formation of tubo-ovarian adhesions.

- *Laparoscopy*–Once tuberculosis is suspected and confirmed by the previously mentioned methods, the value of laparoscopy is limited. The pelvic adhesions with intestinal loops and genital organs prevent observation of the pelvic organs and may even make the procedure dangerous. A phenomenon of "blue uterus" may be seen due to lymphatic intravasation by the intrauterine injected blue dye which colours the uterus and was seen especially in cases of genital tuberculosis.

- *Other tests*–Enzyme-linked immunoabsorbent assay (ELISA), SAFA (Soluble Antigen Fluorescence Antibody) Test, Gas Chromatography and BAC test.

Treatment of Genital TB

Before the advent of antituberculous drug therapy, surgery was often used in the treatment of pelvic tuberculosis. With the advent of effective drug therapy, the surgical treatment for genital tuberculosis has been restricted to specific indications/ four drugs need to be administered daily/three days a week (HRZE) during the intensive phase followed by 2 drugs (Isoniazid + Rifampicin) for 4 months or Isoniazid + Ethambutol for 6 months.

Dosage recommendations are given in table 11.3.

Table 11.3. Treatment of Tuberculosis		
Drug	**Daily**	**Three times a week**
Isoniazid (H)	5 mg/kg	15 mg/kg
Rifampicin(R)	10 mg/kg	10 mg/kg
Pyrazinamide	15-30 mg/kg	50-70mg/kg
Ethambutol	5-25 mg/kg	25-30mg/kg

Surgery: Surgery in the management of patient with pelvic TB should be reserved for specific indications as follows.

1. Persistence or enlargement of an adnexal mass after 4 to 6 months of antitubercular antibiotic therapy. The rare possibility of an ovarian tumour must always be considered even though pelvic tuberculosis is also present. Pelvic ultrasonography is useful in following the response of the adnexal mass to treatment.

2. Persistence of pelvic pain or recurrence of pelvic pain while on medical therapy.

3. Primary unresponsiveness of the tuberculous infection to antibiotic therapy, as shown by persistent spiking temperature, leucocytosis, elevated ESR, and evidence on biopsy specimens of continued endometrial infections.

Surgical options

1. The preferred surgical treatment include total abdominal hysterectomy and bilateral salpingo-oophoectomy. The nature of this inflammatory disease may make the operative procedure technically difficult with an increased risk of injury to the bowel and bladder.

2. For young patients who are eager to attempt future childbearing conservative adnexectomy should be carried out only if it is possible to do so after the extent of the adnexal disease is carefully evaluated and is found to be minimal.

3. Reconstructive tubal surgery has no place in the management of patients whose infertility is the result of bilateral tubal obstruction from tuberculous salpingitis, as pelvic tuberculosis may be reactivated following tubal reconstructive surgery.

Prognosis for fertility Only about 5% of the patients with genital tuberculosis are capable of becoming pregnant and only 2% carry a pregnancy to term. In the presence of tuberculous tubo-ovarian abscess, pregnancy is extremely rare, and conservative surgery for the purpose of preserving fertility is unwarranted.

12

Infertility

The chances of conception for a couple having regular, unprotected intercourse is 80% after 12 and 90% after 18 months. Initiation of an infertility evaluation should be undertaken after 12 menstrual cycles or one year of unprotected intercourse. For women aged 35 years or more, work-up can be started earlier, after 6 menstrual cycles or after 6 months of unprotected intercourse. In situations with significant historical factors that could compromise fertility, such as irregular cycles, pelvic inflammatory disease (PID), and previous infertility, evaluation can be started earlier.

Infertility refers to an absolute inability to conceive.

Subfertility is a relative inability to conceive.

Infertility could be Primary or Secondary depending on the causes:

1. **Primary infertility** when there was no prior conception.

2. **Secondary** when a prior conception has occurred.

Infertility is a two-patient disorder involving either the female, the male partner or both. Both the partners should be interviewed together and explained in detail, with the help of pictures and line diagrams the physiology of conception and the possible causes. The causes of infertility are summarized in table 12.1.

CAUSES IN THE MALE

These are responsible in a third of cases of infertility.

Table 12.1. Causes of Infertility		
Male factor	–	30%
Female factor	–	25%
Both partners	–	25%
Unknown	–	20%

Physiology of male reproduction Understanding the physiology of male reproduction is essential to understand the causes behind it.

Hypothalamus–secretes GnRH releasing hormones which act on the anterior pituitary.

Pituitary gland–secretes FSH and LH which act on the seminiferous tubules and the interstitial cells respectively.

Testis–lie outside the abdominal cavity and have interstitial tissue that secretes testosterone and seminiferous tubules where spermatogenesis occurs under the influence of testosterone. Increase in the level of testosterone inhibits the release of FSH.

Epididymis and vas deferens: The sperms are collected in the epididymis and transported via the vas into the penile urethra.

Seminal vesicles and prostate: cause capacitation of the sperms.

Ejaculation occurs from the penile urethra.

Causes of male infertility

1. ***Hypothalamo-pituitary causes*** severe head injury, meningitis, encephalitis, stress can alter the function of the HPO axis.

2. ***Testicular causes***
   a) Increased scrotal temperature eg. men working in blast furnaces and in sedentary jobs, wearing tight scrotal supports, varicocele, undescended testis
   b) Testicular injury–eg. trauma, inflammation due to mumps (orchitis)

3. ***Epididymal causes*** trauma or inflammatory disease eg. gonorrhoea or tuberculosis

4. ***Causes in the vas deferens*** congenital absence of the vas eg. cystic fibrosis, trauma to the vas

5. ***Causes in the penile urethra*** epi or hypospadias can affect ejaculation

6. ***Systemic causes***
   a) *General illness*–chronic renal or hepatic failure, acute pyrexial illness can affect sperm count for weeks
   b) *Substance abuse*–excessive use of alcohol, tobacco, cannabis can lower the sperm counts
   c) *Drugs*–sulphasalazine used in the treatment of Crohn's disease can lower sperm counts

Evaluation of the male

History The history should include the following:

- Marital history including previous fertility of partners, frequency of intercourse and any problems with erection or ejaculation

- General health including previous chronic illnesses or recent febrile illness (in the past 2-6 months)

- History of gynaecomastia

- Chemical/radiation exposure including smoking history, medications eg. sulphasalzine, past chemotherapy, industrial exposure (especially to organic solvents and heavy metals)

- Genital surgery–hernia repair, hydrocelectomy, retroperitoneal surgery, cystoscopy

- Genital inflammation: past history of tuberculosis-epididymitis, mumps-orchitis, prostatitis

- Genital trauma: especially if associated with scrotal ecchymosis (scrotal haematoma can cause testicular atrophy)

- History of erectile dysfunction.

General examination

- Height and weight – short stature is seen in Klinefelter's syndrome

- Features of systemic illness eg. Tuberculosis

Local examination This should be performed in the upright position.

- Scrotal contents should be assessed for:

  Testes – size and consistency

  Epididymis – size, consistency, any spermatocele is noted.

  Vas deferens – presence, size

  Varicocele – if palpable, size is noted if medium or large.

- Penile abnormalities should be noted.

Investigations in the male

1. **Semen analysis** this is the most important part of the investigation.

   Sample collections: The patient should be instructed on the following specifications for an optimal sample:

   - The sample should be collected in a sterile specimen container obtained from the medical center.

   - The patient should practice abstinence for 2-5 days prior to collection of the sample.

   - He is instructed to masturbate up to the point of ejaculation and not to use lubricants, not even saliva.

- If any of the ejaculate is lost, the sample should be discarded, and another sample should be collected in 2 days. Condoms should not be used.

- The sample should be delivered to the lab within 30 minutes (ideally collected on the site) of collection.

- The sample should be kept at body temperature (55 to 99 degrees F).

Values for normal seminal parameters are not well defined. The World Health Organization (WHO) criteria for semen analysis (Table 12.2) outline the minimal standards for sperm measurements but do not necessarily identify men with male factor infertility. Values are given for sperm concentration, motility, and morphology to classify men as subfertile, of indeterminate fertility, and fertile as shown in the table 12.3.

Table 12.2. Normal semen parameters	
Components	**Normal values**
Volume	1.5 to 5 ml
pH	7.2-8.0
Motile sperm per ejaculate	>20 million (60% forward progression)
Agglutination	none to minimal
Morphology	70% normal forms
Motility–forward progression	grade 3-4 (80-90%)
Liquefaction	Complete in 30 min

Males who have any seminal parameters that fall within the range of subfertile or Indeterminate should have a repeat semen analysis. Men with persistent values in the subfertile or indeterminate range should be referred to a male infertility specialist.

A complete semen analysis also provides information on other factors in the semen. If any of the components of the semen analysis falls outside normal, the results are considered abnormal.

If the first semen analysis is abnormal, a second semen analysis should be ordered to be performed in one month. Careful instructions regarding abstinence, collection, and transportation of the specimen should be repeated. Usually two samples are tested before labelling the seminal analysis as being abnormal.

Abnormalities in the semen analysis

- Increased liquefaction time and viscosity–due to decreased prostatic secretions or a chronic infection in the accessory glands.

- Low semen volume–due to obstruction of the ejaculatory ducts or congenital absence of the seminal vesicles.

- Semen pH of < 7.0 indicates dysgenesis of the vas deferens.

- Sperm count and concentration–the haemocytometer (improved Neubaur counting chamber) is the most frequently used method of assessment of sperm concentration.

   Oligospermia–count of < 20 million/ml

   Azoospermia–complete absence of sperms due to a block in the vas deferens, testicular failure or Klinefelter's syndrome

- Sperm morphology–commonly assessed by the *Papanicolaou stain* or *Shorr's stain*. Atleast 30% of sperms should have a normal morphology.

- Sperm motility–normally should be 60%; decreased in seminal infection or in the presence of sperm antibodies.

- Antisperm antibodies–This test is reserved for samples exhibiting marked agglutination. The commonly used tests are the immunobead and the MAR (mixed antiglobulin reaction) test.

Table 12.3. Categories of semen
Fertile (no evidence of male factor infertility) • Sperm concentration - >48 × 10^6 sperm/ml • Sperm motility - >63% • Sperm morphology (WHO) - >30% normal forms **Indeterminate range** (possible male factor infertility) • Sperm concentration - 13.5 to 48.0 × 10^6 sperm/ml • Sperm motility - 32 to 63% • Sperm morphology (WHO) - <30% normal forms **Subfertile** (previously classified as infertile) • Sperm concentration - <13.5 × 10^6 sperm/ml • Sperm motility - <32% • Sperm morphology (WHO) - <30% normal forms

2. **Testicular biopsy** indicated in patients with azoospermia
   - Normal–indicates obstruction to the vas
   - Abnormal–indicates testicular failure

3. **Endocrine studies** FSH, LH and S Prolactin
   - Increased FSH–testicular failure due to absence of feedback inhibition by testosterone

- Decreased FSH–suggests pituitary failure
- Increased serum prolactin-could be due to a prolactinoma and can cause oligospermia.

4. *Karyotype* indicated in patients with azoospermia as 15-20% have a chromosomal disorder like Klinefelter's syndrome.

CAUSES IN THE FEMALE

The causes are given in the table 12.4.

Evaluation of the female

This includes a detailed history and examination.

History The points to be noted are–

- Her *age* and *time since marriage*. If the age is >35 yrs., investigations should be commenced early.
- *Intercourse*, it's regularity, timing and any dyspareunia.
- *Menstrual cycle*–it's regularity and duration of flow. Regular cycles indicate regular ovulation, irregular cycles are more likely to be anovulatory.
- *Past medical history*–history of tuberculosis, STD, previous treatment for PID, previous appendicectomy indicate tubal block as a possible cause of infertility, any chronic illness eg., liver and renal failure can affect ovulation and cause amenorrhoea.
- *History of medications*–certain drugs have to be stopped when a patient is planning to conceive eg., ethionamide (antitubercular drug), phenytoin, warfarin.
- Previous treatment details.

General examination

- The height and weight (BMI)–Obesity is an indicator of Polycystic ovarian syndrome (PCOS) and Cushing's syndrome.

Table 12.4. Causes of female infertility	
Vulva	Vaginismus, perineal scars
Vagina	Vaginal septum, vaginitis
Tubal	Pelvic inflammatory disease due to chlamydia, gonorrhoea, tuberculosis, endometriosis,
Ovarian	Chronic anovulation (PCOS)
Hypothalamo-pituitary	Stress, Prolactinomas (by causing anovulation)

- Acne and hirsuitism are suggestive of PCOS.

- *Acanthosis nigricans*–hyperpigmented thickening of the skin folds seen with PCOS and obese women.

- Breasts–for the stage of development and any galactorrhoea.

- Any thyromegaly and signs of hypo or hyperthyroidism are noted.

- Cardiovascular or respiratory system for any evidence of disease. Blood pressure should be checked as anaesthesia may be required at a later stage; hypertension is seen in cushing's syndrome.

Local examination

- Note any vaginismus or perineal scarring which may cause dyspareunia.

- Speculum examination–to note any vaginal infection, this needs to be treated first.

- Size of the uterus, any adnexal tenderness or mass may suggest PID or endometriosis.

The points to be noted in examinationare summarized in table 12.5.

Table 12.5. Examination of the female – Key points	
• Signs of endocrine disorders	– Acne, hirsuitism, balding – Acanthosis nigricans – Virilization – Signs of thyroid disease
• BMI • Blood pressure • Fitness for possible anaesthetic	
• Breast examination	– Galactorrhoea, any lumps
• Abdomen	– Scars, masses, hirsuitism
• Pelvic examination	– Vaginismus – Adnexal mass/ tenderness – Nodules in the POD (of endometriosis)

Investigations in the female

These include

1. **Baseline investigations** to know the general health and fitness

   - The tests commonly performed are: haemogram with ESR, chest x-ray, urine analysis, random blood sugar, serum VDRL of both husband and wife, as the incidence of syphilis and tuberculosis is still high in our country.

2. **Tests for ovulation**

   i) *Basal Body Temperature (BBT) × 3 cycles* The rationale is the rise in basal body temperature by 0.2-0.5 degrees centigrade is due to the effect of progesterone. Patients are instructed to take their temperatures using a digital thermometer before rising in the morning. Lately, urinary luteinizing hormone (LH) kits have become available, which may be used to document the luteinizing hormone surge prior to ovulation, but these kits are expensive. The days when intercourse occurs should also be marked down so that coital frequency can be noted. A rise in the basal body temperature indicates ovulation. However, 10-15% of ovulatory cycles fail to show an adequate rise in the BBT.

ii) *Cervical mucus* One may also document ovulation by looking for the presence of a ferning pattern of the cervical mucus Fig. 12.1 in a patient in her midcycle (estrogen effect causes ferning and progesterone effect does not).

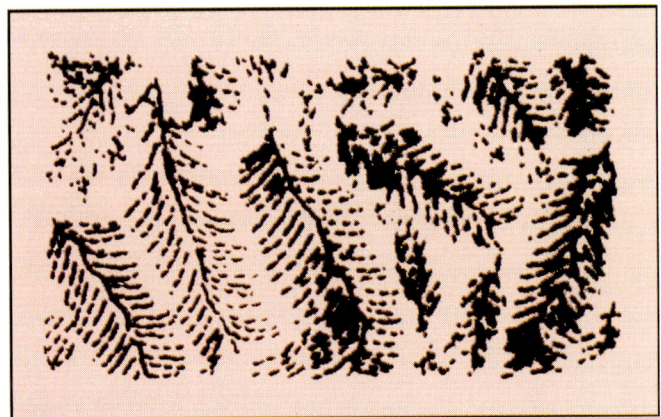

Fig. 12.1.   Microscopy of cervical mucus showing the ferning pattern at ovulation

iii) *Endocrine profile*

- *Serum progesterone levels* A normal day 21 serum progesterone (use day 21 if a 28 day cycle, or check at 7 to 8 days post basal body temperature shift if the cycle is longer or shorter) confirms normal corpus luteal production of progesterone, which is associated with normal ovulation. Day 21 progesterone levels > 30 nm/l are indicative of ovulation.

- *Gonadotropin levels (LH/FSH)* these are commonly performed on the third day of the cycle. FSH is the best indicator of ovarian function. A level of >10 iu/l on more than one occasion indicates anovulation. A level of >25 iu/l suggests premature ovarian failure. A high LH (>10iu/l) compared to FSH suggests that the patient has PCOS.

- *Serum prolactin* This is increased in 15% of women with PCOS. Levels of >1000 miu/l indicate a pituitary adenoma.

- *Androgens-serum testosterone and dehydroepiandrosterone sulphate (DHEAS)* are indicated in women with acne and hirsuitism.

iv) *Pelvic ultrasound* A baseline transabdominal ultrasound scan is carried out to inspect the pelvic structures, detect asymptomatic fibroids, ovarian cysts and visualise the abdominal viscera. A transvaginal ultrasound is preferred for ovulation studies to a transabdominal one as it obviates the need for a full bladder and allows high frequency probes (5-7 mhz) to be used so that higher resolution and greater precision can be achieved. USG is also useful in detecting PCOS and ovarian cysts.

- *Polycystic ovarian syndrome* (PCOS) is characterised by enlarged, sclerocystic ovaries with amenorrhoea, infertility and hirsuitism which was first described by Stein and Leventhal in 1935. The ovaries are polycystic with 10 or more cysts, 2-8 mm in diameter arranged around a dense stroma (Fig. 12.2).

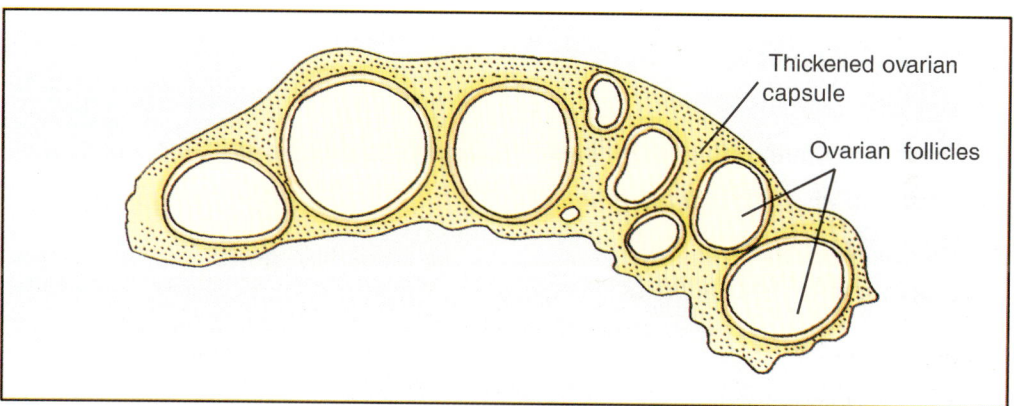

Thickened ovarian capsule

Ovarian follicles

Fig. 12.2. The ovary in PCOS—note the multiple follicles with a thickened ovarian cortex

- *Ovulation studies* In spontaneous cycles, small follicles can be visualised 10 days before the day of ovulation (day 4). By day 5, there is usually a dominant follicle which grows at the rate of approximately 2-3 mm/day until the day of ovulation. Ovulation is indicated by a corpus luteum which is either ovoid or irregular in outline with a cystic, echo-free interior and fluid in the pouch of douglas.

- *Endometrial changes also indicate ovulation* In the follicular phase, the endometrium is a single hypoechoeic line of 4-6 mm. In the peri-ovulatory phase the estrogenised endometrium takes on a "triple-line" appearance. In the luteal phase, the functional layer becomes hyperechoeic due to stromal edema and is about 14mm thick.

- *Doppler ultrasound* Doppler studies of the ovarian circulation are still at a research stage. The ovarian blood flow on the side of the dominant follicle is increased with a reduced resistance to arterial blood flow. Assessment of uterine blood flow helps in assessing endometrial receptivity prior to implantation.

v) *Endometrial biopsy* Although the western countries have given up this invasive procedure as a test for ovulation, it has a role in India where the resources are limited. The presence of secretory endometrium in the pre-menstrual phase indicates ovulation. Pre-menstrual endometrium is also sent for AFB staining and culture to exclude endometrial tuberculosis. Endometrial dating is of little value.

3. Tests for tubal patency

i) *Hysterosalpingogram (HSG):* Hysterosalpingography involves injection of a radiopaque dye through the uterus with fluoroscopic visualization of the uterine cavity and tubal lumina. The resulting hysterosalpingogram (HSG) is also useful in detecting uterine anomalies in women with a history of repetitive spontaneous abortions or infertility.

Contraindications to HSG

- Possible pregnancy
- Abnormal uterine bleeding, abnormal last menstrual period (rule out pregnancy)
- Acute pelvic inflammatory disease
- Recent curettage
- Active genital tract infection

Timing Optimally within 10 days of a menstrual cycle. Contraception should be used for the rest of the cycle in which an HSG is performed. If a woman is oligomenorrhoeic, a withdrawal bleed is induced with progesterone after a negative pregnancy test.

Prophylactic antibiotics are routinely used as there is a possibility of silent infection with chlamydia. The dye used is a water soluble contrast medium which is usually absorbed after an hour. Pre-procedure analgesia is optional and includes nonsteroidal anti-inflammatory drugs given orally or as an injectable. An antispasmodic is also prescribed and the procedure performed under image intensification fluoroscopy

Usually four radiographs are obtained documenting the following anatomy:

a) A complete view of the endometrial cavity and cervical canal should be obtained where the uterine cavity is not over distended with the dye and is oriented parallel to the x-ray film.

b) Bilateral proximal tubal anatomy with special emphasis to rule out salpingitis isthmica nodosum

c) Distal tubal anatomy with care being given to assess for the presence of rugal folds, tubal diameter and evidence of spillage

d) Complete dispersion of the dye ruling out evidence of peri-adnexal adhesions

- *Normal findings:* The cavity of the body of the uterus is usually triangular with the diameter of the cornual portion approximately 35 mm. The fallopian tubes are 56 cm long and free spill of the contrast into the peritoneal cavity should be seen if the tubes are patent.

- *Hydrosalpinx* appears as a large sacculated structure that is often convoluted or retort shaped.

- *Salpingitis isthmica nodosa* is seen as multiple small diverticula of the proximal 2 cm of the fallopian tubes.

- Tubal blockage after *TB salpingitis* appears as tubes with a ragged outline or a beaded appearance. Occasionally, the tubes are rigid with a "*pipe stem appearance*".

ii) *Ultrasound contrast hysterosalpingography (hysterosalpingocontrast sonography, Hycosy)* A hysterosalpingogram is performed using ultrasono-graphy, using an ultrasound contrast medium which contains galactose microparticles and is therefore free of the possible risks of radiation. It is undertaken in the same manner and at a similar time in the cycle as the conventional HSG. The tubal patency is assessed; additionally the ovarian morphology is visualised and any fibroids or congenital uterine anomalies also detected. The advantage is that it avoids the need for radiation, however, the drawbacks are the time taken to perform the test and trained personnel needed for the procedure.

iii) *Laparoscopy* It is often the final diagnostic procedure in an infertility evaluation. It should be performed in the post-menstrual phase. An assessment of the pelvis is made with an endoscope. Careful inspection of the peritoneal surfaces of the uterus, bladder, bowel, the peri-appendicular area, the sub-diaphragmatic surface of the liver are carried out as any adhesions may indicate chlamydial or gonococcal pelvic inflammatory disease in the past (*Fitz-Hugh Curtis syndrome*).

The ovaries are inspected for signs of follicular activity and ovulation. Endometriosis often occurs on the undersurface of the ovary and in the ovarian fossa. Any endometriotic spots are fulgurated using a diathermy probe.

Methylene blue dye (methyl trioninium chloride) is injected transcervically and the fimbrial ends of the fallopian tubes observed for any spill.

iv) *Hysteroscopy* Many practioners carry out a hysteroscopic evaluation in addition to evaluate the endometrial cavity and cannulate the cornual ends of the fallopian tubes on both sides.

Postcoital test It has lately been suggested that the post-coital test should be deleted from the basic infertility evaluation. This conclusion is based on:

- A limited correlation to fertility

- Confusion about standardized normal values

- Controversies in treatment

- An abnormal test tends to create further testing without an apparent significant effect on the pregnancy rate

– The work-up of an infertile couple is given in table 12.6

Table 12.6. Basic work-up of an infertile couple	
Investigations in the male	• Semen analysis
	• Serum VDRL
Investigations in the female	
General	• Haemogram and ESR
	• Chest x-ray
	• Montoux test
	• Urine routine and microscopy
	• Random blood sugar
	• Serum VDRL
Tests for ovulation	• BBT charting
	• LH/FSH and D 21 serum progesterone
	• Endometrial biopsy
Tests for tubal patency	• Hysterosalpingogram
	• Diagnostic laparoscopy

MANAGEMENT OF THE SUB-FERTILE COUPLE

It is essential that both partners are counselled together. It should be emphasized to them that neither of them are guilty or should be held resposible for the delay in conception.

General measures which apply from partners are:

• Stoppage of smoking, reduction in alcohol intake

• Regularity of intercourse and timing–this may mean changing a job or changing one's lifestyle.

• Rubella status of the female partner should be checked and if sero-negative, rubella vaccination offered and the woman advised not to become pregnant within one month of immunisation.

• Folic acid supplementation of the female partner is necessary at the dose of 1 mg / day to prevent neural tube defects. If there is a previous history of neural tube defects, the dose is increased to 5 mg /day.

Management of the female

Management depends on the cause detected.

1. ***Anovulation*** The following measures can be adopted:

- *Exercise and weight loss* reduce the androgen excess in PCOS and helps in regulating ovulation. Conservative measures should be strongly advocated before starting ovulation inducing agents as prolonged usage can be potentially carcinogenic.

- *Clomiphene citrate* This is the agent of first choice. It is a synthetic, weak estrogen which acts by competing with endogenous circulating estrogens for estrogen binding sites on the hypothalamus and blocks the negative feedback of endogenous estrogen. This results in an increased release of LH and FSH from the anterior pituitary resulting in better oocyte maturation and ovulation. The drug is usually given from day 2 for 5 days starting at 50 mg per day. Ovulation if checked by a rise in the BBT, measurement of an elevation of day 21 serum progesterone or follicular study using ultrasound. If ovulation / conception does not occur, the dose is sequentially increased by 50 mg increments upto a maximum of 250 mg per day.

- *Gonadotropins* These are indicated in patients who do not respond to clomiphene. The gonadotropins commonly used are–hMG (human menopausal gonadotropin which has both LH and FSH), pure FSH and human chorionic gonadotropin (hCG).

- *Pulsatile GnRH* This is indicated in patients with hypothalamo-pituitary dysfunction; sub-cutaneous or intravenous injection results in a pulsatile release of FSH and LH.

2. ***Management of tubal factors***

- *Endometriosis:* If mild to moderate, fulguration of endometriotic spots and adhesiolysis improves the fertility rate. Severe endometriosis needs excision of the endometriomas followed by Invitro fertilization (IVF).

- *Pelvic Inflammatory Disease*–Adhesiolysis is carried out either by laparoscopy or by open surgery for distal tubal disease (Fig. 12.3). In case of proximal tubal disease or hydrosalpinx with chronic PID, IVF is indicated.

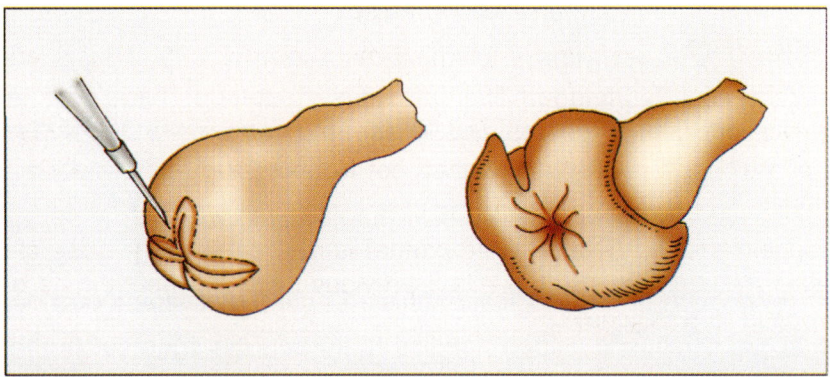

Fig. 12.3. Salpingostomy for distal tubal block (a) Distal end of the fallopian tube incised and (b) Mucosa everted to create an opening

3. *Unexplained infertility*–When the cause cannot be found, IVF is carried out.

Management of the male

General measures

- Education about coital frequency, fertile period and timing of intercouse.
- Stoppage of smoking, tobacco chewing and alcohol intake can significantly improve the sperm count
- Reduce scrotal heat by wearing loose cotton underwear.

Specific measures

- Azoospermia and Oligospermia–need referral to a urologist
- Varicocele–Varicocelectomy should be carried out to improve the semen quality
- Retrograde ejaculation–needs artificial insemination of husband's semen (AIH)
- Astheno-zoospermia–could be due to genital tract infection, needs treatment with antibiotics for 6 weeks
- Medical treatment with clomiphere citrate, testosterone or synthetic androgens mesterolone is indicated in oligoasthenozoospermia

Assisted reproductive techniques (ART)

In 1978, Dr. Patrick Steptoe conceived Louise Brown, the first 'test tube' baby in a laboratory in England. With Dr. Steptoe's technique, called IVF (In Vitro Fertilization) couples who otherwise had no problems that could be fixed surgically now had another option. Currently, the most popular methods of ART involve IVF, GIFT, ZIFT, AI and ICSI.

IVF-In vitro fertilization

This is the legacy of Dr. Steptoe. The infamous "test-tube" baby was actually first conceived by the mixture of sperm and eggs in a laboratory dish. This technique involves:

- *Ovulation induction,* for better egg retrieval which could result in a higher pregnancy rate.
- *Ultrasound* evaluation of the follicles stimulated during ovulation induction.
- *Egg retrieval,* via ultrasound-guided needles to suction the eggs out of the follicles.
- *Insemination* in a dish, with resulting conception of one or more embryos.
- *Embryo transfer.*

GIFT-Gamete intrafallopian transfer

In this technique, eggs and sperm are injected into a woman's fallopian tube(s), where fertilization takes place.

ZIFT-Zygote intrafallopian transfer

In this technique, a fertilized egg via the IVF technique is injected into the fallopian tube, as in GIFT. Conception takes place in the lab. The fertilized egg i.e. the zygote rolls down toward the intrauterine cavity, like in normal fertilization.

AI-artificial insemination

This is a technique established long before Louise Brown or Patrick Steptoe. Sperm are injected into the uterus from a vaginal approach. Fertilization still takes place in the fallopian tube. This procedure is indicated in conditions where sperm deposition is a problem eg. in ejaculatory failure, gross hypospadias, erectile dysfunction.

ICSI-Intracytoplasmic sperm injection

In this process, a single sperm is injected into the egg, is used when the sperm count is low or only a small percentage of sperms are healthy.

13

Benign Diseases of the Vulva and Vagina

BENIGN LESIONS OF THE VULVA

1. Lichen Sclerosus

- Constitutes 0.3-1 per 1000 of all new patients attending the outpatient clinics.

- Aetiology: unknown, associated with vulval carcinoma in 2.5-5%.

- Clinically: the lesion appears as thin, pearly white crinkly plaques with areas of lichenification, echymosis and pigmentation. The labia minora may become adherent with narrowing of the introitus.

  Involves the pudendum as a figure of eight lesion involving the vestibule, clitoris, labia minora and inner aspect of labia majora (Fig. 13.1a) and is usually bilateral and symmetrical.

- Histology: reveals epidermal atrophy, dermal edema, hyalinization of the collagen, sub-dermal chronic inflammatory infiltrate and blunting and widening of the rete ridges (Fig. 13.1b).

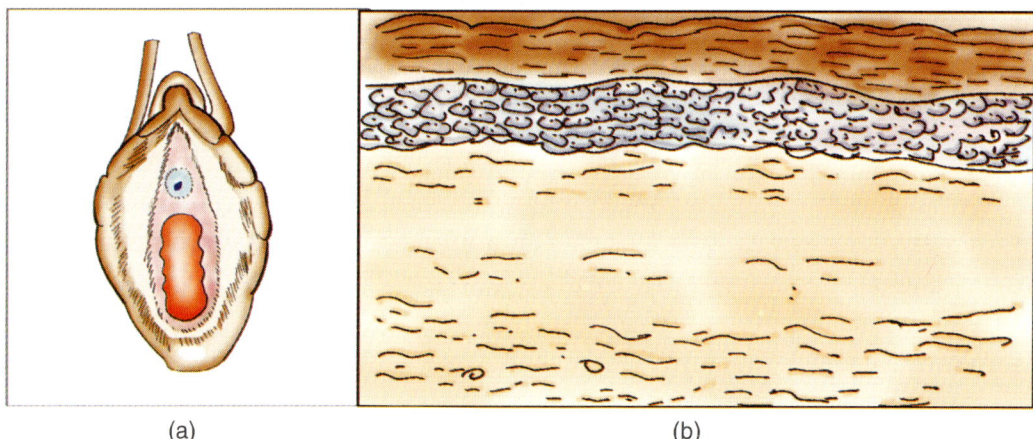

(a) (b)

Fig. 13.1ab. Lichen Sclerosis (a) Clinical appearance, (b) Histology–Note the epidermal atrophy, blunting and widening of the rete ridges

- Treatment: Topical steroids for upto 3 months.

2. Dermatoses

They are generalized cutaneous lesions also seen on the vulva. These are found in 60% of the patients with chronic vulval pruritus.

Lichen simplex chronicus

- In this condition, there are symmetrical lesions on the vulva where the skin becomes dry, thick, scaly white but sometimes fissured due to the trauma of constant scratching.
- Treatment: Low to moderate potency topical steroids with sedatives at night.

Lichen planus

- These lesions are seen on the inner surfaces of the wrists, lower legs, vulva and may extend into the vagina.
- They are usually red or purple, flat topped nodules or papules with an overlying white lacy pattern.
- Histology reveals liquefactive degeneration of the basal epidermal layer, long and pointed rete-ridges and dense inflammatory infiltrate.
- Treatment is with topical and systemic steroids.

Contact dermatitis

- This occurs is an allergic response to various allergens, creams and perfumes.
- Clinically presents with diffuse erythema and edema with superimposed infection or lichenification.

Eczema

- This is associated with generalized chronic eczema.
- Treatment is with moisturizers and mild steroids.

Psoriasis

- Presents as salmon-pink lesions with a sharp but irregular outline.
- Treatment is with local and systemic steroids.

3. Vulval infections

The infection could be primarily vulval or secondary to an infection in the vagina. The mode of transmission could be sexual or non-sexual.

Candidiasis

- Seen more commonly in diabetics.
- Present with curdy white discharge and white plaques in the vagina and vulva. Severe infection leads to erythema and edema of the vulva with superficial maceration.
- Treatment: Topical imidazoles—Clotrimazole pessary once at night for 3-6 days. For extensive and recurrent infections, Fluconazole 150 mg is given as a single dose.

Tinea versicolor

- This is a fungal infection presenting as small circular lesions involving the trunk, limbs and the vulva.

Genital warts/condyloma acuminata

- They are caused by *human papilloma virus (HPV)*. They are usually elevated and discrete and cover large areas.
- These are associated with involvement of the vagina and cervix.
- Treatment: Application of 25% Trichloracetic acid and 25% Podophyllin.

Pediculosis

- Caused by the pubic louse *Pthirus pubis.*
- Involves the hair bearing areas of the vulva and causes pruritus.
- Treatment is with topical malathion and carbaryl.

Scabies

- Causative agent is the mite *Sarcoptes Scabei.*
- Commonly involves the hands, axillae, buttocks and genitalia.
- Treatment: Gamma-benzene hexachloride (Lindane) or Benzyl Benzoate.

Threadworms

- *Enterobius vermicularis* live in the large bowel and lay eggs on the anal margins, causing pruritus-ani and vulvae
- Treatment: Mebendazole and Piperazine

4. Premalignant lesions of the vulva–vulval intraepithelial neoplasia (VIN)

Classification is based on the degree of dysplasia of the vulval epithelium.

Commonly seen in women < 41 yrs. of age and are asymptomatic in 20-45%.

Clinically present as raised multifocal lesions with a rough surface. The lesions could be white/red/dark brown due to melanin deposition. Following acetic acid application, the lesion turns white and punctation with mosaicism are visible.

Treatment Spontaneous regression is seen in young women with asymptomatic multifocal lesions. Suspicious cases need close observation and biopsy. Symptomatic treatment is necessary if the patient has symptoms.

Medical therapy Topical steroids-bid for 6 months provide relief.

Surgery Excisional biopsy is sufficient for small lesions. Multifocal lesions need a skinning vulvectomy with skin grafting.

DISEASES OF THE VAGINA

Anatomy of the vagina

- The upper 2/3 of the vagina is derived from the mullerian ducts and the lower 1/3 is derived from the ectoderm of the cloaca.

- Relations of the vagina

  1. Anteriorly–bladder above, urethra below

  2. Posteriorly–peritoneum of the pouch of douglas–upper 1/3

     Mid 1/3–anterior wall of the rectum

     Lower 1/3–Perineal body

  3. Laterally–Supported by the lower portion of the cardinal ligaments. Lower part by the medial part of lavator ani muscles. Ureters run close to the cervix on either sides of the vault (*see* Fig. 1.2 and 1.3 in chapter 1).

Histology of the vagina

Lined by stratified squamous epithelium which is characterized by the absence of glands. The epithelium is thick and rich in glycogen. Doderlein's bacillus is a normal commensal. The vaginal pH is usually acidic and prevents the growth of bacteria.

Doderlein's bacilli

↓

Glycogen of vaginal epithelium

↓

Lactic Acid

↓

Acidic vaginal pH4.5

↓

Prevents bacterial growth

Age related changes in the vagina

1. Neonate–Epithelium is well developed under the influence of maternal oestrogens. Doderlein's bacilli are present and vaginal acidity is similar to adults.
2. Childhood–Maternal oestrogen levels disappear, pH rises to 7 and the epithelium atrophies.
3. Puberty–There is an increase in oestrogen levels, increased glycogen content of vaginal epithelium with an increase in Doderlein's bacilli resulting in an acidic pH.
4. Menopause–Oestrogen levels decline, vaginal mucosa becomes thin and atrophic and the pH increases to 7.

Natural defence mechanisms of the vagina

1. Mucosa is stratified squamous devoid of glands and crypts and provides a smooth unbroken surface.
2. Acidic pH prevents bacterial growth. Doderlein's bacilli are the only bacteria surviving at a low pH.

Normal vaginal flora in the upper vagina are Doderlein's bacilli, both saprophytic and parasitic organisms are present in the lower 1/3rd.

In the puerperium and menopause, vaginal acidity is decreased and pathogens can grow.

Vaginal discharge

Normal healthy women have some discharge due to escape of vaginal and cervical secretions. If the woman complains that the amount and character of the discharge have altered from the usual pattern, it needs attention.

Vaginal secretions are derived from

1. The sweat, sebaceous and bartholin's glands of the vulva.
2. Transudate from the vaginal epithelium with desquamated cells of the squamous epithelium.
3. Secretions of endo-cervical glands and endometrial glands.

Causes of excessive vaginal discharge (earlier term Leucorrhoea) (Flow chart 1)

1. *Physiological* Clear or whitish, non-offensive, non-irritant. Seen in the pre-ovulatory phase, women on oral contraceptive pills and during pregnancy.
2. *Ectropion* on the cervix.

3. *Vaginitis* Candidal, Trichomonal or Bacterial vaginosis. (Discussed in chapter on STD)

4. *Malignancy* Tumours of the cervix, vagina or uterus cause a blood stained discharge.

5. *Foreign body* A forgotten tampon, a pessary, a wood-apple (used by rural women to push prolapses inside).

6. *Oestrogen deficiency vaginitis* Seen in children and post menopausal women.

   Vulvovaginitis in children could be also be due to:

   • Atrophic vaginitis

   • Foreign body or threadworms

   • Sexual abuse

   • Vaginal tumour

   Senile vaginitis is a patchy granular vaginitis with an associated low grade chronic urethritis.

7. *Non-specific vaginitis* is due to excessive usage of chemicals, douches and tampons which alter the pH of the vagina making it more alkaline and favouring non-specific infections.

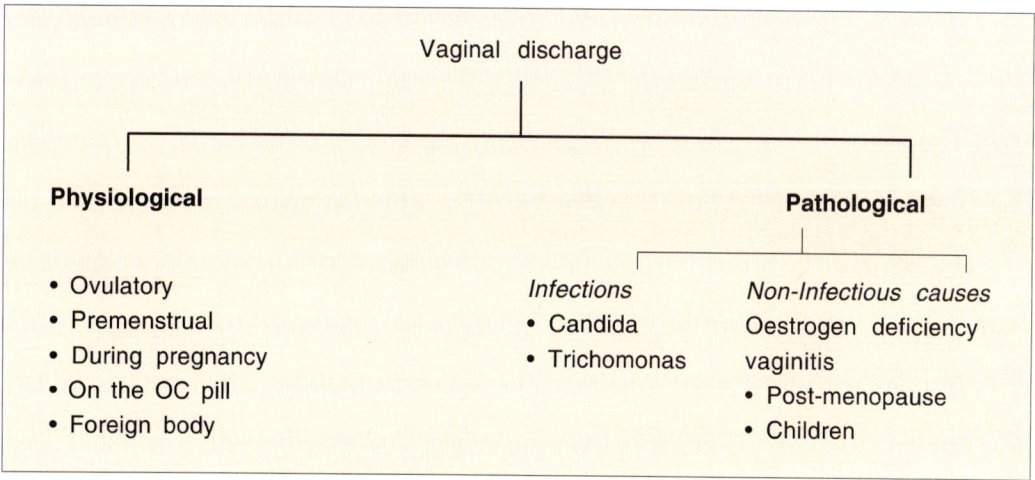

Flow chart 1. Causes of vaginal discharge

Investigation of a patient with vaginal discharge

History

• Onset and duration, any recent change indicates infection

• Associated features—offensive with vulval pruritis indicates an infective cause

- Blood stained discharge–seen in malignancy or with a foreign body.
- Associated dysuria–indicates STD i.e., gonorrhoea.
- History of diabetes–suggests the discharge could be due to candidal.

Examination

- General examination–evidence of sexual abuse may be found in children.
- Examination of the external genitalia for evidence of inflammation and erythema.
- Speculum examination to note
  1. Character of discharge *Candidal infection*–cheesy, *trichonomas*–greenish with strawberry vagina, *bacterial vaginosis*–scanty
  2. Any growth or foreign body in the vagina.
  3. Cervix for evidence of erosion (ectropion) or malignancy.
  4. High vaginal swab is taken with a wet film for gram stain and culture.

Treatment

- Depends on the cause identified.
- Infective vaginitis needs specific treatment (see chapter on STD).
- Oestrogen deficiency in children–Topical oestrogens used externally on the vulva for 2 weeks.
- Senile vaginitis needs oestrogen replacement therapy to reverse the symptoms of end organ failure.

Dyspareunia

Painful Intercourse

Causes

Depending on the onset

Primary From the onset of sexual activity due to psychological problems.

Secondary Onset later on in life, commonly due to organic disease, could be superficial or deep.

Based on the site of pain

Superficial (when the initial penile entry is painful)–due to vulval disease, vulval scars due to episiotomy, radiation induced atrophic vaginitis.

Deep due to endometriosis, chronic pelvic inflammatory disease (PID), retroversion of the uterus.

Examination

- Spasm of the levator-ani muscles indicates a psychological cause
- Tender perineal scars may be present
- Vaginal adhesions, vaginitis or atrophic changes may be present
- Bimanual examination may reveal a retroverted uterus, evidence of endometriosis or PID
- Diagnostic laparoscopy is necessary to diagnose endometriosis or PID.

Treatment Depends on the cause

Superficial

- Psycho-sexual counselling regarding the correct coital technique
- Steroid creams for lubrication. K-Y jelly (water based)
- Surgery to excise perineal scars.

Deep dyspareunia—treatment of the underlying condition is necessary.

Benign tumours of the vagina

The common tumours are

1. Condyloma acuminata/Genital warts–frond-like surface is characteristic.
2. Endometriotic deposits
3. Mesonephric (Gartner's) cyst from the remnant of the mesonephric duct.
4. Vaginal adenosis–multiple mucus–containing vaginal cysts with a *cocks-comb* cervix seen in women with intrauterine exposure to di-ethylstilbesterol, it is of no clinical significance.

14

Endometriosis

Endometriosis is the occurrence of endometrial tissue (glands and stroma) at sites outside the endometrial cavity. Ectopic endometriotic implants have structural and functional differences to those which are intrauterine. Common sites include the uterosacral ligaments, the pouch of douglas, the ovaries and ovarian fossae. Other rare sites are the umbilicus, lung, brain, bowel and various other parts of the body.

Adenomyosis is endometrial tissue deep in the uterine wall.

PREVALENCE AND EPIDEMIOLOGY

• Endometriosis is a common disorder, having a prevalence of 15-25% in most reported series.

• More common in caucasian women, although this may simply reflect diagnosis rather than true incidence.

• More common in the reproductive years, but also reported in post-menopausal women possibly due to the use of exogenous oestrogens.

• More frequent among women being investigated for infertility (24-85%).

• The incidence of endometriosis is 15% among those being investigated for chronic pelvic pain, while among those undergoing abdominal hysterectomy, it can be as high as 25%.

PATHOGENESIS

Despite decades of research, the aetiology of endometriosis remains an enigma and various theories are postulated.

Sampson's theory is the most popular and widely held theory and was hypothesized by Sampson back in 1927.

He proposed the aetiology of endometriosis to be implantation of endometrial cells transported from the endometrial cavity by retrograde menstruation (the *retrograde menstruation hypothesis*).

Retrograde menstruation is common, occurs in at least 90% of women; viable endometrial cells can be recovered from the peritoneal fluid during menstruation, suggesting an obvious route of introduction of ectopic endometrium into the pelvic cavity. So why do the majority of women not develop endometriosis? It has been suggested that women who develop endometriosis may have aberrant cellular clearance mechanisms or intrinsic genetic factors which might affect ectopic endometrium or pelvic peritoneal surfaces allowing for adhesion, proliferation, and invasion of ectopic implants.

Meyer's hypothesis suggested that coelomic metaplasia and transformation of embryonic cell rests results due to prolonged exposure to oestrogens (*coelomic metaplasia theory*). It could also explain why endometriosis is seldom reported before menarche and after menopause.

CLINICAL PRESENTATION

- The majority of women with endometriosis are asymptomatic.

- Symptoms associated with the condition are not specific and may be present in a variety of other gynaecological conditions (table 14.1).

- **Common complaints** are

    - Dysmenorrhoea which is of secondary onset and premenstrual. Dysmenorrhoea occurs due to the local production of prostaglandins within the endometrial implants.
    - Non-cyclical pelvic pain not controlled with analgesics
    - Deep dyspareunia
    - Infertility and menorrhagia.

- **Rarer symptoms** include

    - Pain on defecation (dyschezia)
    - Loin pain
    - Pain on exercise
    - Low back pain
    - Cyclical rectal bleeding or cyclical haematuria can occur due to rectal or bladder involvement (in 1-2%) and is pathognomonic of the disease.

- There is little correlation between the extent of endometriosis and the severity of symptoms. Studies have shown that 15% of women examined for pelvic pain had endometriosis.

Table 14.1. Clinical features of endometriosis
Symptoms
Dysmenorrhoea
Deep dyspareunia
Non-cyclical pelvic pain
Infertility
Menorrhagia
Dyschezia
Loin pain
Pain on exercise
Low back pain
Cyclical rectal bleeding
Cyclical haematuria
Signs
Pelvic tenderness
Adnexal mass
Restricted uterine mobility
Retroverted fixed uterus
Nodules in the pouch of douglas

Staging of endometriosis

The American Society for Reproductive Medicine has developed a staging system for endometriosis (table 14.2). This is a useful classification for research and allows the monitoring of disease progression and response to therapy. However, it has limitations in the consultation room as there is often little, if any, correlation between the stage of disease and the symptoms experienced by the patient. Thus some women with extensive endometriosis report little in the way of symptoms, while others with few lesions experience considerably greater discomfort. The location of the endometriotic lesions might also influence the symptomatology.

Table 14.2. American Fertility Society (AFS) classification of endometriosis		
Stage I	Minimal	Few, superficial lesions on one ovary, uterosacral ligaments or peritoneum
Stage II	Mild	Superficial lesions on two or more of the above or extensive involvement of one ovary
Stage III	Moderate	Ovarian cysts, adhesions and scarring
Stage IV	Severe	Deeply invasive lesions and/or severe adhesions

In the AFS system, points are assigned for the severity of endometriosis based on the size and depth of the implant and the severity of adhesions (Fig. 14.1). Points are summed, and patients are assigned to one of four stages:

Stage I–minimal disease, 1 to 5 points

Stage II–mild disease, 6 to 15 points

Stage III–moderate disease, 16 to 40 points

Stage IV–severe disease, more than 40 points. Although the new classification scheme does not alter the staging of the disease, it does allow for the inclusion of atypical lesions in the point system.

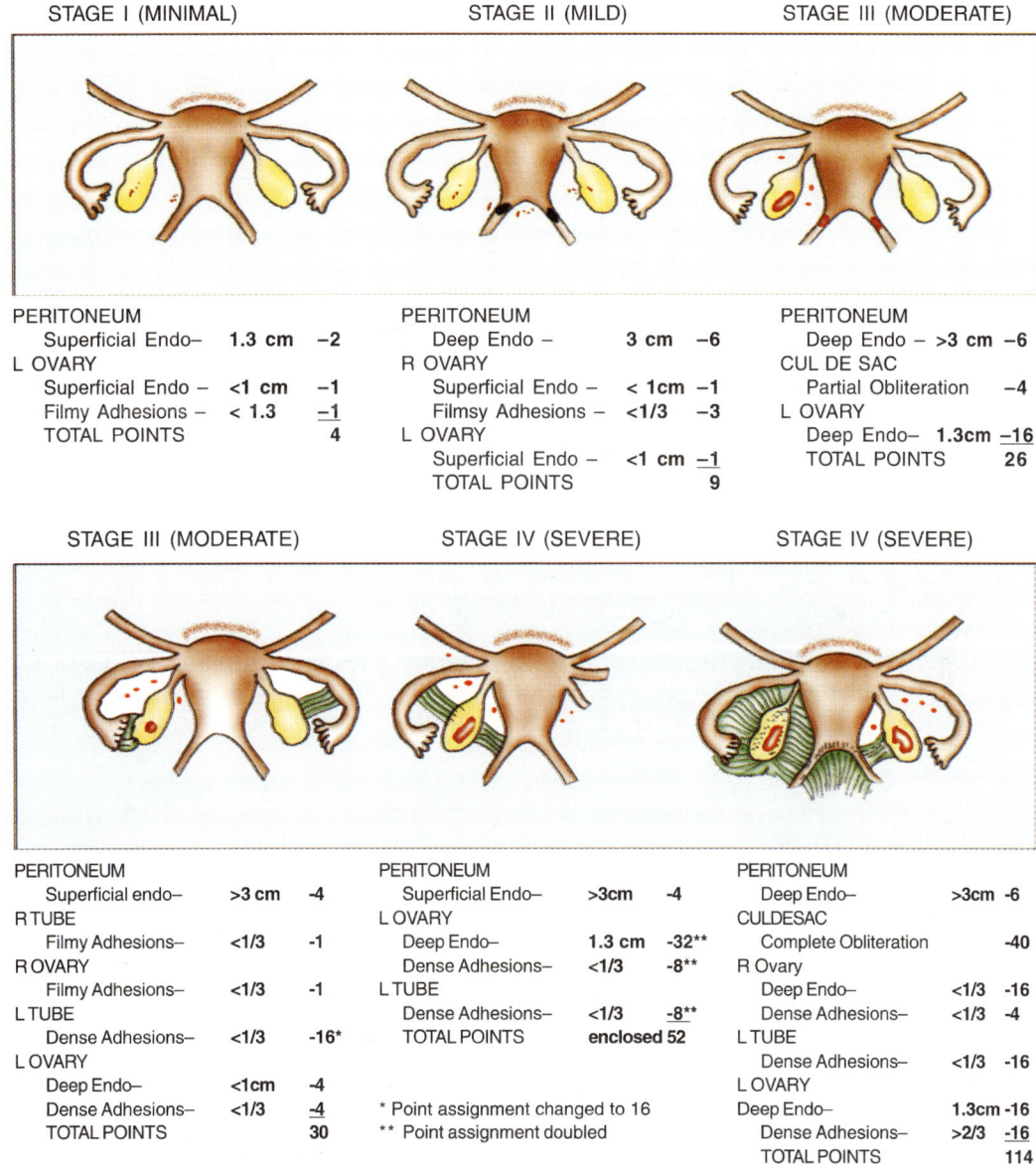

STAGE I (MINIMAL)

PERITONEUM
    Superficial Endo–   **1.3 cm**   –2
L OVARY
    Superficial Endo –   <1 cm   –1
    Filmy Adhesions –   < 1.3   <u>–1</u>
    TOTAL POINTS   4

STAGE II (MILD)

PERITONEUM
    Deep Endo –   3 cm   –6
R OVARY
    Superficial Endo –   < 1cm   –1
    Filmsy Adhesions –   <1/3   –3
L OVARY
    Superficial Endo –   <1 cm   <u>–1</u>
    TOTAL POINTS   9

STAGE III (MODERATE)

PERITONEUM
    Deep Endo –   >3 cm   –6
CUL DE SAC
    Partial Obliteration   –4
L OVARY
    Deep Endo–   1.3cm   <u>–16</u>
    TOTAL POINTS   26

STAGE III (MODERATE)

PERITONEUM
    Superficial endo–   >3 cm   –4
R TUBE
    Filmy Adhesions–   <1/3   –1
R OVARY
    Filmy Adhesions–   <1/3   –1
L TUBE
    Dense Adhesions–   <1/3   –16*
L OVARY
    Deep Endo–   <1cm   –4
    Dense Adhesions–   <1/3   <u>–4</u>
    TOTAL POINTS   30

STAGE IV (SEVERE)

PERITONEUM
    Superficial Endo–   >3cm   –4
L OVARY
    Deep Endo–   1.3 cm   -32**
    Dense Adhesions–   <1/3   -8**
L TUBE
    Dense Adhesions–   <1/3   <u>-8**</u>
    TOTAL POINTS   **enclosed 52**

* Point assignment changed to 16
** Point assignment doubled

STAGE IV (SEVERE)

PERITONEUM
    Deep Endo–   >3cm   -6
CULDESAC
    Complete Obliteration   -40
R Ovary
    Deep Endo–   <1/3   -16
    Dense Adhesions–   <1/3   -4
L TUBE
    Dense Adhesions–   <1/3   -16
L OVARY
    Deep Endo–   1.3cm   -16
    Dense Adhesions–   >2/3   <u>-16</u>
    TOTAL POINTS   114

Fig. 14.1.   American Fertility Society classification of endometriosis (examples and guidelines)

Endometriosis and infertility

- The incidence of infertility attributed to endometriosis is difficult to assess; about 30% to 50% of women with endometriosis have some degree of infertility.

- Infertility in severe disease results due to distortion of the pelvic anatomy resulting in impaired egg release, distortion of the fallopian tubes, and inhibited ovum pick-up.

- The mechanism of subfertility in less severe cases may be due to altered immunological function, chronic inflammatory states and altered endometrial function.

DIAGNOSIS

History and examination

- A careful history and thorough pelvic examination will often establish the diagnosis.

- The presentation could be with dysmenorrhoea or nonspecific symptoms of malaise and sleep disturbance and could be seen by other specialists initially.

- Painful symptoms which have a cyclical element in women of childbearing age may be caused by endometriosis. All doctors should be alert to this possibility even when the patient presents with apparently non-gynaecological symptoms.

- The presentation could be with pelvic pain, dysmenorrhoea, dyspareunia and subfertility.

- Signs of endometriosis include pelvic tenderness, adnexal mass, reduced uterine mobility, retroverted fixed uterus and nodules in the pouch of douglas.

- Patient may be completely asymptomatic and pelvic examination may be completely normal.

Investigations

1. *Laparoscopy*

- Laparoscopy is considered the 'gold standard' for the diagnosis of endometriosis as diagnosis is made only on visualisation of these lesions.

- Lesions identified at laparoscopy have been described as: (Fig. 14.2)

  - Red flame lesions
  - Blue black lesions
  - Brown lesions
  - Peritoneal windows
  - Powder burns
  - Yellow lesions
  - White lesions
  - Red polypoid lesions

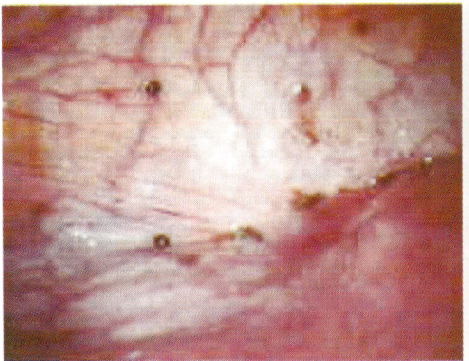
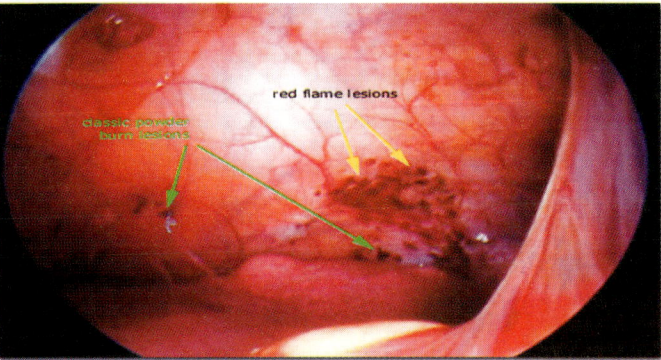

Brown lesions   Red flame lesions

Fig. 14.2. Laparoscopic appearance of endometriosis

- Associated features are ovarian endometriomas and pelvic adhesions. An *ovarian endometrioma* arises from a free superficial implant which is in contact with the ovarian surface and is sealed off by adhesions. A pseudocyst is thus formed by accumulation of menstrual debris from shedding and bleeding from the small implant resulting in fluid collection. Progressive invagination of the ovarian cortex occurs and the associated inflammatory reaction causes thickening around the inverted cortex. The contents of the cyst are to a large extent, fluid which represents debris from cyclical menstruation from the ovarian implants I. Laparoscopic features of a typical endometrioma include ovarian cysts not greater than 12 cm in diameter, adhesions to the pelvic side-wall and/or the posterior broad ligament with associated powder burn, red or blue spots with puckering. The cyst is filled with characteristic tarry, thick chocolate coloured fluid content (*Chocolate cysts*) (Fig. 14.3).

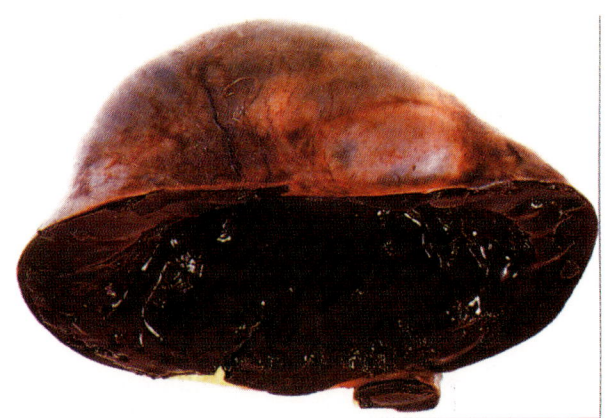

Fig. 14.3. Ovarian endometrioma

- The overall positive predictive value (PPV) for laparoscopic diagnosis of endometriosis and histological confirmation is 43-45%.

2. ***Serum CA 125*** is elevated in endometriosis. However, it is a nonspecific test and has limited value both as a screening and diagnostic test.

3. ***Ultrasonography*** is useful in the presence of an adnexal mass. Ovarian endometriomas appear as cystic structures containing low level homogeneous internal echoes consistent with old blood. Transvaginal ultrasonography is useful in diagnosing as well as excluding endometriomas.

4. ***Magnetic resonance imaging (MRI)*** may have some value for the detection of deeply infiltrating endometriosis of the posterior *cul de sac* and uterosacral ligaments; however it lacks sensitivity in detecting rectal involvement. It has the ability to characterise the lesion, to study extraperitoneal locations and the contents of pelvic masses. MRI is not used routinely in most centres except where there may be a suspicion of an ovarian malignancy.

TREATMENT OF ENDOMETRIOSIS

Principles of treatment

- There is no cure for endometriosis, the therapeutic options are aimed at symptom control.
- Factors to be taken into consideration at the outset are:
  - Fertility plans of the patient
  - Severity of symptoms especially pelvic pain and dysmenorrhoea
  - Severity of the condition and the stage of the disease
  - Patients personal preference of the method of treatment and its side effects.

Women with pain and endometriosis associated infertility may have to decide which is the major priority as all the medical treatments interfere with conception. Identifying the presence of endometriosis does not automatically warrant intervention, if the patient is asymptomatic. There is no permanent cure for endometriosis and none of the options can be guaranteed to prevent a recurrence.

Medical treatment

Symptomatic endometriosis can be managed medically or surgically. The rationale behind both types of treatment is to remove the endometrial tissue that has been implanted outside the uterus. The first line of treatment should be medical, surgery being reserved for cases where medical treatment fails or for severe disease. The various modalities of medical treatment available and their modes of action with side-effects are given in table 14.3. Most medical treatment are based on the consensus that endometriosis is a hormonally responsive disease. Two physiologic conditions, pregnancy and menopause, are often associated with resolution of the signs and symptoms of endometriosis.

Table 14.3. Medical treatment of endometriosis

Drug	Effect on the endometriotic implants	Side-effects
NSAIDs (Non Steroidal Anti-Inflammatory Drugs) eg. Diclofenac, Ibuprofen, Mefenamic acid	Inhibit the production of prostaglandins	Gastric irritation
Progestogens (Dydrogesterone, Medroxyprogesterone acetate, Norethisterone)	Secretory activity, necrobiosis and resorption of endo-metriotic implants	Bloating, fluid retention, breast tenderness, nausea
Synthetic androgens (Danazol, Gestrinone)	Atrophy & regression of endometriotic implants	Seborrhoea, acne, weight gain, muscle cramps,
Combined estrogens & progestogens	Decidualisation of endometriosis	Similar to those of combined pill
Gonadotropin releasing hormone analogues (GnRHa)- Leuprorelin acetate, Goserlin, Buserelin, Nafarelin	Hypo-estrogenic state resulting in endometrial atrophy	Menopausal symptoms including osteoporosis

All medical treatments seem to be equally effective in managing endometriosis. About 80-85% of patients have improvements in their symptoms. The difference is in their side effects with some treatments being more acceptable than others.

Therapeutic Trial: If a woman is not trying to conceive and there is no evidence of a pelvic mass on examination, there may be a role for a therapeutic trial of a combined oral contraceptive (monthly or tricycling) or a progestogen only to treat pain suggestive of endometriosis without performing a diagnostic laparoscopy. Those patients who do not respond to such intervention should undergo a laparoscopy.

- *Non steroidal anti inflammatory drugs* like ibuprofen can be taken for pain relief. Women reporting excessive menstrual bleeding have higher levels of endometrial prostaglandins. Mefenamic acid, a prostaglandin synthetase inhibitor is also useful in relieving pain as well as in reducing menstrual flow.

- The *Intrauterine system (IUS)*, Mirena coil originally developed as a contraceptive, is effective in reducing menstrual blood loss and can also lead to reversible amenorrhoea. The IUS releases 20µg levonorgestrel per 24 hrs. into the endometrial cavity, thus suppressing endometrial proliferation and has been used successfully.

- *Gestrinone* is a synthetic trienic 19 nor-steroid (13 ethyl-17α ethinyl-17 hydroxy-gona-4, o, II-triene-3-one). Several trials have shown it to be effective in the treatment of endometriosis. Gestrinone has mild androgenic, marked antiprogestogenic and antioestrogenic, as well as moderate antigonadotropic properties. One effect of these actions is to produce progressive endometrial atrophy. These tablets taken twice a week in doses of 2.5-5mg work by interacting with receptors for progesterone and oestrogen in the hypothalamus and anterior pituitary, thus decreasing the secretion of LH and FSH. As a result the release of oestrogen and progesterone by the ovary is suppressed. Side effects are moderate and dose dependant.

- *Danazol* is a synthetic derivative of the naturally occurring male hormone testosterone. It abolishes the release of LH and FSH by binding to androgen receptors, resulting in atrophy of the endometrium. It also directly inhibits ovarian steroidogenesis and causes an increase in the free testosterone levels. If given in a dose of 400-800 mg daily for 6 months, it results in symptomatic improvement in 85%. Despite its side-effect profile, it is easily available and currently widely used.

- *Gonadotropin releasing hormone analogues (GnRHa)* result in continuous stimulation of the Gonadotropin receptors in the anterior pituitary leading to an initial release and then depletion of FSH and LH (down regulation of receptors). They cannot be taken orally as they are denatured by gastric enzymes. They are administered daily as nasal spray or monthly by intramuscular or subcutaneous injections for a period of three to six months. Implants are also available. If longer treatment is required, GnRH agonist use can be extended safely with 'add-back' therapy to counter the side-effects due to a pseudo-menopause eg. hot flushes, vaginal dryness, atrophic vaginitis and reduced libido.

Surgical treatment

Surgical treatment may be conservative or radical.

- *Conservative surgery* aims to preserve the reproductive potential of the patient. The procedures carried out laparoscopically are: fulguration of endometriotic spots, division of adhesions, excision of endometriomas and deroofing of endometriotic cysts. However, surgery may be more extensive with dissection of the urinary tract, bowel and the rectovaginal space. It can be carried out by laparotomy, or laparoscopically. The benefit of conservative surgery is seen to be greater in the group with most severe disease. Addition of postoperative medical therapy significantly prolongs the symptom free interval.

- *Radical surgery* includes hysterectomy with bilateral salpingo-oophorectomy. Although this is generally considered as definitive surgery, recurrence of disease has been reported following hysterectomy for endometriosis in 5-10% of cases, especially in women who go on to use hormone replacement therapy.

- *Laparoscopic uterine nerve ablation (LUNA)* is based on the premise that destruction of the efferent nerve fibres in the uterosacral ligaments will diminish the pain arising from the uterus. Presacral neurectomy (PSN) is designed to interrupt efferent sympathetic pathways from the uterus. Both procedures are only effective in relieving the pain of endometriosis in selective cases. LUNA is currently being evaluated in a multi-centre study in the United Kingdom.

Ovarian endometriomas Surgery is the appropriate approach to evaluate and treat women suspected of having ovarian endometrioma. Small cysts may be excised but most should be drained and tissue obtained for histological evaluation.

Combined medical and surgical therapy Medical therapy is given for 3 months preoperatively to reduce the size of the endometriotic spots and 3-6 months postoperatively to eliminate any residual macro or microscopic disease.

Management of infertility associated with endometriosis

The value of surgery for women with minimal or mild disease who have reduced fertility is yet to be established. There is no role for medical therapy with hormonal drugs as all the drugs have a contraceptive effect. Laparoscopic ablation of minimal-mild endometriosis has been shown to improve fertility rates. Surgery and assisted conception are indicated in moderate and sever disease.

Ovarian hyperstimulation using gonadotropins with IUI and IVF are the other options.

Benign Tumours of the Uterus–Leiomyoma

Leiomyoma or myoma, commonly called as fibroid uterus, is the most common tumour in women. It is a benign tumour of smooth muscle cells of the uterus and is common in women during the reproductive years.

INCIDENCE

- Upto 20% of women in reproductive age have a uterine leiomyoma.
- Maximum incidence is between 35-45 years of age.
- It is more common in nulliparous infertile women.

AETIOLOGY

The exact aetiology is unknown but oestrogen may have some role in its causation. The following observations suggest that leiomyomas are oestrogen dependent:

- Their rarity before puberty and cessation after the menopause.
- Growth during pregnancy.
- Increase in size with exogenous hormones.
- Presence of oestrogen receptors in leiomyomatous cells.
- Higher incidence of myomas in women with hyperoestrogenic states like polycystic ovarian disease (PCOD) and granulosa cell tumour of ovary. Often myomas are associated with endometrial hyperplasia and endometrial cancer.
- Higher incidence in nullipara.
- Reduction in size following administration of GnRH analogues.

SITES OF OCCURRENCE OF LEIOMYOMA

Most common site of leiomyoma is body of the uterus, in 1-4% of cases it arises in the cervix and rarely it may occur in extrauterine sites like the vagina, vulva, round ligament etc. (Flow chart 1).

194

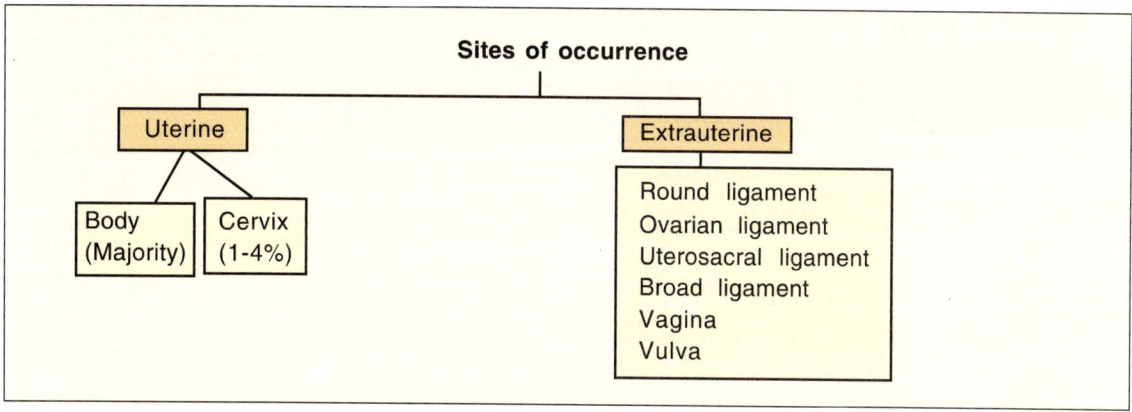

Flow chart 1. Sites of occurrence of leiomyoma

TYPES OF LEIOMYOMAS

Based on the location of a myoma in the uterus, leiomyomas are classified as intramural, submucous or subserous (Fig 15.1).

* **Intramural or interstitial myomas** lie within the myometrial wall. Most of the myomas (approximately 75%) are intramural.

* **Submucous** 5% of the myomas are submucous. When the myoma grows towards the cavity of the uterus and is lined by the endometrium it is called a submucous leiomyoma. It may develop a pedicle and become a myomatous polyp, or grow downwards and protrude through the cervix into the vagina. This may cause inter-menstrual bleeding or get infected and ulcerated. The uterus is usually not enlarged unless other fibroids are also present.

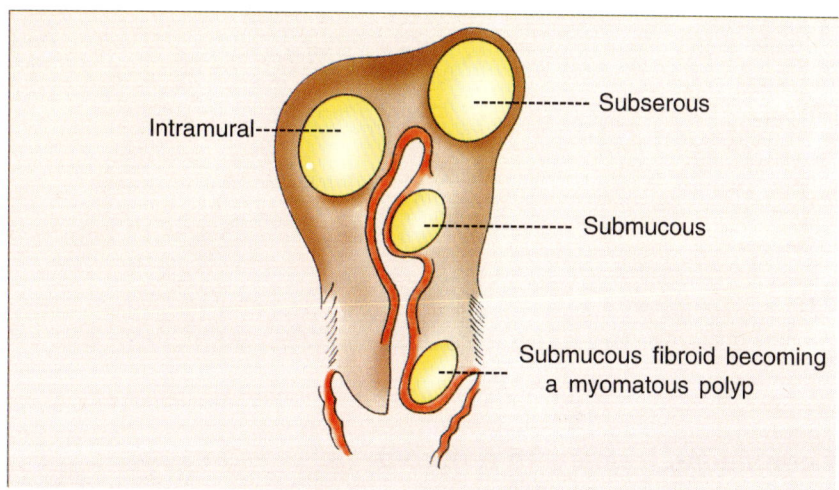

Fig. 15.1. Types of myoma

- **Subserous myomas** grow towards the serosa of the uterus and form about 10% of uterine myomas. These also may become pedunculated. Rarely a pedunculated subserous fibroid gets attached to a surrounding vascular organ and becomes a parasitic or a wandering fibroid.

PATHOLOGY

Gross

- Myomas are well circumscribed, firm tumours with a *pseudo-capsule*, which consists of condensation of surrounding myometrial tissue. The pseudo-capsule provides a plane of easy cleavage during myomectomy.
- Myomas may be single or multiple; cervical and broad ligament myomas are usually single. Size of the myoma varies from microscopic to a very large tumour.
- On cut section, the myoma appears white and has a whorled appearance as compared to the adjacent pink myometrium (Fig. 15.2a).
- Blood supply to the myoma comes from the periphery, hence cystic changes takes place in the center and calcification occurs at the periphery. In a subserous fibroid, blood vessels are seen over the fibroid beneath the peritoneum.

Microscopically

A myoma consists of bundles of plain muscle cells and varying amount of interlacing fibrous strands (Fig 15.2b). A cervical fibromyoma has more of fibrous tissue than submucous and intramural myomas.

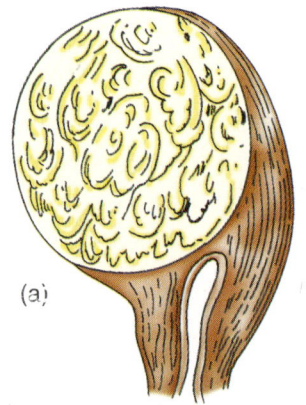
(a)

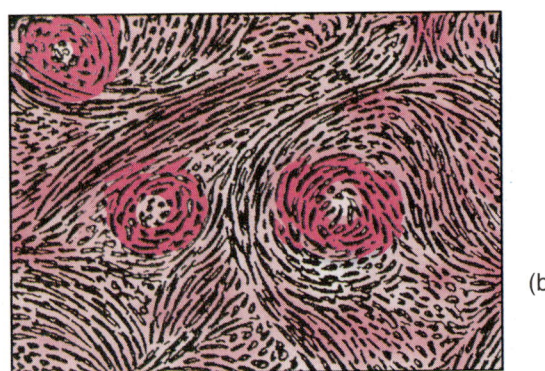
(b)

Fig. 15.2ab. (a) Gross appearance of a leiomyoma (b) Microscopic appearance of a leiomyoma

Associated conditions found with a fibroid

- Hypertrophy of the myometrium due to associated hyperoestrogenism

- A distorted and enlarged uterine cavity due to the presence of intramural or submucous myomas.

- Endometrial hyperplasia

- At times, the ovaries are enlarged, cystic and hyperaemic.

- In 15% of cases there is evidence of salpingo-oophoritis.

Secondary changes in fibroids

1. *Atrophy*

   Following menopause and in the postpartum period, the tumour atrophies due to decreased vascularity, shrinks in size and becomes firm and fibrotic.

2. *Hyaline degeneration*

   - Commonest type of degeneration. Usually seen in tumours more than 4 cm.
   - Asymptomatic
   - The tumour loses the typical whorled appearance and its cut surface becomes smooth and homogenous. Muscle cells are replaced by hyaline material.

3. *Cystic degeneration*

   - Generally seen in the centre of a large intramural or subserous fibroid.
   - Liquefaction of hyaline material following hyaline degeneration leads to cystic spaces in the fibroid.
   - Tumour becomes soft due to the cystic degeneration and is asymptomatic.

4. *Calcareous degeneration*

   - Occurs in long standing fibroids in old women and causes no symptoms.
   - There are deposits of calcium in the periphery, along the course of the blood vessels resulting in 'egg-shell' calcification; or the whole fibroid may become calcified when it is sometimes called a 'womb stone'.

5. *Red degeneration*

   - Is a degenerative change occurring during pregnancy or in the postpartum period.
   - The exact cause is not known but it may be due to increased vascularity during pregnancy.
   - Fibroid appears purple and thrombosis of the vessels of capsule and the tumour is usually found.
   - Clinically there is pain and fever with marked uterine tenderness. The condition has to be differentiated from other causes of acute abdomen like appendicitis, ovarian torsion or accidental haemorrhage.

- Management is conservative with analgesia and maintenance of hydration.

6. *Fatty change*
   - Occurs usually after menopause and is not very common.
   - Fat cells are found among muscle cells.

7. *Sarcomatous change* Seen in 1 in 1,000,000 myomas.
   - Occurs in women over 40 years of age.
   - Clinically presents with rapid growth of the fibroid with irregular bleeding and acute pain in the peri or postmenopausal age group.
   - Such myomas are highly malignant and rapidly metastasize through the blood stream.
   - Grossly, the tumour becomes soft and friable; with the pseudocapsule merging with the myometrium. On cut section, the tumour is yellowish grey and haemorrhagic.
   - Very often, however, the diagnosis is made only after histopathological examination of the removed tumour or the uterus.

The secondary changes in fibroids are summarized in table 15.1

Table 15.1. Secondary changes in fibroids
• Atrophy • Hyaline degeneration • Cystic degeneration • Calcareous degeneration • Red degeneration • Fatty change • Sarcomatous change

COMPLICATIONS OF LEIOMYOMA

1. *Torsion* Torsion or rotation of a pedunculated subserosal fibroid at its attachment to the uterus occurs sometimes giving rise to acute abdominal pain. Rarely axial rotation of the whole uterus can occur along with the fibroid.

2. *Inversion of uterus* A submucous fibroid attached to the fundus of the uterus may sometimes cause inversion of uterus. It usually occurs in a long standing fibroid. Clinically, the woman presents with intermittent lower abdominal pain with irregular blood stained offensive discharge, irregular vaginal bleeding or a mass protruding through the cervix or the introitus.

The condition may be confused with uterine prolapse (neglected), cervical fibroid or with a myomatous polyp. Presence of a cup shaped depression or inability to palpate the fundus of the uterus on bimanual examination suggests the diagnosis of inversion. Diagnosis is confirmed on sounding the uterus or on ultrasonography.

3. **Capsule rupture** Rarely results due to rupture of a surface vessel causing intraperitoneal haemorrhage.

4. **Inflammation and infection** Usually seen in a submucous or myomatous polyp. Infections from the vagina infect the already thin epithelium of the myoma causing sloughing and blood stained discharge or irregular bleeding. Vascular disturbance at the pedicle causes congestion of the fibroid making it more vulnerable to infection. The complications due to fibroids are summarized in Flow chart 2 given below.

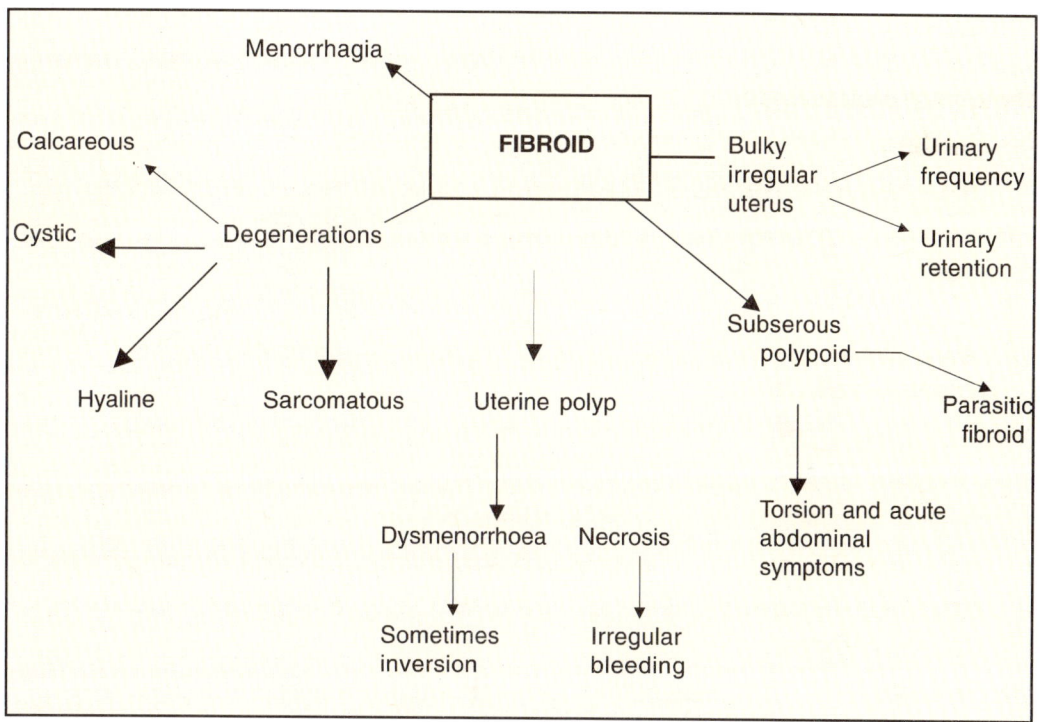

Flow chart 2. Complications of leiomyoma

CLINICAL FEATURES

Asymptomatic A fibroid may not produce any symptoms and may be detected incidentally on examination or on ultrasonography. Around 50% of the tumours are asymptomatic.

Symptomatic The clinical features of a fibroid depend on the location, the size and the number of tumours present. A small submucous fibroid may be more symptomatic than a large subserous fibroid.

Symptoms

The leiomyomas may cause one or more of the following symptoms.

1. Menstrual disturbances
2. Pain
3. Infertility
4. Abdominal lump
5. Pressure symptoms
6. Non-specific symptoms

1. Menstrual disturbances

Menorrhagia

- This is the most commonly encountered symptom seen in 30-50% of women.
- The woman typically gives history of increased bleeding starting from day two that continues for 8-10 days.
- Causes of menorrhagia in a leiomyoma include increased surface area of uterine cavity (normal surface area is about 15 cm sq.), endometrial hyperplasia and increased vascularity.

Polymenorrhoea

- It is often seen in large intramural myomas and is due to hyperaemia and pelvic congestion affecting the ovarian function.
- Associated PID and cystic ovaries are also responsible for polymenorrhoea.
- More often the menstrual cycles are short along with excessive menstrual flow (Polymenorrhagia).

Metrorrhagia

- Usually seen in a myomatous polyp or in an infected submucous fibroid. However, if irregular bleeding is seen in women of child-bearing age, pregnancy should be ruled out and if seen in women over 40 years malignancy (endometrial carcinoma) needs to be excluded.

2. Pain

- Second commonest symptom.
- It may be in the form of dysmenorrhoea, acute pain abdomen or dull aching pain.

Dysmenorrhoea–Both spasmodic and congestive dysmenorrhoea is common in fibroid uterus. Congestive dysmenorrhoea is due to increased vascularity and congestion of the uterus and adnexa. Spasmodic pain occurs due to uterine contractility in an attempt to extrude the myomatous polyp.

Acute pain may occur due to torsion, red degeneration, infection or sarcomatous change.

Heaviness in the lower abdomen causing dull aching pain can occur due to the pressure of a large fibroid on the surrounding structures.

3. Infertility

Although fibroids are often encountered in pregnancy, infertility is sometimes attributed to a fibroid. The exact cause of infertility is not known; the probable causes are:

- Cornual block or tubal block due to mechanical obstruction.
- Distortion of the uterine cavity interfering with sperm ascent.
- Failure of nidation if the fertilized ovum happens to implant on the submucous fibroid.
- Associated pelvic inflammatory disease (PID).

4. Abdominal lump

Myoma may present as an abdominal lump although it takes a long time to grow. If the lump grows rapidly, malignancy should be suspected. A fibroid can grow up to the xiphisternum.

5. Pressure symptoms

The myoma may cause symptoms due to pressure on the bladder, bowel and blood vessels. A fibroid on the anterior wall of the uterus causes frequency of micturition, which could be more pronounced pre-menstrually due to congestion. A cervical fibroid can cause retention of urine. A fibroid on the posterior wall of uterus may get impacted in the pouch of douglas and cause frequency and later acute retention of urine and constipation. Edema of feet can occur due to pressure on the vessels. A broad ligament fibroid can cause hydroureter and hydronephrosis.

6. Other symptoms

- Palpitations, dyspnea and weakness due to anaemia.
- Shock may occur due to capsular rupture and intraperitoneal bleed.

The presenting symptoms in a patient with fibroid are summarized in Table 15.2.

Table 15.2. Presenting symptoms in a patient with fibroid	
Menstrual	• Menorrhagia • Polymenorrhoea • Metrorrhagia
Pain	• Dysmenorrhoea • Acute pain abdomen • Dull aching pain
Infertility	• Primary • Secondary
Abdominal lump	
Pressure symptoms	• Frequency • Retention of urine • Constipation • Edema feet
General	• Palpitations and weakness (secondary to anaemia)

Signs

* On general examination signs of anaemia may or may not be present.

* On *abdominal examination,* a lump arising from the pelvis is palpable if the uterine size is more than twelve weeks gestational size. It feels firm in consistency and is mobile (unless there is associated PID or if there is broad ligament fibroid).

* On *bimanual examination,* uterus may be uniformly or irregularly enlarged due to the presence of multiple fibroids. The fibroid feels firm to hard in consistency. The position of the uterus varies according to the site of tumour; if tumour is anterior, the uterus is retroverted. It is deviated to the opposite side if it is a broad ligament fibroid.

* In case of a cervical fibroid, the cervix is ballooned out and the uterus is felt on top of the mass. If a polyp is present in the cervical canal, the cervical os may be open and the polyp may be felt through the os.

Differential diagnosis

Usually, the clinical symptoms and signs are typical and confirmative of fibroid, however, the following conditions should be kept in mind.

1. *A full bladder* Full bladder may appear as a soft suprapubic mass (catheterisation helps in making a diagnosis).

2. *Pregnancy* Symptoms and signs of pregnancy are present. A proper history and careful clinical examination helps in making a correct diagnosis. Pregnancy test and ultrasound are confirmatory.

3. *Ovarian tumour* A pedunculated subserous fibroid with no menstrual disturbances may be mistaken for an ovarian tumour. Ultrasound may be of value in differentiating between the two.

4. *Adenomyosis* Adenomyosis causes a symmetrical enlargement of the uterus to not more than 14 weeks and is associated with progressive dysmenorrhoea. In a uterine fibroid of similar size, dysmenorrhoea is infrequent. If the adenomyosis is localized, it causes asymmetrical enlargement of uterus with tenderness; myomas of similar size are not tender.

5. *Endometriosis or chocolate cysts of the ovary* The presentation is similar to fibroids with menorrhagia, dysmenorrhoea and infertility. Ultrasound may be helpful, but diagnostic laparoscopy clinches the diagnosis.

6. *Pelvic inflammatory disease* A chronic tubo-ovarian mass adherent to the uterus makes the uterine contour feel irregular and may be difficult to differentiate from multiple fibroids. The presence of adnexal tenderness and fixity of the uterus points towards PID.

7. *Endometrial cancer* Abnormal uterine bleeding in a patient with fibroid may be because of associated endometrial cancer. In 3% of cases endometrial carcinoma may be associated. Thus, in an elderly woman with a fibroid uterus and menstrual abnormality, D&C is mandatory.

8. *Chronic inversion of uterus* Inversion of the uterus may be confused with a myomatous polyp, uterine sounding and ultrasonography helps in diagnosis. The other differentiating features are presence of a dimple at the uterine fundus and failure to visualize the cervical ring on speculum examination.

DIAGNOSIS

Investigations are required to confirm the diagnosis, to know the general condition of the patient and plan the optimum line of management.

Investigations to confirm the diagnosis

1. *Ultrasonography (USG)* is done to confirm the diagnosis, check the number, location and size of the fibroids and for any associated lesion. On USG, a fibroid appears as a well-defined, hypo-echoic lesion. It appears cystic in the presence of cystic degeneration.

2. *Sonohysterography* Sonography with saline infusion in the uterine cavity delineates intrauterine lesions better. The exact site and the size of a submucous fibroid or polyp can be made out on sonohysterography and the treatment planned accordingly.

3. *Hysterosalpingography (HSG)* helps in diagnosis and location of a submucous fibroid

or polyp and in testing tubal patency. A myomectomy in an infertile woman is only indicated if the fibroid is interfering with tubal patency.

4. *Hysteroscopy* helps to confirm the site and number of submucous fibroids and can be combined with operative hysteroscopy for removal. If >50% of the volume of a fibroid is protruding into the cavity, it can be removed by hysteroscopic resection.

5. *Laparoscopy* is sometimes required to differentiate between endometriosis, ectopic pregnancy, pelvic inflammatory disease (PID) and uterine inversion.

6. *Intravenous pyelogram (IVP)* should be done in cases of a very large cervical fibroid causing pressure symptoms, and routinely in a broad ligament fibroid to know the position of ureters. It can also help in differentiating a broad ligament fibroid from a pelvic kidney.

7. *MRI* rarely needed and has no place in the routine investigation of a patient in the fibroids. In a woman with a suspected uterine sarcoma or adenomyosis, it provides an excellent view of it's relation to the endometrial cavity.

Other relevant investigations

8. *Pap smear* should be carried out in all sexually active females to exclude pre-malignant and malignant lesions of cervix.

9. *Dilatation and curettage* D&C or endometrial sampling is done to exclude endometrial malignancy in women >40 yrs. old with menstrual disorders and a fibroid.

10. *Complete blood count* anaemia needs to be corrected prior to surgery. Progesterone or GnRH analogues can be given for 3-4 months to control the bleeding and improve the anaemia.

11. *Blood group and Rh typing* as blood needs to be cross-matched at the time of surgery

12. *Urine analysis* urinary tract infection, if present, is to be treated prior to surgery.

13. *Blood urea and serum creatinine, fasting and postprandial blood sugar*

14. *X-Ray chest PA view and ECG* for pre-anaesthetic check up.

Management

Management of a woman with fibroid uterus depends on

- The presence or absence of symptoms.
- The age of the woman.
- The size and site of the fibroid.
- The desire for preservation of reproductive function.

1. Conservative management

- This is indicated in a woman with a fibroid of <12 weeks size, which has been detected on routine clinical examination, ultrasonography or during a caesarean section.
- Women in the perimenopausal age group should be explained about the possibility of regression after the menopause.
- Young, nulliparous women should be explained that it doesn't need removal unless it is causing tubal block; they should also be explained the possibility of it undergoing red degeneration during pregnancy.
- Follow-up is required every six months to one year.

2. Medical management

Medical management is used to treat anaemia, reduce bleeding and to temporarily reduce the size of the fibroid. Medical management of a fibroid helps:

- To defer surgery if the woman is unfit eg. due to anaemia.
- Reducing the size of the fibroids facilitates removal of the uterus by the vaginal route.
- Surgery can be performed by a Pfannenstiel (transverse) incision which has a lower risk of scar dehiscence.
- As the fibroid shrinks in size, the blood loss at surgery is reduced.
- Decrease in size and vascularity of the tumour facilitates minimally invasive surgery (laparoscopic or hysteroscopic).
- It helps to avoid surgery in a woman with symptomatic fibroids who is nearing menopause as fibroids regress after menopause.

Medical treatment The options are:

1. GnRH analogues

- These are the most commonly used hormones.
- *Mechanism of action:* They have a biphasic gonadotropin-gonadal steroid response with an initial surge in gonadotropins followed by a sustained desensitization phase with suppression of gonadotropin release and low oestrogen levels. The lack of oestrogen stimulation results in regression of the size of fibroids.
- *Preparations available:*

    Goserelin (3.6mg) and Leuprolin (3.75mg): given as monthly subcutaneous depot injections

    Buserelin (900-1200 μg daily) and Nafarelin (800 μg daily) as an intranasal spray

- *Disadvantage of GnRH analogues:* They cause a state of hypogonadism resulting in menopausal symptoms like hot flushes, insomnia, headache, and myalgia if used for a longer period, bone loss and osteoporosis may occur. To prevent such adverse effects, oestrogen is added after three months as 'add-back' therapy.

- The other disadvantage of using this drug is the regrowth of fibroid after stopping this drug. 'Recurrence' of fibroid is noticed after surgery as the very small fibroids shrink and can get missed during surgery.

2. *GnRH antagonists* They directly inhibit the action of GnRH on the anterior pituitary, resulting in immediate gonadal suppression with rapid reduction in the uterine volume with avoidance of the stimulatory phase seen with the agonists eg. Cetrorelix and Ganirelix.

3. *Mifepristone (RU-486)* The action is similar to GnRh agonists but with less profound oestrogen suppression. 50 mg daily for 3 months causes amenorrhoea and shrinkage of the fibroid by 50%.

4. *Progestogens* Norethisterone or Medroxyprogesterone, 5-10 mg from day 5 to 20 help in reducing menorrhagia.

5. *Androgens* Testosterone proprionate in doses of 25-50 mg. IM daily for 2-3 days is sometimes used to stop excessive bleeding in a perimenopausal woman awaiting surgery. This treatment should not be given in a young woman because of the androgenic side effects.

6. *Anti-fibrinolytic drugs* Tranexamic acid, 2-4 gm daily for three to five days during periods is used for controlling menorrhagia.

7. *Anti-anaemic treatment* Iron therapy is supplemented for improving anaemia.

The various drugs available are given in table 15.3.

Table 15.3. Options for medical management of fibroids
• GnRH analogues • GnRH antagonists • Antiprogesterones (Mifepristone) • Progestogens (Norethisterone, Medroxyprogesterone) • Androgens (Testosterone propionate) • Antifibrinolytics (Tranexamic acid)

Surgical management The surgical options available are:

1. *Myomectomy* This technique has been developed by Victor Bonney in the 19th century. This involves surgical removal or enucleation of myoma from the uterus leaving behind a potentially functioning organ capable of future reproduction. If myomectomy is

being done for infertility, all other causes of infertility must be excluded as the myoma may not be the causative factor.

Indications of myomectomy: Myomectomy is indicated in young women with symptomatic fibroids who are infertile, those who have not completed their family, and wish to preserve their reproductive function. All women undergoing a myomectomy should be counselled about the potential risk of hysterectomy especially those with multiple fibroids.

Myomectomy can be done by abdominal or vaginal route or by laparoscopy or hysteroscopy.

Abdominal myomectomy (Fig. 15.3a-c): This is generally the preferred approach especially in multiple or large fibroids, as haemostasis and reconstruction of uterus is better. Since the main purpose of myomectomy is to retain or improve fertility, proper reconstruction of uterus and prevention of postoperative adhesions is essential. A pregnancy rate following myomectomy is usually around 40%. However, the risk of recurrence is 5-10%, persistent menorrhagia is 1-5% and need for re-laparotomy and hysterectomy is 20-25%.

Laparoscopic myomectomy: Laparoscopic myomectomy is performed in selected cases where myoma is less than 5 cm and is subserous or intramural. Myomas which are more than 5 cm are preferably treated with GnRH agonists before laparoscopic removal. Broad ligament myomas have also been removed laparoscopically. The advantages of laparoscopic surgery are faster recovery, reduced hospital stay and avoidance of complications associated with major open abdominal surgeries.

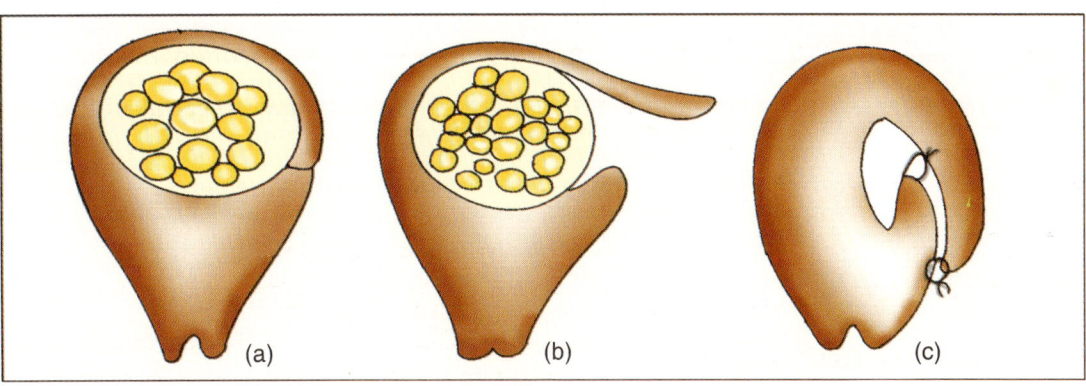

(a) A transverse incision is made across the capsule of the fibroid as low down and anteriorly as possible

(b) The capsule is lifted up and the fibroid enucleated

(c) The redundant myometrium is trimmed and sewn over the uterus as a "hood" so that the apex of the lower end lies in the uterovesical space

Fig. 15.3a-c. Steps of Bonney's Myomectomy

Hysteroscopic myoma resection: This is indicated if there is a submucous myoma less than 5cm in size and projecting more than 50% in the cavity. Pedunculated submucous myoma can be removed by cauterizing and cutting the pedicle hysteroscopically.

Vaginal myomectomy: Pedunculated myoma can be removed vaginally by tying the pedicle and cutting it or simply by twisting the pedicle if it is thin. If the pedicle is not accessible, a vertical incision on the cervix after reflecting the bladder can reveal the base of the pedicle, which can then be tied and cut thus removing the myoma.

2. **Hysterectomy** Hysterectomy is the treatment of choice in women over 40 years of age with symptomatic or large fibroids. It is also indicated in cases with rapid growth of fibroid (as it may be due to malignancy). Rarely uncontrolled haemorrhage and unforeseen surgical difficulties during myomectomy may require a hysterectomy. Hysterectomy can be done by laparotomy or laparoscopically. A large myoma can be morcellated and removed laparoscopically.

Newer techniques The following methods have been tried and are being done in the context of research trials

1. *Laparoscopic myolysis:* Destruction of the myoma (myolysis) by laser (Nd:YAG), bipolar cautery or cryo are being tried. Myolysis results in shrinkage and marked devascularisation of the myoma. It is recommended only after the family is completed.

2. *Uterine artery embolisation:* Bilateral uterine artery embolisation as a treatment of myoma was introduced in 1995 and has been used in more than 5000 women. The aim of the procedure is to cause avascular necrosis and shrinkage of the fibroid by occluding the feeding artery (uterine) with polyvinyl alcohol particles introduced through percutaneous femoral artery catheterisation. Although it is a simple procedure and is done under IV sedation, complications have, however, been reported.

The management options in a patient with fibroid are summarized in table 15.4.

Table 15.4. Fibroid uterus-management options	
Patient desirous of retaining uterus	**Patient not desirous of retaining uterus**
• Myomectomy (abdominal / vaginal / laparoscopic / hysteroscopic) • Laparoscopic myolysis • Laser myolysis • Uterine artery embolisation	• Hysterectomy (abdominal / vaginal)

Section III
Gynaecological Cancers

16

Carcinoma of the Cervix

Carcinoma of the cervix is the commonest cancer in Indian women with an incidence of 24.2 per 100,000 women. It is also the commonest genital tract cancer in Indian women. Like oral cancer, cervical cancer can be diagnosed by regular visual inspection by simple speculum examination. It has an appreciably long pre-invasive stage which can be diagnosed by cervical cytology. Routine universal screening by pap smear cytology has markedly reduced the incidence and mortality due to this disease in most of the developed countries; however in India, 80% of women report to the hospital with advanced stage disease when the treatment is very difficult and expensive.

AETIOLOGY AND RISK FACTORS

The major risk factors for carcinoma cervix are:

- Human papilloma virus 16 and 18; which are the most common viruses in India.

- Women with multiple sexual partners.

- Promiscuity of the husband–several potent immunosuppressive agents are present in human seminal plasma which reduce the local immune response and increase the risk of HPV.

- Early age at first intercourse–as the adolescent cervix is more vulnerable to potential oncogenic agents.

- Immunosuppression and HIV–the incidence of CIN and squamous cell carcinoma is increased.

- Smoking in both partners–smoking reduces the number of Langerhans' cells in the cervical epithelium resulting in a local immunodeficiency.

- Oral contraceptive pills–recent evidence shows an increased risk of adenocarcinoma of the cervix in women on long term oral contraceptive usage.

PATHOLOGY

The squamo-columnar junction lies just inside the external cervical os and is the site of origin of most pre-invasive and invasive cervical cancer. There are two main histological types of cervical cancer:

1. *Squamous cell carcinoma (85%)* This is the commonest and easily diagnosed type. Depending on the cell type, it could be of two types—

   - Large cell keratinizing (LCK) (good prognosis type)
   - Small cell non-keratinizing (SCNK) (poor prognosis type)

Grading of cervical cancer   Based on the degree of differentiation, the tumour could be

Grade I–well differentiated (mainly squamous cells)

Grade II–moderately differentiated (mainly transitional cells)

Grade III–poorly differentiated (mainly small basal cells)

2. *Adenocarcinoma cervix (15%)* Arises from the endocervical epithelium. Since it is not visible on the ectocervix, it is more difficult to diagnose by examination and colposcopy. Endocervical smears with a cytobrush and endocervical curettings are necessary for diagnosis.

   Grossly, the tumour may be *exophytic*, growing out from the surface as a papillary or polypoidal excrescence, *ulcerative* or mainly *endophytic* and infiltrating the surrounding structures (Fig. 16.1a-c).

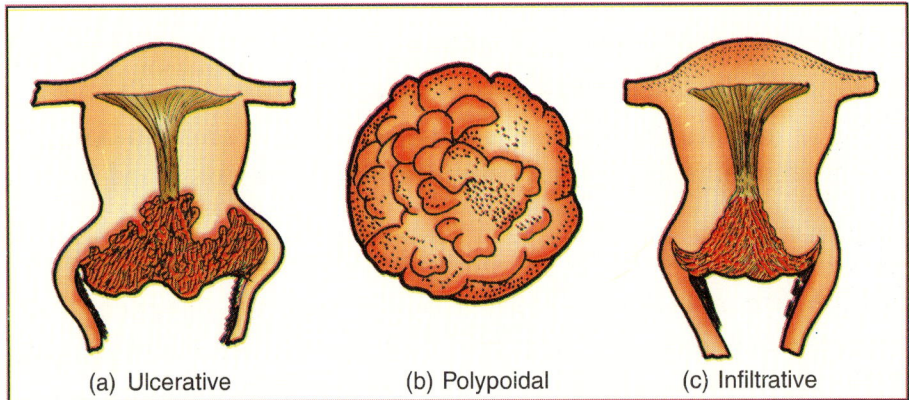

(a) Ulcerative	(b) Polypoidal	(c) Infiltrative

Fig. 16.1a-c.   Types of growth in carcinoma cervix

Mode of spread

1. *Direct spread* Anteriorly to the bladder, posteriorly to the rectum, inferiorly to the vagina and superiorly to the endometrium and myometrium. Laterally, the tumour can

spread to the fallopian tubes, ovaries and the parametrium including the ureters. Metastasis to the ovaries are seen in 1% of cases. Parametrial involvement is initially via lymphatics, later by direct spread and can be detected by palpating the parametrium on rectal examination. Occlusion of the ureters leads to hydronephrosis and renal failure.

2. *Lymphatic spread* The tumour spreads initially to the small lymphatic glands in the parametrium, then to the obturator, external iliac, internal iliac and rarely to the para-aortic nodes, mediastinal and cervical lymph nodes. Retrograde lymphatic spread leads to distant vaginal metastasis.

3. *Spread by blood stream* Occurs in advanced stages commonly to the lungs, liver and bones and rarely to the kidneys and brain.

CLINICAL FEATURES

Early symptoms

- Haemorrhage–the types of bleeding patterns seen are
    - Metrorrhagia or intermenstrual bleeding–there is no definite menstrual pattern.
    - Post-coital bleeding or trickle of blood after straining hard at defaecation.
    - Postmenopausal bleeding
- Vaginal discharge–the types of discharge which should raise a suspicion are
    - Any discharge in a postmenopausal woman
    - Any discharge which is offensive
    - Any blood stained vaginal discharge
- Asymptomatic–The early stages of cervical carcinomas (both squamous and adenocarcinomas) are asymptomatic and can be detected by visual inspection or by a pap smear. As there is a regular screening programme in the western countries, they are picked up in the early stages.

It is very important to remember the early symptoms to diagnose cervical cancer at its early stage. Unfortunately, the early symptoms go unrecognized. The irregular pattern of menstrual bleeding is mostly ignored as a normal pattern in the perimenopausal age.

Late symptoms

- Anaemia and malnutrition
- Loss of appetite
- Loss of weight
- Referred pain can occur due to involvement of the nerves. Involvement of the obturator

nerve leads to referred pain in the knees, involvement of the sacral plexus causes pain along the back of thighs.

- Urinary symptoms–haematuria and incontinence are seen in late stages when the disease has spread to the bladder.
- Pyometra–due to cervical stenosis can give rise to fever and malaise
- Painful defaecation can occur due to spread to the rectal wall.
- Symptoms due to secondaries in the lungs, bone or liver.

Clinical examination

General

Depending on the degree of spread, there could be anaemia, icterus, supra-clavicular lymphadenopathy, enlarged liver or kidneys and enlarged inguinal lymph nodes.

Pelvic examination

- *Speculum examination* The following signs may be noted.
  - Bleeding on touch and friability seen with exophytic growths and warrant a gentle examination.
  - The cervix may be ulcerated and excavated in an ulcerative growth
  - In an infiltrative growth there is restricted mobility of the cervix due to parametrial infiltration
  - In an endocervical growth, the cervix is hard to feel and may be barrel shaped.
- *Bimanual examination* The uterus may be enlarged and tender due to pyometra, resulting from stenosis and blockage of the cervical canal by the malignant growth.
- *Rectovaginal examination* is carried out to assess parametrial and posterior spread and involvement of the rectal mucosa. In case of parametrial spread, the parametrium feels hard and indurated.

Thus, from these symptoms and signs, the diagnosis of cervical cancer should not be difficult and must be confirmed by taking a punch biopsy from the growth with a part of the normal tissue of cervix and sent for histopathology.

DIAGNOSIS

Early stages A diagnosis can be made by a combination of the factors given below in Flow chart 1.

Differential diagnosis

Polypoidal growth arising from the cervix can also be seen with

- cervical polyps
- ulcerated myomatous polyps
- grapelike sarcoma of the cervix

Ulcerative lesion on the cervix also seen in

- *Ectropion* seen in puberty, pregnancy, and women on oral contraceptive pills. This occurs due to eversion of the columnar epithelium of the endocervix so that the squamocolumnar junction lies on the ectocervix.
- *Syphilitic ulcer of cervix (chancre)* this can occur anywhere on the ectocervix and typically produces a rounded ulcer with a firm base and a slightly elevated edge.
- *Tuberculous ulcer* very rare, but could be seen in developing countries like India.

The diagnosis should be confirmed by a cervical punch biopsy. If this is not confirmatory, a cone biopsy should be taken.

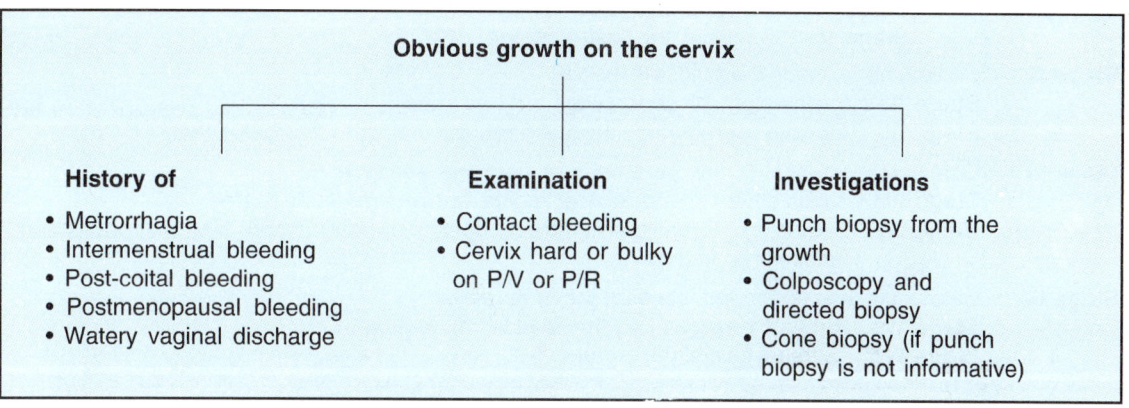

Flow chart 1. Diagnosis of cervical carcinoma

STAGING OF CERVICAL CARCINOMA

According to the International Federation of Gynaecology and Obstetrics (FIGO), carcinoma of the cervix is divided into four clinical stages depending on the extent of spread of the disease.

Broadly speaking, there are four stages of invasive cervical cancer as given in table 16.1 and depicted diagrammatically in Fig. 16.2a-f.

In short, the important points to remember about staging is that–

- When the carcinoma involves only the cervix it is stage I–In stage Ia it cannot be appreciated by simple speculum examination with the naked eye. If it is enlarged enough to be seen as a friable exophytic, ulcerative or an endophytic growth with the cervix giving an 'eaten up' appearance, it is stage Ib.

- If the cancer spreads beyond the cervix to the upper vagina or upper or medial half of parametrium, it becomes stage II.

- If whole of the parametrium upto lateral pelvic wall and lower third of vagina also get involved, it is stage III.

- In stage IV, the cancer spreads outside the pelvis or even to the distant organs.

Table 16.1. FIGO staging of cervical cancer	
Stage 0	Carcinoma in situ, CIN III
Stage I	Carcinoma strictly confined to the cervix

	Stage Ia : Pre-clinical carcinomas, diagnosed only by microscopy
	   Stage Ia 1 : Stromal invasion <3 mm deep, < 7 mm wide
	   Stage Ia 2 : Stromal invasion 3-5 mm deep < 7 mm wide

	Stage Ib : Clinical lesions, all grossly visible lesions, or pre-clinical lesions greater than Ia
	   Stage Ib 1 : Size of the lesion is < 4 cm
	   Stage Ib 2 : Size of the lesion is ≥ 4 cm

Stage II	Carcinoma extends beyond the cervix **Stage IIa** : Involvement of upper vagina **Stage IIb** : Obvious parametrial involvement, but not upto the pelvic wall
Stage III	Carcinoma extends to the parametrium upto the pelvic wall **Stage IIIa** : Involvement of the entire vagina but parametrium is free **Stage IIIb** : Extension to the parametrium upto the pelvic wall/ hydronephrosis/non-functioning kidney
Stage iV	Carcinoma has extended beyond the true pelvis **Stage IVa** : Spread of growth to the bladder or rectum **Stage IVb** : Spread to distant organs

Thus it is very important to understand and learn to stage the disease clinically by vaginal, rectal or rectovaginal examination. The lateral extension to the parametrium can be appreciated only by rectal or rectovaginal examination. Sometimes examination under anaesthesia may be required to properly stage the disease.

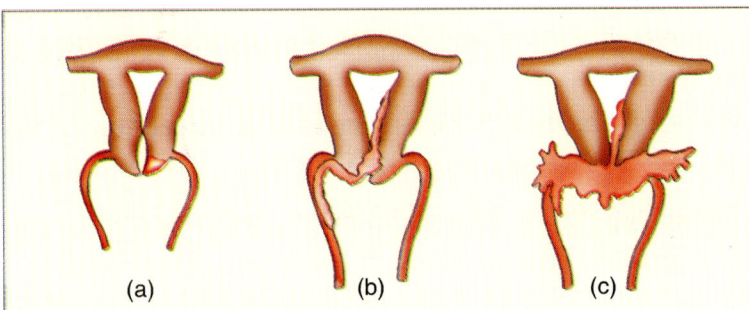

(a)   (b)   (c)

Fig. 16.2a-c. Stages of carcinoma cervix (a) Stage I–Growth confined to cervix (b) Stage IIa–Spread to upper vagina (c) Stage IIb–Spread to the medial parametrium

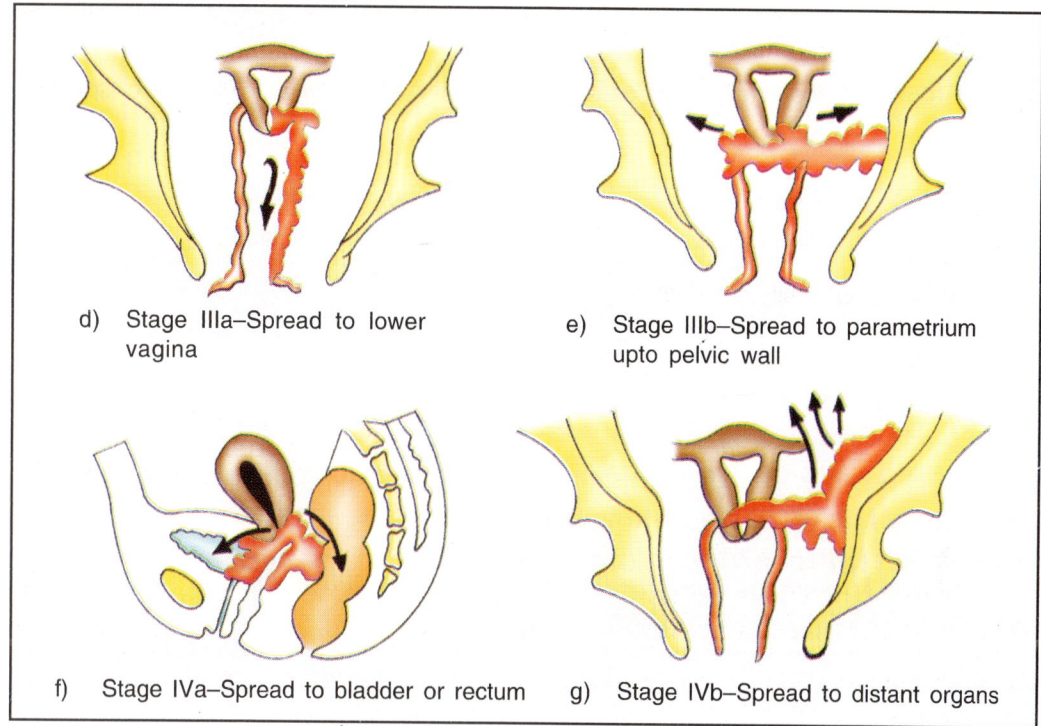

d) Stage IIIa–Spread to lower vagina

e) Stage IIIb–Spread to parametrium upto pelvic wall

f) Stage IVa–Spread to bladder or rectum

g) Stage IVb–Spread to distant organs

Fig. 16.2d-g. Stages of carcinoma cervix

MANAGEMENT

Management comprises of investigations and the specific treatment.

Investigations in a patient with suspected carcinoma cervix are:

General

- *Haemogram*
- *Blood group and Rh type* blood may need to be cross-matched and transfused if the patient is anaemic.
- *Renal and liver function tests* indicate involvement of these organs.
- *Chest x-ray PA view* to exclude metastases.
- *Urine cytology* presence of red cells or malignant cells indicates bladder involvement.

Specific

- *Examination under anaesthesia (EUA)* to stage the disease and plan the mode of treatment.

- *Cervical punch biopsy* multiple punch biopsies are taken from all the quadrants of the cervix and any vaginal extension.

- *Cone-biopsy of the cervix* if the punch biopsy reveals necrotic tissue or dysplasia only and is not informative, a cone shaped piece of the cervix including the squamo-columnar junction is taken with a diathermy loop or a cold knife. A cone biopsy is mandatory in the diagnosis and classification of stage Ia disease

- *Proctosigmoidoscopy* to assess involvement of the rectum if clinically suspected

- *Cystoscopy* to assess involvement of the bladder. The bladder washings can also be sent for cytology to look for malignant cells. Bullous edema of the bladder mucosa indicates lymphatic obstruction

- *Colposcopy* is indicated only if the lesion is small, the cervix is stained with Schiller's iodine and a directed biopsy taken from iodine negative areas.

- *Ultrasound pelvis and abdomen* is carried out to assess involvement of the bladder, presence of hydronephrosis or hydroureter and to detect any secondaries in the liver.

- *Intravenous urography (IVU)* to know the presence of hydronephrosis or hydroureter and the position of ureters. The presence of hydronephrosis puts the patient in stage IIIb

- *CT scan abdomen and pelvis* is useful to detect enlarged lymph nodes in the pelvis and retroperitoneum

- *MRI pelvis* this is a new modality useful to detect parametrial invasion

- *Lymphangiography* is accurate in only 75% of the patients and is useful for determining the completeness of lymphadenectomy at surgery

Treatment   The treatment modalities available are:

1. Surgery
2. Radiotherapy–primary or in combination with chemotherapy
3. Neoadjuvant chemotherapy–primary chemotherapy followed by surgery

   The treatment options stagewise are given in table 16.2. In stage I disease, the five year survival is similar with both surgery and radiotherapy.

1. *Surgery for carcinoma cervix*

The patients suitable for surgery are:

1. Young patients <40 yrs. of age
2. FIGO stage Ia to IIa
3. Associated conditions like fibroids, ovarian tumours, prolapse
4. Patient not willing for radiotherapy

Table 16.2. Treatment options in cervical cancer

Disease Stage	Treatment
Ia1	• Cervical conization (young patient desirous of preserving fertility) • Hysterectomy (completed family)
Ia2, Ib & IIa	Radical hysterectomy with bilateral pelvic lymphadenectomy
Ib & IIa poor surgical risk	Full external and intracavitary RT
Large bulky barrel shaped lesions	Full external and intracavitary pelvic RT+ extra fascial abdominal hysterectomy+ para-aortic node biopsy
IIb, IIIa & IIIb IVa & IVb	• Full external and intracavitary pelvic irradiation • Pelvic exenteration is carried out in centrally placed stage IVa carcinoma involving the bladder or rectum

Structures removed in radical hysterectomy and bilateral pelvic lymphadenectomy:

1. Uterus and cervix
2. Upper third of vagina
3. Parametrium upto the pelvic wall (only medial half in modified radical hysterectomy)
4. Lymph nodes–external and internal iliac, obturator and the common iliac group

Complications of radical hysterectomy are:

1. Injury to the bowel, bladder and uterus
2. Injury to the pelvic vessels causing haemorrhage
3. Venous thromboembolism due to the prolonged surgery
4. Urinary retention and UTI due to bladder dissection causing bladder hypotonia
5. Ureteric and bladder fistulae seen in 1-2% of cases.

Radical Trachelectomy

This involves excision of the cervix and para-cervical tissues with laparoscopic lymphadenectomy. This procedure conserves the uterus and is reserved for young women with very early disease and desirous of preserving fertility.

2. Radiotherapy

The patients selected for radiotherapy are–

1. FIGO stage IIb and IIIb

2. Older patients

3. Associated medical illnesses

4. Patient not willing for surgery

Principles of radiotherapy High dose gamma ray irradiation from intra-cavitary sources is given along with external RT with high energy megavoltage proton beams to the midplane of the pelvis, including the uterus, broad ligament and lateral pelvic wall. The details are given in the chapter on radiotherapy.

Advantages of radiotherapy

* Less primary mortality and morbidity

* Successful in all stages of cancer

* Possible in those unfit for anaesthesia

* Less risk of blood loss and transfusion

Drawbacks of radiotherapy

* Narrowing of the vagina

* Proctosigmoiditis resulting in rectal ulcers and strictures

* Intestinal injuries

* Radiation cystitis

* Ureteric fibrosis and obstruction

Post-op RT is indicated in patients with large tumours and those with positive pelvic lymph nodes

RT to para-aortic lymph nodes is indicated in patients with several positive pelvic lymph nodes

3. Chemoradiotherapy

Indicated in stage IIb and IIIb disease. Chemotherapeutic agents, eg. Cisplatin, Bleomycin and Methotrexate are given to cause tumour regression before RT. Trials have shown good response to chemoradiotherapy.

Follow-up

The follow-up is life-long. After any modality of treatment by–

* Pap smear every 3-4 months for the first three years.

* For the next 2 years, pap smear and a pelvic examination is performed every 6 months

- Annual health maintenance visits for general medical problems, mammography and hormone replacement therapy whenever necessary.

CERVICAL CANCER IN PREGNANCY

Approximately 2.7-3.5% of cervical cancers occur in pregnant women. The diagnosis of cancer is not so easy during pregnancy and treatment options must consider safety of the fetus as well. Therapeutic recommendations should be individualized based on the FIGO staging, size of the growth and the desire to continue the pregnancy.

Malignant Tumours of the Uterus

The tumours of the body of uterus could be carcinomas arising from the endometrium or sarcomas arising from the stroma. Carcinoma endometrium is more common than sarcoma.

CARCINOMA ENDOMETRIUM

Endometrial carcinoma is the third commonest cancer (commonest is cervix followed by the ovary) of the female reproductive tract in Indian women. Globally, however, its prevalence is on the rise mainly because of increased longevity. In developed countries the prevalence of endometrial cancer is higher than cervical cancer; however, it is less common in Indian women with a mean incidence of 1.73 per 100,000 women as compared to 24.2 per 100,000 for cervical cancer. More than 90% of patients are postmenopausal at the time of diagnosis.

Risk factors

The risk factors known to be associated with endometrial carcinoma are:

1. *Nulliparity* is associated with a 2-3 fold increased risk, the risk falls with increasing number of children.

2. *Early menarche and late menopause* are known to increase the risk.

3. *Obesity* leads to increased peripheral conversion to oestrogens leading to increased serum levels of oestrone and oestriol, which results in hyperplasia of the endometrium

4. *High oestrogen levels* seen in feminizing ovarian tumours, oestrogen only hormone replacement therapy cause proliferation of the endometrium. Addition of cyclical progesterone prevents this proliferation.

5. *Diet and exercise* Diets rich in fat and low in complex carbohydrates and fibre are associated with an increased risk independent of body weight. Exercise lowers oestrogen levels, a sedentary life-style increases the risk.

6. *Gene defects* involving the genes MSH2 and MLH1 cause an increased risk of cancers of the colon, endometrium, ovary, stomach, small intestine and renal tract.

7. *Endometrial hyperplasia* Simple glandular hyperplasia is not pre-malignant, however atypical hyperplasia has a 50% risk of developing carcinoma.

8. *Tamoxifen therapy* Tamoxifen, an anti-oestrogen used for treatment of breast cancer has an increased risk of causing endometrial polyps and endometrial hyperplasia

Pathology

This malignancy is derived from the endometrial glandular cells (a tumour of the stroma is stromal sarcoma). The histological types are:

1. *Adenocarcinoma*–glandular pattern resembles proliferative endometrium. This is the most common histological type.

2. *Adenoacanthoma*–malignant glands have islands of benign squamous change in the stroma

3. *Adenosquamous carcinoma*–malignant glands with a malignant squamous component

4. *Clear cell carcinoma*–have large clear cells with glycogen and are associated with poor prognosis

The tumour is further graded depending on the degree of differentiation of the glandular epithelium (Fig. 17.1a-c).

Grade I–well differentiated

Grade II–moderately differentiated with infiltrating cell columns

Grade III–poorly differentiated with solid masses of malignant cells with little or no stroma and numerous mitoses

Grossly, the tumour could be in the form of papillary excrescences, a localized polypoidal growth or an ulcerated necrotic growth.

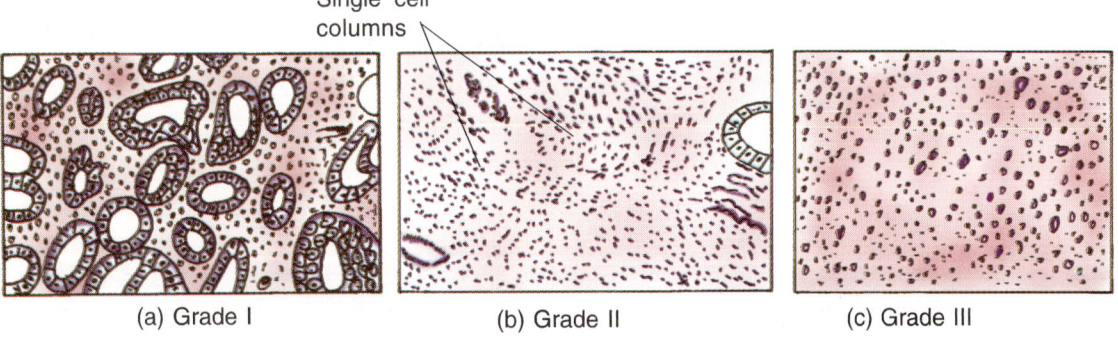

Single cell columns

(a) Grade I   (b) Grade II   (c) Grade III

Fig. 17.1a-c. Histological grades of endometrial carcinoma

Spread of endometrial carcinoma (Fig. 17.2)

Direct Spread

 – Myometrium
 – Fallopian tubes and ovaries
 – Endocervix

Lymphatic Spread

 – Fallopian tubes
 – Ovaries
 – Para-aortic lymph nodes (direct spread can also occur)
 – Pelvic lymph nodes
 – Superficial inguinal lymph nodes (via the round ligaments)
 – Supraclavicular lymph nodes (rarely)

Haematogenous

 – Lower vagina
 – Lungs
 – Liver

A growth in the fundus spreads more often to the para-aortic nodes while a growth in the cervix is more likely to cause pelvic node metastasis.

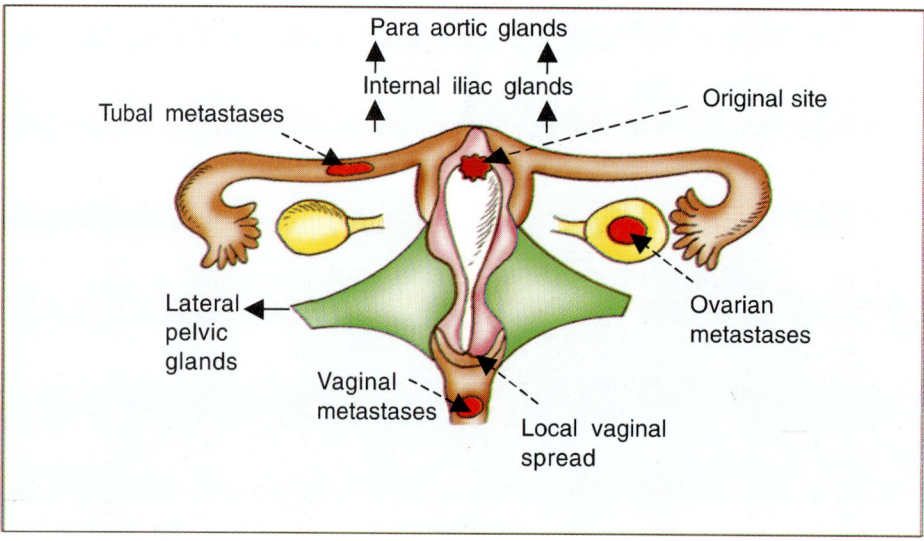

Fig. 17.2.   Spread of endometrial cancer

FIGO staging of endometrial cancer

The staging is surgical and given in table 17.1 and shown diagrammatically in Fig. 17.3a-f.

Table 17.1. Staging of endometrial cancer		
Stage	Ia	Tumour limited to endometrium
	Ib	Invasion to less than one-half of myometrium
	Ic	Invasion to more than one-half of the myometrium
Stage	IIa	Endocervical glandular involvement only
	IIb	Cervical stromal invasion
Stage	IIIa	Tumour invades serosa and / or adnexa and / or positive peritoneal cytology
	IIIb	Vaginal metastasis
	IIIc	Metastasis to pelvic and / or para-aortic lymph nodes
Stage	IVa	Tumour invasion of bladder and / or bowel mucosa (bullous edema does not put the patient in this category)
	IVb	Distant metastasis including intra-abdominal and / or inguinal lymph nodes
Based on the histology of the endometrium, the tumour could be graded as		
Grade I well differentiated		
Grade 2 moderately differentiated		
Grade 3 poorly differentiated		

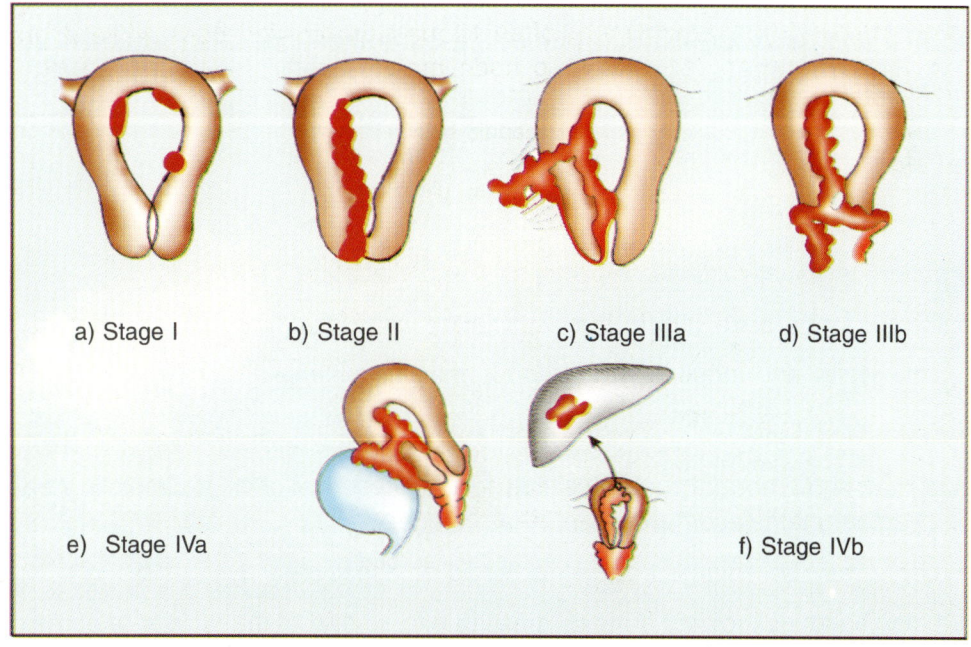

a) Stage I b) Stage II c) Stage IIIa d) Stage IIIb

e) Stage IVa f) Stage IVb

Fig. 17.3a-f. Stages of endometrial cancer

Prognostic factors–factors determining the prognosis are:

*   Stage of the disease
*   Presence/absence of myometrial invasion
*   Grade of the tumour
*   Size of the tumour
*   Age of the patient
*   Peritoneal cytology

Clinical features

Symptoms

*   *Vaginal bleeding* The most common symptom is postmenopausal bleeding. Of all the causes of postmenopausal bleeding, 15% are due to endometrial carcinoma. The other causes of postmenopausal bleeding and the differential diagnosis is given at the end of the chapter.
*   *Vaginal discharge* is a rare symptom and seen if the growth becomes polypoidal and protrudes from the cervical os.
*   *Pelvic pain* is due to spread of the disease causing nerve compression. Suprapubic pain, fever and malaise could also be due to pyometra.
*   *Dyspnoea and haemoptysis* due to metastases in the lungs.
*   *Asymptomatic* (5%)

Physical signs

General examination

*   The patient is usually obese, hypertensive and diabetic (30-50%).
*   Hirsuitism may be seen due to the association with polycystic ovarian disease.
*   Supra-clavicular and inguinal lymph nodes may be enlarged.

Pelvic examination

*   Vagina may show normal rugosities due to the presence of high circulating oestrogen levels. Vaginal metastases are seen in late stages.
*   The uterus may be enlarged due to a fibroid or associated pyometra.
*   There may be an associated adnexal mass due to spread of the tumour or an associated feminizing ovarian tumour.

Investigations in a confirmed case of carcinoma endometrium

General These are carried out to know if the woman is fit for surgery.

- Haemogram, blood grouping and Rh typing
- Blood sugar-fasting and postprandial
- Blood urea and serum creatinine
- Urine routine examination and microscopy
- Serum bilirubin and liver enzymes
- X-ray chest PA view and ECG

Specific

- MRI of the pelvis to detect spread to the cervix and myometrium
- CECT (contrast enhanced CT scan) of the pelvis detects enlarged pelvic and para-aortic lymph nodes

Management of endometrial cancer

Exploratory laparotomy is essential for surgical staging of all patients diagnosed as carcinoma of the endometrium.

Stage I disease

Surgery

- Total abdominal hysterectomy and bilateral salpingo-oophorectomy (TAH+BSO) is the treatment of choice. The adnexae are removed because of the risk of involvement with the tumour. A midline infraumbilical incision is given, saline washings taken from the pelvis and abdomen for cytology. The liver, omentum, uterine adnexae and retroperitoneal node bearing areas are palpated for any enlarged lymph nodes. An infracolic omentectomy may also be performed as 8% of cases contain microscopic disease.
- Vaginal hysterectomy and bilateral salpingo-oophorectomy performed in suitable cases has a lower complication and mortality rate with an equivalent 5 yr. survival.
- Pelvic lymphadenectomy: Although practised routinely by some surgeons, there is no clear data demonstrating a therapeutic benefit.
- Role of laparoscopy: Laparoscopic removal of adnexae can be performed if vaginal removal is unsuccessful. Laparoscopic lymphadenectomy is shown to be inadequate and not recommended in the routine management of patients with this cancer.

Post-op Radiotherapy

- Grade 1 and 2 tumours with superficial invasion are given brachytherapy to the vagina with 15-18 Gy in 2-3 fractions to reduce the incidence of vault recurrence.
- Grade 3/deep invasion are given brachytherapy to the vagina with 4 Gy in 2 fractions followed by teletherapy to the pelvis (45 Gy in 25 fractions).

Stage II disease (Involvement of the cervix)

- Stage IIa–there is microscopic involvement of the glands, the prognosis is similar to stage I and managed similarly.
- Stage IIb (cervical stromal involvement)–Radical hysterectomy with bilateral pelvic lymphadenectomy is carried out if the woman is fit for surgery. If unfit, radiotherapy is given.

Stage III disease

- Extrauterine spread to the parametrium and adnexae except the ovaries: Intracavitary and external radiotherapy give a cure rate of 70%.
- Ovarian metastases indicate exploratory laparotomy, total abdominal hysterectomy with bilateral salpingo-oophorectomy omentectomy and para-aortic lymphadenectomy.

Stage IV disease

- Isolated lung metastases–Hysterectomy with bilateral salpingo-oophorectomy is performed and progestins given post-operatively.
- Associated other metastases–Radiotherapy to the primary and secondary growth are given.

Post-op hormone replacement therapy

Oestrogens are contraindicated as they may cause recurrence.

Medroxyprogesterone acetate, Selective Oestrogen Receptor Modulators (SERMs) (Raloxifen) may provide some relief of menopausal symptoms.

Recurrent disease

- Vaginal recurrence–needs wide excision with radiotherapy.
- Hormones-commonly used hormones are progesterone analogues, medroxy progesterone acetate (MPA) 200mg bd/tds. The response rate is 70%.
- Tamoxifen and aminoglutithimide are used in some cases with limited success.
- Cytotoxic agents have a limited role and are indicated if there is no response to progesterone.

Follow-up

The follow-up is every 3 monthly for the first year and 6 monthly for the next 3 years. The mode of follow-up is outlined in Flow chart 1.

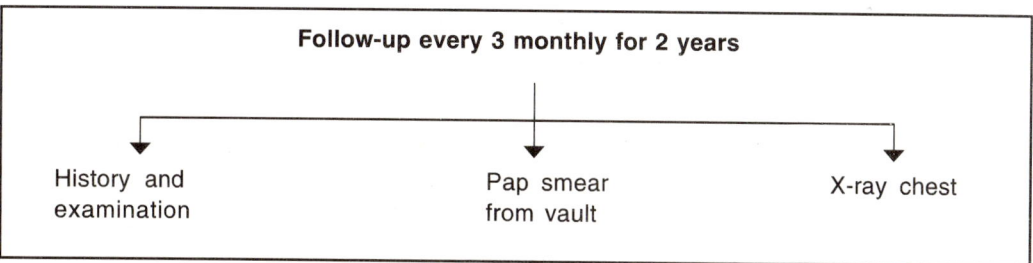

Flow chart 1. Follow-up of endometrial cancer

Annual checkup for lifelong should also include mammography and other imaging techniques to rule out recurrence, if facilities are available.

Overall 5 yr survival rate: 70%

UTERINE SARCOMAS

- Highly malignant tumours with an incidence of 2/1,00,000 women above 20 years of age.
- Increased incidence has been seen in women on oral contraceptive pills, obese women and women of afro-carribean origin.
- **Histological types** Based on the cell of origin they could be of four different types:
  1. *Endometrial stromal tumours* which are derived from the stromal cells of the endometrium and could be of low-grade or high-grade.
  2. *Adenosarcoma* has both epithelial and stromal components, of which the epithelial component is benign and the stromal component is malignant.
  3. *Malignant mixed mullerian tumour* (carcinosarcoma) is composed of malignant glands in a malignant stroma.
  4. *Leiomyosarcoma* is the malignant counterpart of the leiomyoma and is the commonest pure sarcoma of the uterus with an incidence of 6.7 per 10,000 women or 2-3 women per 1000 women with a leiomyoma.

Clinical presentation

- They usually present with menorrhagia, metrorrhagia, postmenopausal bleeding, vaginal discharge, pelvic pain and weight loss.
- Rapidly increasing fibroid could suggest a leiomyosarcoma.

- They could be asymptomatic and be detected only on histology of a hysterectomy specimen.

Treatment

- TAH+BSO+omentectomy and pelvic lymphadenectomy if cut section of the uterus shows areas of necrosis and haemorrhage.
- If there is invasion into the pelvic structures and parametrium, palliative chemotherapy is given.

POSTMENOPAUSAL BLEEDING (PMB)

The causes of PMB are outlined in Flow chart 2. The evaluation of a patient includes a detailed history, examination and investigations as given below and summarized in table 17.2.

Table 17.2. Evaluation of PMB

History–   Age, parity
               Medical history
               Drug intake–oestrogens, tamoxifen
               History of discharge or mass abdomen
 	
General examination–
Examination of external genitalia and cervix
Pelvic examination
Pelvic USS
Endometrial aspiration and/or D & C
Hysteroscopy
Colposcopy and directed biopsy

History The points to be noted are:

- Age, parity
- History of diabetes, hypertension, polycystic ovarian disease
- History of exogenous oestrogen intake
- History of tamoxifen usage
- Any associated symptoms like discharge, pelvic pain or pelvic mass

Examination

General: Presence of pallor, icterus, lymphadenopathy, hepatosplenomegaly, pedal edema indicate advanced endometrial cancer. Presence of purpura or bruising indicates a bleeding disorder.

Pelvic examination

- The external urethral meatus and anus are carefully inspected for any urethral caruncle or external haemorrhoids respectively, as bleeding per urethra or bleeding PR may be mistaken for vaginal bleeding.
- Vulva, vagina and cervix are carefully inspected and a cervical smear taken.
- Bimanual examination is carried out to assess the size of the uterus and detect any adnexal pathology.

Investigations

- *Transvaginal ultrasound* The endometrial thickness is measured and any associated adnexal pathology is picked up. The patient is reassured if the endometrial thickness is <5mm as endometrial malignancy is very unlikely.
- *Outpatient endometrial biopsy* This is taken with a narrow plastic cannula (Pipelle, Karman's). If the endometrial thickness is <5mm on ultrasound scan, and the biopsy is benign, one can reassure the woman that an intrauterine malignancy is very unlikely.
- *Hysteroscopy* A hysteroscope can detect endometrial polyps and submucous fibroids. A thorough evaluation of the endocervix and endometrium can also be performed.
- *Colposcopy and cervical biopsy* are carried out if the cervix is found to be unhealthy and suspicious of cervical cancer.

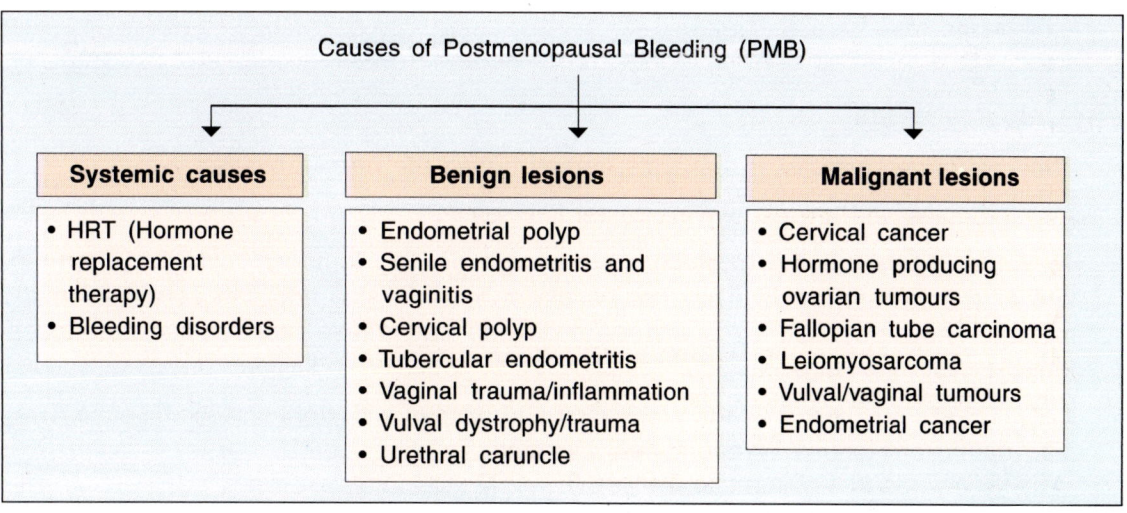

Flow chart 2. Causes of Postmenopausal Bleeding (PMB)

18

Tumours of the Ovary

Tumours of the ovary could be benign, borderline or malignant based on their nature. Of all the ovarian tumours majority are benign; malignant ovarian tumours constitute 13% of all ovarian tumours in premenopausal and 45% of all ovarian tumours in postmenopausal women.

PATHOLOGICAL CLASSIFICATION OF OVARIAN TUMOURS

Based on their nature, they are classified as benign or malignant; further sub-classification is based on the cell of origin. **Borderline** tumours are those which, while having some of the features of malignancy, lack any evidence of stromal invasion and mostly remain confined to the ovaries. The classification defined by WHO, given in the table 18.1, is based on the cell of origin.

BENIGN OVARIAN TUMOURS

Physiological cysts

- They are large versions of the cysts formed during the normal ovarian cycle
- Asymptomatic and are usually incidental findings
- *Follicular cysts* are the most common benign ovarian tumours caused by non-rupture of a dominant follicle. They are usually < 5 cm in size and can persist for many months. They are lined by granulosa cells and can cause menstrual disturbances. Multiple cysts are an occasional complication of ovulation induction.
- *Luteal cysts* are seen in early pregnancy and women with trophoblastic disease. They can rupture and cause intraperitoneal bleeding.

Benign Epithelial Tumours

Origin

They arise from the ovarian surface epithelium and are essentially mesothelial in nature,

Table 18.1. Classification of ovarian tumours

Common epithelial tumours (benign, borderline or malignant)
- Serous tumours
- Mucinous tumours
- Endometroid tumours
- Clear cell (mesonephroid) tumour
- Brenner tumour
- Mixed epithelial tumours
- Undifferentiated carcinomas
- Unclassified tumours

Sex cord stromal tumours
- Granulosa cell tumour
- Androblastoma-Sertoli-Leydig cell tumour
- Gynandroblastoma
- Unclassified tumour

Lipid cell tumours

Germ cell tumours
- Dysgerminoma
- Endodermal sinus tumour (yolk sac tumour)
- Embryonal cell tumour
- Polyembryoma
- Choriocarcinoma
- Teratoma
- Mixed tumours

Gonadoblastoma

Soft tissue tumours not specific to the ovary

Unclassified tumours

Metastatic tumours

as they are derived from the coelomic epithelium overlying the embryonic gonadal ridge. As the gonadal ridge has the capacity to differentiate into mullerian and wolffian structures, the tumours could develop into mucinous cystadenomas (from endocervical cells), endometroid (from endometrial cell), serous (from tubal cell) and brenner (from uroepithelial cells) Table 18.2.

Table 18.2. Cell of origin of epithelial tumours

Cell of origin	Type of tumour
Endocervical cell	Mucinous cystadenomas
Endometrial cell	Endometroid
Tubal cell	Serous
Uroepithelial cell	Brenner

Age at presentation They are most common in women >40yrs.

1. Serous cystadenomas

- Most common benign epithelial tumour
- Bilateral in 10%
- Usually unilocular with papilliferous processes on the inner surface.
- Occasionally have concentric psammoma bodies (intracellular calcification).

2. Mucinous cystadenomas

- This is the second most common benign epithelial tumour
- It is a large, unilateral, multilocular cyst which may reach the size of a full term gravid uterus filled with thick gelatinous fluid.
- *Pseudomyxoma peritonei:* Well differentiated mucinous cystadeno-carcinomas or borderline tumours can result in seedling growths in the peritoneal cavity secreting mucin causing matting and obstruction of the bowel loops. The 5 year survival rate is 50%.

3. Brenner tumours

- Account for 1-20% of all ovarian tumours
- More common in women >40 yrs., half of them occur as incidental findings
- Majority are <2 cm
- Origin–from wolffian metaplasia of the surface epithelium
- Microscopically-consist of islands of transitional epithelium (*Walthard rests*) in a dense fibrotic stroma
- Some of them secrete oestrogens and cause vaginal bleeding.

4. Endometroid cystadenoma These are difficult to differentiate from endometriosis.

Sex cord stromal tumours

- Represent 4% of benign ovarian tumours
- Can be seen at any age including children and postmenopausal women
- They are hormone secreting and of four histological types, theca cell, granulosa cell, fibromas and Sertoli-Leydig cell tumours.

- *Granulosa cell tumours* are all malignant tumours, are slow growing and largely solid. The pathognomic features are the *Call-Exner bodies*.
- *Theca cell tumours* Almost all are benign, solid and unilateral
  - Present at 60-70 yrs.
  - Oestrogen secreting and can cause precocious puberty, postmenopausal bleeding, endometrial hyperplasia or cancer
- *Fibromas* They are derived from stromal cells of the ovary
  - Present around 50 yrs. of age
  - Grossly are hard, mobile with a glistening white surface
  - Bilateral in < 10%
  - Are mostly associated with ascites
  - *Meig's syndrome* is a syndrome in which fibromas are associated with ascites and pleural effusion; is seen in 1% of fibromas
- *Sertoli-Leydig cell tumours* They are commonly androgen secreting tumours causing virilization
  - They are of low grade malignancy
  - They are usually seen at about 30 yrs. of age
  - Usually small and bilateral

Germ cell tumours

- Most common ovarian tumours in women <30 yrs.
- They arise from totipotent germ cells and may contain elements of all the three germ layers.

  ### Mature cystic teratoma (Dermoid cyst)
  - Accounts for 40% of all ovarian tumours
  - Most common in young women with a median age of 30 yrs.
  - Bilateral in 11% of cases
  - Grossly: They are unilocular cysts <15cm with predominant ectodermal structures lined with epithelium like the epidermis and containing skin appendages eg. teeth, sebaceous material, hair and nervous tissue (Fig. 18.1).
  - May contain thyroid tissue (*struma ovarii*)
  - Malignant component is seen in 2% of women >40 yrs. and is usually a squamous cell carcinoma.
  - *Clinical features:*
      Asymptomatic in 60%

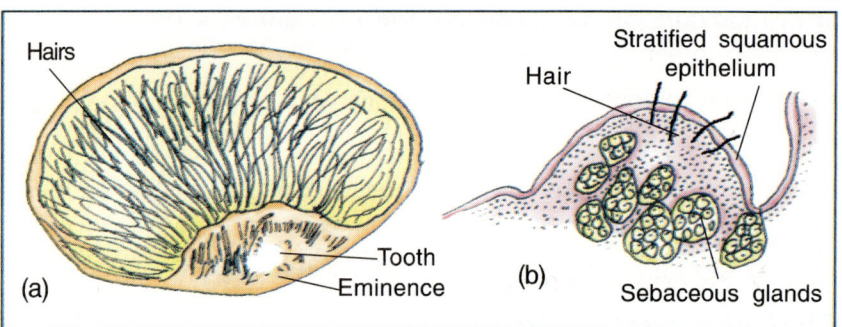

Fig. 18.1. Mature cystic teratoma (a) Gross appearance (b) Microscopic appearance

3.5-10% can undergo torsion around its pedicle (Fig. 18.2), which causes a sharp, constant pain caused by ischaemia of the cyst.

1-4% can rupture and present as an acute abdomen with chemical peritonitis. Rupture is more common during pregnancy due to external pressure from the gravid uterus or trauma during delivery.

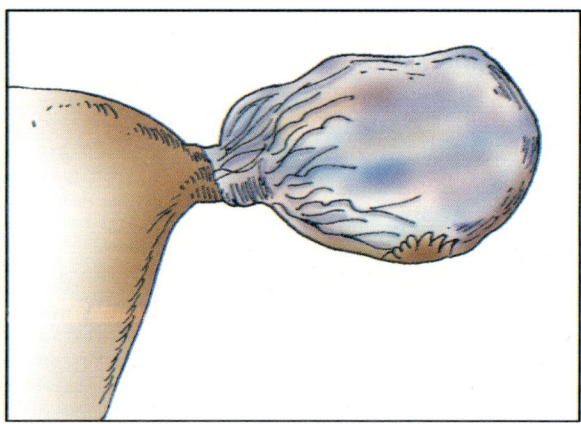

Fig. 18.2. Twisted ovarian cyst–Torsion occurs around the pedicle

MALIGNANT OVARIAN TUMOURS

Ovarian cancer is the fourth most common cancer in women worldwide accounting for 6% of deaths in women. It is the second commonest cancer of the genital tract in Indian women with an annual incidence of 6.1 per 100,000 women. They have a maximum incidence between 50-60 yrs. of age.

Risk factors

• Early menarche, late menopause and nulliparity are associated with an increased risk due to the theory of '*incessant ovulation*' causing repeated epithelial damage and reconstruction. Use of oral contraceptive pills and pregnancy suppress ovulation and decrease the risk.

- Infertility treatment—prolonged treatment with ovulation inducing agents increases the risk.

- *Family history* Inheritance plays a role in 5% of epithelial ovarian cancers. With one affected relative in the family, the risk is 4%; if the affected relative is the mother, the risk is 7%. With more than one affected relative, the risk increases to 14%. The ovarian cancer genes are BRCA 1 and 2 located on chromosome 17. Mutations in these genes increase the risk of breast and ovarian cancer.

Classification of malignant ovarian tumours

The WHO classification of ovarian tumours is as shown in the table earlier:

Pathology

1. Malignant epithelial tumours

As described earlier, they are derived from the ovarian surface epithelium and sub-classified according to the epithelial cell type into serous, mucinous, endometroid and clear cell tumours. Stage for stage there is no difference in survival in the different epithelial sub-types. However, mucinous and endometroid cancers are more likely to present at an earlier stage and be of a lower grade than serous tumours. The gross and microscopic appearance is summarized in the table 18.3.

Table 18.3. Summary of gross and microscopic appearance of malignant epithelial tumours

Pathology	Serous Tumours	Mucinous Tumours	Endometroid Tumours	Clear cell Tumours
Gross	Solid and cystic Bilateral in 50-90%	Multiloculated thin walled cysts filled with mucinous fluid; are largest tumours of the ovary having a smooth surface	Cystic unilocular and contain turbid brown fluid with a rough internal surface with rounded poly-poidal projections	Thick walled unilocular cysts filled with blood stained fluid and having solid poly-poidal projections on the internal surface. Bilateral in 10%
Microscopic appearance	Papillary pattern of glands seen with stromal invasion. Psammoma bodies (calcified bodies) commonly seen	Lined by mucinous cells, tall picket-fence cells with stromal invasion	Epithelium is tall and columnar with a high nuclear-cytoplasmic ratio	Well differentiated glandular pattern lined by clear cells

Borderline Tumours

These tumours border in between the benign and malignant types. Microscopically, they show varying degrees of nuclear atypia and an increase in mitotic activity with multilayering of neoplastic cells, and no stromal invasion. They remain confined to the ovaries.

2. *Germ cell tumours*

The common malignant germ cell tumours are

*   Dysgerminoma
*   Embryonal carcinoma
*   Immature teratoma
*   Yolk sac tumours (Endodermal sinus tumour)
*   Choriocarcinomas

Germ cell tumours are derived from the primordial germ cells of the ovary. The origin of the tumours and their tumour markers are given as shown in Fig. 18.3a-c.

*   *Dysgerminoma*
    *   This accounts for 2-5% of all primary malignant ovarian tumours. It is most commonly seen in women <30 yrs. of age.

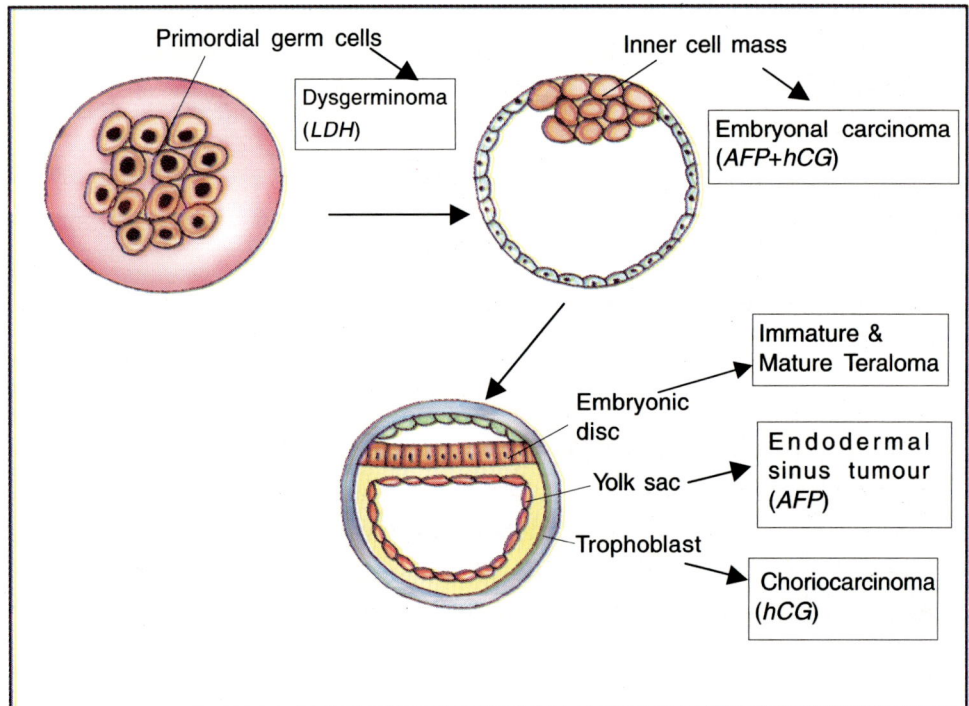

Fig. 18.3a-c.   Origin of germ cell tumours and their tumour markers

– Pathology: Grossly, they have a smooth or nodular bosselated external surface and are soft or rubbery in consistency. They are bilateral in 10% of cases. Microscopically, they are made up of large, round tumour cells separated by fibrous tissue and infiltrated with lymphocytes. The cells have abundant cytoplasm, are rich in glycogen and alkaline phosphatase (Fig. 18.4).

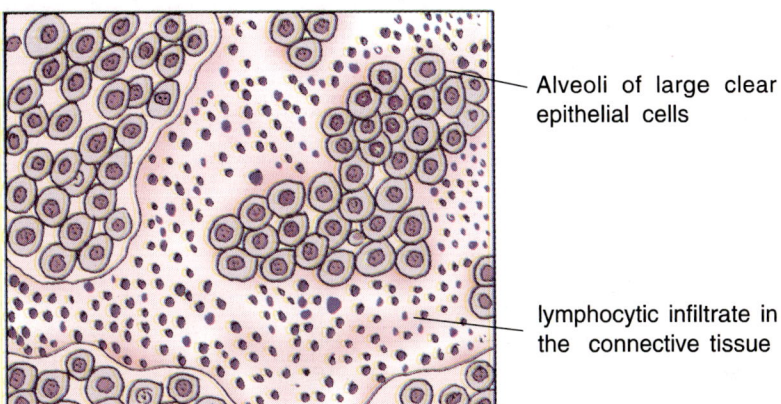

Alveoli of large clear epithelial cells

lymphocytic infiltrate in the connective tissue

Fig. 18.4. Microscopic appearance of Dysgerminoma–Note the masses of large, clear epithelial cells with large nuclei, in cords or alveoli; the connective tissue is infiltrated by lymphocytes

Immature teratomas

– Comprise 1% of all ovarian teratomas.

– Grossly, they are unilateral solid masses with solid tissue. Areas of bone and cartilage may be seen.

Yolk sac tumours (Endodermal sinus tumours)

– They are well encapsulated and solid with areas of necrosis and haemorrhage. They are soft to firm in consistency and the cut surface is slippery and mucoid.

– Microscopically, the characteristic feature is the endodermal sinus (*Schiller-Duval body*)

3. *Malignant sex cord stromal tumours*

– Malignant sex cord tumours have both theca and granulosa cells.

– They are bilateral in 5%.

– Grossly they are generally solid but may have cystic areas. The cut surface is yellow, due to the presence of neutral lipid with areas of haemorrhage.

– They express alpha inhibin.

Spread of ovarian cancer

Ovarian cancer spreads by direct, lymphatic and blood spread. The FIGO staging of ovarian cancer is given in table 18.4.

- *Direct spread* occurs to other pelvic and intraabdominal organs, the omentum and under surface of the diaphragm.

- *Lymphatic spread* occurs along the lymphatics running along with the ovarian vessels to the para-aortic lymph nodes at the level of the renal vessels. These nodes are involved in 20% of stage I and II and 60% of stage III and IV. Spread to the mediastinal and cervical lymph nodes occurs from the para-aortic nodes. Inguinal lymph nodes may be involved by retrograde spread via the ovarian ligaments. Dysgerminoma usually spreads by lymphatics.

- *Blood spread* occurs to the liver, lung and occasionally to the bone and brain. Teratomas are more likely to spread by this mode.

Table 18.4. FIGO staging of ovarian carcinoma		
Stage I		**Growth limited to ovaries**
	Ia	Growth limited to one ovary, no ascites, capsule intact
	Ib	Growth limited to both ovaries, no ascites, capsule intact
	Ic	Growth involving one or both ovaries with either one of the following: tumour on the surface / capsule ruptured / ascites containing malignant cells / positive peritoneal washings
Stage II		**Growth involving one or both ovaries with pelvic extension**
	IIa	Extension and/or metastases to the uterus or tubes
	IIb	Extension to other pelvic tissues
	IIc	Tumour of either stage IIa or IIb, but tumour on the surface of one or both ovaries; or with capsule ruptured; or with ascites containing malignant cells; or with positive peritoneal washings
Stage III		**Growth involving one or both ovaries with peritoneal implants outside the pelvis or positive retroperitoneal or inguinal nodes.** (Superficial liver metastases equals stage III)
	IIIa	Tumour grossly limited to the true pelvis with negative nodes but with histologically confirmed microscopic seeding of abdominal peritoneal surfaces
	IIIb	Tumour with histologically confirmed implants on abdominal peritoneal surfaces, none exceeding 2 cm in diameter. Nodes are negative
	IIIc	Abdominal implants greater than 2cm in diameter or positive retroperitoneal or inguinal nodes
Stage IV		**Growth involving one or both ovaries with distant metastases.** If pleural effusion is present there must be positive cytology to allocate a case to stage IV. Parenchymal liver metastasis equals stage IV.

EVALUATION OF A PATIENT WITH AN ADNEXAL MASS

The evaluation includes a detailed history, a thorough physical examination and investigations.

History The points to be noted are

- *Age* If the age is <40 yrs., the mass is more likely to be benign, inflammatory or of germ cell variety. In prepubertal girls, germ cell and sex cord stromal tumours are more common. If the age of the patient is >40 yrs., the mass has a higher chance of being malignant.

- *Family history* A family history of tuberculosis favors a diagnosis of encysted ascites due to tuberculosis (as it can many times mimic an ovarian tumour). A family history of breast, ovarian, endometrial and colonic cancers increases the risk of epithelial ovarian cancer due to the presence of ovarian cancer genes. The number of children born is also important to note to plan the management.

- *Previous history of contraceptive usage* Oral contraceptives decrease the risk of ovarian cancer due to suppression of ovulation.

- *Previous history of ovulation inducing agents* increases the risk.

- *Abdominal pain* Neoplastic tumours are generally painless. A painful mass is more likely to be inflammatory or endometriotic. Sudden onset of pain in a painless tumour could be due to torsion, rupture, haemorrhage or infection of the tumour.

- *Distension, dyspepsia, anorexia* are pointers in favour of malignancy in ovarian tumours; which could be due to ascites or omental caking. A mucinous cystadenoma may completely fill the abdomen and cause distension.

- *Menstrual irregularities* are usually seen in inflammatory masses (eg. PID), endometriosis or chronic ectopic pregnancy. However, oestrogen secreting ovarian tumours can cause precocious puberty and postmenopausal bleeding.

- *Unilateral edema, unilateral varicose veins, or deep vein thrombosis* point towards a malignant ovarian tumour with spread to the pelvic vessels and lymph nodes.

- *Altered bowel habit, rectal bleeding* point to a GI primary with secondaries to the ovaries (*Krukenberg's tumour*).

- *Urinary frequency, constipation* could be related to the pressure effects of the tumour on the bladder and rectum.

Examination

- *General examination* the points to be noted are

  - Lymphadenopathy (which could be due to metastatic disease or associated tuberculosis)

  - Breast examination–for any lump, as the ovarian mass could be secondary to a primary in the breast (*Krukenberg's tumour*).

  - Chest examination–could reveal a pleural effusion which indicates metastatic spread.

  - Jaundice–could be due to spread to the liver.

- Anaemia–could be due to haemorrhage into an ovarian tumour or a benign condition like chronic ectopic pregnancy.

- Pedal edema–unilateral is due to pressure effects of the tumour. Bilateral edema is more likely to be nutritional.

- Hirsuitism and signs of virilization–indicate a virilizing ovarian tumour

• *Abdominal examination* The best way to detect a mass arising from the pelvis is to palpate with the radial border of the left hand and working caudally (Fig.18.5).

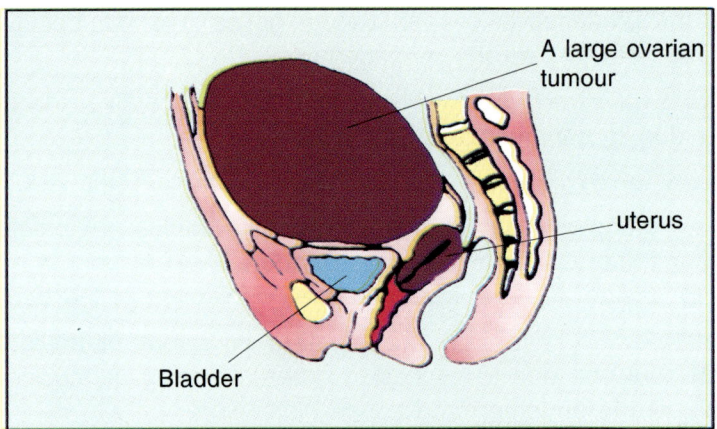

A large ovarian tumour

uterus

Bladder

Fig. 18.5.   A large ovarian cyst occupying the abdomen

- Ascites-points in favour of a malignant ovarian tumour. Ascites is also seen in tuberculosis. Ascites without a pelvic mass could be the only presentation of a malignant ovarian tumour. Differentiation of ascites from a large ovarian cyst is shown in Fig. 18.6.

- Periumbilical nodules suggests a malignant ovarian tumour with cutaneous depos-

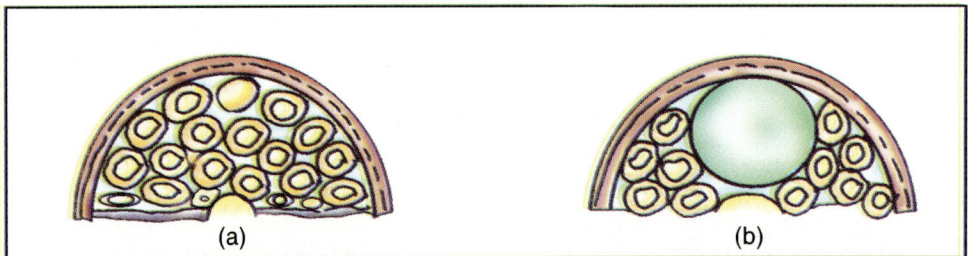

(a)   (b)

Fig. 18.6.   Differentiation between ascites and a large ovarian cyst (a) Ascites pushes the bowel loops forward with dullness in the flanks (b) An ovarian cyst pushes the bowel loops laterally and is dull in the centre

its.

Pelvi-rectal examination A pelvic combined with a rectal examination gives accurate

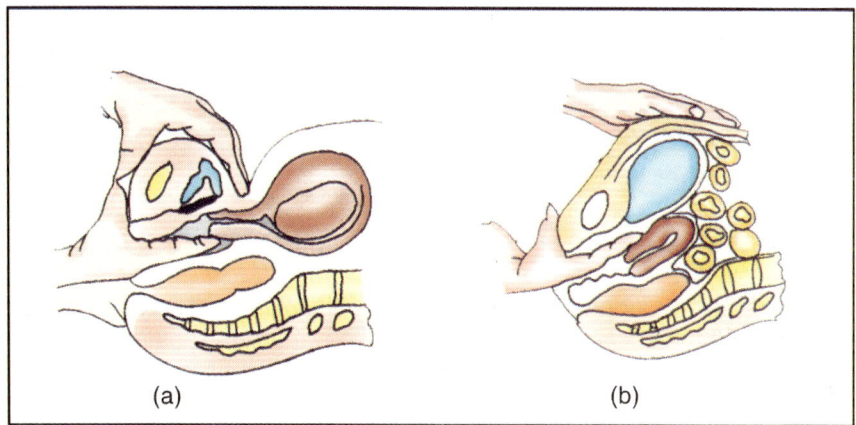

Fig. 18.7. Differentiation of a uterine from an adnexal mass (a) A uterine mass moves with the cervix (b) An adnexal mass does not move with the cervix

information regarding the mass. Fig. 18.7 shows the technique of differentiation of a uterine and adnexal mass.

- A fixed cystic mass could be a hydrosalpinx, encysted ascites (due to tuberculosis) or a neoplastic cyst which is adherent to the surrounding structures.
- A fixed nodular mass indicates malignancy
- Nodules in the Pouch of Douglas (POD) suggest a malignant tumour. Nodules can also be palpated in endometriosis.

Investigations

General investigations

These are carried out to assess the fitness of the woman for surgery and detect any metastases.

- Haemogram
- Liver function tests
- Renal function tests
- Serum electrolytes
- Chest x-ray PA view
- ECG

Specific

- *Ultrasound abdomen and pelvis* provides information regarding the pelvic mass, whether it is uterine or adnexal, it's nature (cystic or solid). A thin walled cyst indicates a benign cyst, whereas a thick walled cyst with septae or a solid ovarian tumour indicates it is malignant. The addition of colour Doppler gives more information regarding the nature of the tumour; increased blood flow in the ovarian vessels indicates a malignant ovarian tumour.

- *CECT scan of the abdomen and pelvis*–is helpful when ultrasound is not informative and in advanced stage disease for staging.

- *Tumour markers* The tumour markers useful in the differential diagnosis of an ovarian mass.

  CA 125–the normal level is <35 IU/l; the level is increased in malignant epithelial ovarian tumours, also in benign conditions eg. endometriosis or PID.

  CEA (Carcinoembronic antigen)–increased levels are seen in GI malignancies.

  AFP and beta HCG–increased levels are seen in malignant teratomas and choriocarcinoma respectively.

  Alkaline phosphatase and lactate dehydrogenase (LDH)–levels are increased in dysgerminoma.

  Testosterone–levels are increased in androgen secreting tumours.

- *Cytology of pleural fluid and Fine Needle Aspiration Cytology (FNAC)* of any clinically suspicious lymph nodes–a positive cytology indicates stage IV disease.

MANAGEMENT

The management is tailored for each patient taking into consideration the age of the patient, the type of ovarian tumour, the presence or absence of symptoms and if malignant, the stage of the disease.

Conservative management

Simple ovarian cysts <8 cm in diameter with normal CA125 should be observed and re-examined after 3-6 months. Surgery is indicated if the cyst significantly increases in size.

Surgery for ovarian tumours

The ***aims of surgery*** are

- Diagnostic–to know the nature of the tumour and to stage the disease
- Therapeutic–to excise benign lesions and debulk the malignant ones

Exploration of the abdomen: A vertical incision is given to allow exploration of the upper abdomen. A sample of ascitic fluid or peritoneal washings with normal saline should be taken for cytology. Scrapings should be taken from the undersurface of the diaphragm for cytology. Frozen section histology of the tumour is of limited value as thorough examination of the tumour is required to exclude invasive disease.

The *surgical options* are:

* Women <35 yrs.

    - Unilateral tumour (benign appearing)–*ovarian cystectomy* (excision of the cyst from the ovary) or *salpingo-oophorectomy* (removal of the tube and ovary) should be carried out.

    - If suspicious of malignancy–unilateral salpingo-oophorectomy is carried out and the peritoneal washings are taken for cytology. If the cytology is positive, chemotherapy is given in the postoperative period.

* Women 35-40 yrs.–treatment should be individualised based on the completeness of her family and the appearance of the tumour at surgery.

    Benign appearing–ovarian cystectomy or salpingo-oophorectomy.

    - If her family is complete, *total abdominal hysterectomy with bilateral salpingo-oophorectomy with omentectomy* is carried out, along with peritoneal washings for cytology.

    - If her family is not complete–conservative surgery can be carried out after thorough staging and counselling regarding the risk of recurrence.

* Advanced stage ovarian cancer–maximal cytoreductive surgery should be the aim to reduce the volume of residual disease to <1 cm.

* *Interventional debulking surgery*–A biopsy is taken at initial surgery followed by chemo-therapy and repeat surgery. It is still undergoing clinical trials at present.

* *Second-look surgery*–planned laparotomy at the end of chemotherapy has not been shown to improve survival and is not recommended routinely.

* *Laparoscopic surgery*–The indications are for diagnosis, when the nature of the pelvic mass is uncertain, or for the management of a benign simple ovarian cyst. The types of procedures performed are aspiration of fluid and fenestration of the cyst, cystectomy (enucleation of the cyst without cyst puncture), oophorectomy or salpingo-oophorectomy. The disadvantages of laparoscopic surgery are inability to stage the disease and the possibility of dissemination.

Adjuvant chemotherapy

Patients with residual epithelial ovarian cancer of >1cm following surgery and patients with stage Ic and higher, need adjuvant therapy to halt progression and prevent a relapse. The agents used are Carboplatin+Paclitaxel (CP) or Cisplatin+ Doxorubicin+ Cyclophosphamide (CAP) are given parenterally every three weekly for 6 cycles.

Newer therapies

Immunotherapy using a radio labelled antibody has shown response in small trials.

Management of non-epithelial ovarian tumours

- *Sex cord stromal tumours*–radical surgery is indicated in all stages due to the high risk of recurrence
- *Germ cell tumours–laparotomy with salpingo-oophorectomy* sparing fertility is the rule as even malignant germ cell tumours are very sensitive to chemotherapy. A combination of Bleomycin, Etoposide and Cisplatin (BEP) and Cisplatin, Vincristine, Methotrexate and Bleomycin (POMB) are used.

Survival rates

The five year survival rates for ovarian malignancies are
- Epithelial ovarian cancer
    - Stage I – IIa - 75-80%
    - Stage IIb – IV - 20-25%
- Germ cell tumours
    - Stage I - 95%
    - Advanced stage - 75%

19

Malignancies of the Vulva and Vagina

CARCINOMA VULVA

- Accounts for 3-5% of all female genital tract cancers.
- It is of two distinct types:
  - I. Well differentiated associated with lichen sclerosus and squamous hyperplasia.
  - II. Associated with VIN/HPV and preneoplastic lesions on the cervix, vagina and anus.

Aetiology–risk factors

- Poor genital hygiene and chronic irritation increase the risk
- HPV, 11 and 18, and HSV2 have been identified as the aetiological agents
- Smoking is identified as an important cofactor in HPV related vulvar tumours

Pathology

The commonest site is the anterior two-thirds of labium-majus. The clitoris and labia-minora may be involved. The lesion can present in 4 different forms.

- Ulcerative
- Fungating papillomatous (Fig. 19.1)

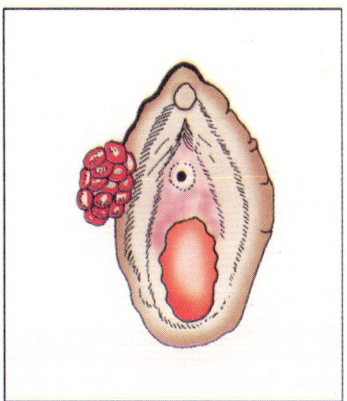

Fig. 19.1. Carcinoma vulva–polypoidal growth on the labia

247

- Flat plaque like
- Hypertrophic

Histological types

- Well differentiated squamous cell cancer (95%)
- Melanoma (4%)
- Adenocarcinoma (1%)
- Basal cell cancer <1%

Spread

- Direct (to urethra, vagina, rectum and the pelvic bones)
- Lymphatic spread (commonest)
- Haematogenous spread (rare)

Lymphatic spread

The spread is mainly by embolisation. Spread by lymphatics occurs to the ipsilateral side (Fig. 19.2). However, contralateral spread occurs in 25% of cases, especially if the tumour is involving the midline structures. Hence, bilateral groin node dissection is essential in all cases where the growth involves the clitoris, fourchette or anus.

Symptoms

- Pruritus
- Vulval swelling

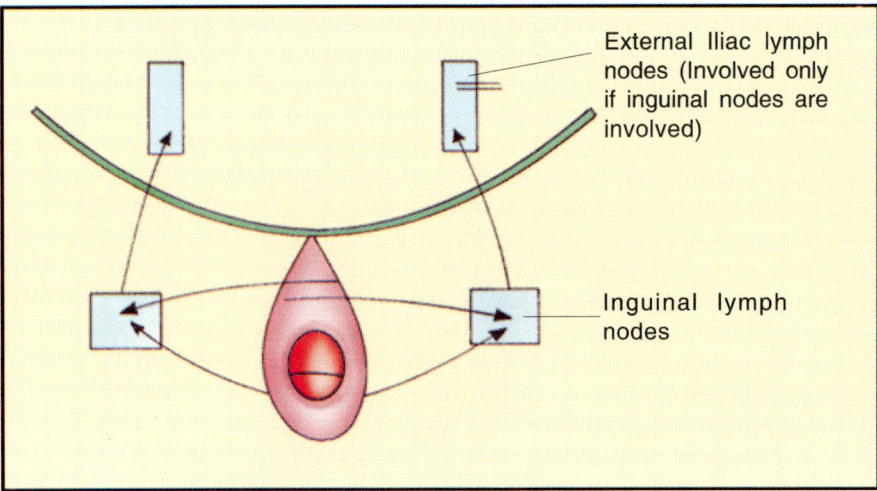

Fig. 19.2. Lymphatic drainage of the vulva

- Foul smelling discharge or bleeding
- Difficulty in urination

Signs

- Ulcerated or proliferative growth on the vulva
- Offensive discharge
- Enlarged inguinal lymph nodes
- Coexistent cancer of cervix, vagina or rectum
- Vulval and pedal edema

Investigations

1. *Cervical cytology* should be carried out in all patients due to the multicentric nature of genital cancer and the possibility of CIN.
2. *FNAC* of suspicious groin nodes.
3. *Chest X-ray* to detect metastases.

Diagnosis

- By typical clinical features
- Excisional biopsy by knife or punch biopsy forceps under local anaesthesia

Differential diagnosis

- Condyloma acuminata presents as warty, fleshy lesions
- Syphilitic ulcer–presents as presents as punched out lesions
- Tuberculous ulcer–edges can be undermined and are pigmented
- Soft sore (Chancroid)–presents as multiple superficial lesions

FIGO staging the staging of Ca vulva is as shown in the table 19.1.

Table 19.1. Clinical staging based on FIGO (1995)	
Stage 0	: Ca-in-situ, VIN3
Stage Ia	: Lesion confined to the vulva and <2 cm in diameter, stromal invasion <1mm
Stage Ib	: Confined to the vulva < 2 cm, stromal invasion is >1mm
Stage II	: Tumour confined to vulva > 2 cm, groin nodes not palpable
Stage III	: Tumour of any size with adjacent spread to the lower urethra / vagina / anus/ with unilateral regional lymph node metastasis
Stage IVa	: Tumour invades the upper urethra, bladder mucosa, rectal mucosa, pelvic bone or bilateral regional lymph nodes
Stage IVb	: Any distant metastases including pelvic lymph nodes

Causes of death

- Uraemia from ureteric obstruction due to enlarged common iliac and para-aortic nodes.
- Rupture of femoral vessels by enlarged inguinal lymph nodes
- Sepsis

Management of carcinoma vulva

Prevention

- Adequate therapy for non-neoplastic epithelial disorders
- Adequate therapy for persistent pruritus vulvae especially in postmenopausal women
- Maintaining good perineal hygiene
- Liberal use of simple vulvectomy in postmenopausal women with VIN where follow up facilities are not available.

Surgery

All patients with carcinoma vulva should be offered surgery regardless of their age and general condition. The options for surgery as per the stage of the disease are given in Flow chart 1. Prospective studies of women with tumour thickness of <1mm concluded that the safest course is to perform ipsilateral groin node dissection in all cases of clinical carcinoma, regardless of the depth of invasion or thickness of the tumour. The steps of modified radical vulvectomy, inguinal lymphadenectomy and wide excision are shown in Fig. 19.3a-c and 19.4.

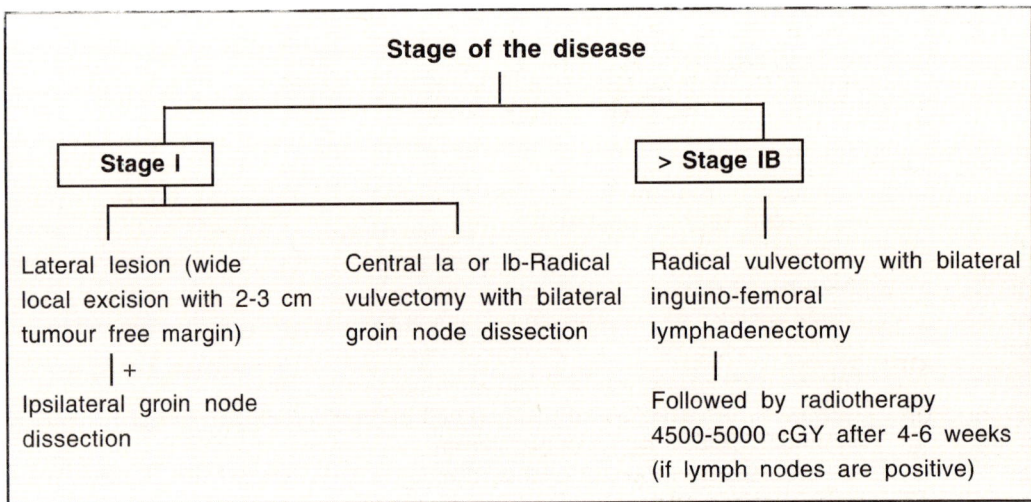

Flow chart 1.   Options for surgery in carcinoma vulva

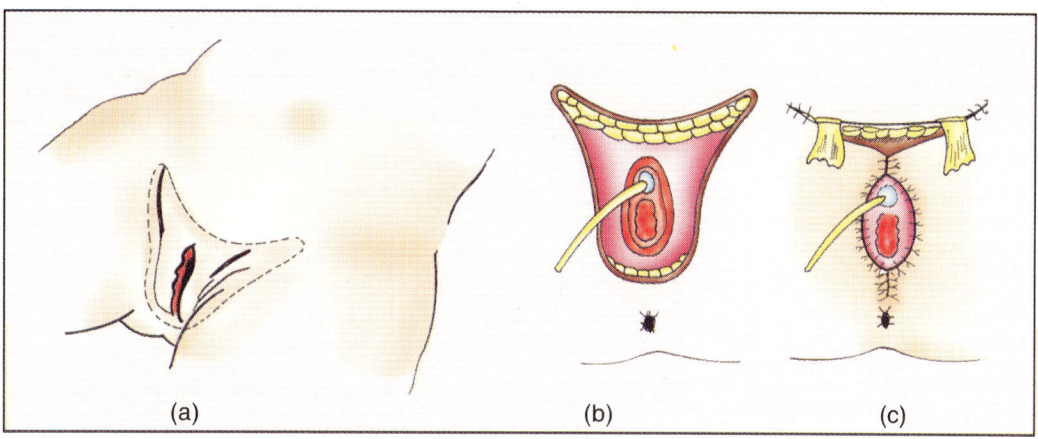

Fig.19.3a-c. Technique of modified radical vulvectomy (a&b) The whole vulval space skin and subcutaneous tissue are excised upto the periosteum (c) Closure of the wound with mobilisation of the skin

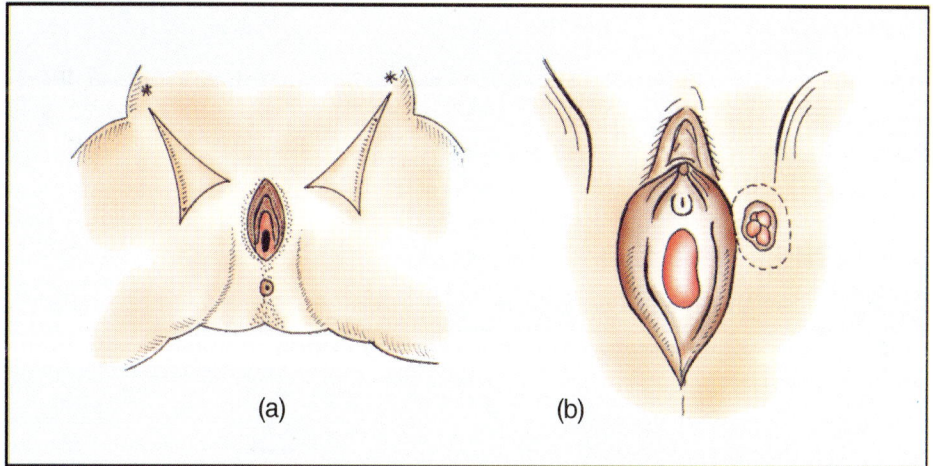

Fig. 19.4ab. (a) Inguinal lymphadenectomy using separate groin incisions (b) Wide excision of a lateral lesion

Post-op radiotherapy to the groin and pelvic nodes is given in patients with positive groin nodes (after an inguino-femoral lymphadenectomy).

Complications of vulvectomy

- Wound breakdown and infection–the commonest complication. Treatment is with liquid honey packs
- Osteitis pubis
- Venous thromboembolism

- Secondary haemorrhage
- Chronic leg edema
- Numbness and paraesthesia over the anterior thigh due to division of small cutaneous branches of the femoral nerve.
- Loss of body image and impaired sexual function.

Adjuvant therapy

- Primary radiotherapy is given in patients unfit for surgery.
- Neoadjuvant chemotherapy before surgery (Cisplatin and 5 FU) is given in patients with large tumours involving the urethra, vagina or anus, to facilitate surgery and reduce morbidity.
- *Chemoradiation:* Pre-op chemotherapy with Cisplatin followed by radiotherapy for advanced disease in the groin nodes or vulva produces complete response in upto 30% of patients and reduces the need for radical surgery. The recurrence rates with this modality are very high at present.

MELANOMA

- Second most common cancer of vulva.
- Overall prognosis is poor.
- Presents as patchy diffusely pigmented raised areas.
- Radical surgery is the mainstay of treatment.
- Radiotherapy and chemotherapy are not effective.

CARCINOMA OF THE VAGINA

Least common of the genital tract malignancies, accounts for 1-2% of all genital tract cancers.

Aetiology The theories postulated are:

1. Immunosuppresion with multicentric neoplasia of cervix, vagina and vulva suggests infection with HPV.
2. Chronic irritation due to vaginal pessaries or procidentia.

Pathology

- 92% squamous cell cancers

- Upper vagina commonest site.
- Spread–is initially by local invasion. Lymphatic spread by tumour embolisation to the pelvic nodes from the upper vagina and pelvis and vaginal nodes from the lower vagina. The staging of carcinoma vagina is given Table 19.2.

Clinical features

Criteria to make a diagnosis of primary vaginal cancer.

- The primary site of growth should be in the vagina.
- Uterine cervix should not be involved.
- There is no clinical evidence that the vaginal tumour is metastatic disease.

Symptoms

- Vaginal bleeding–commonest symptom
- Vaginal discharge
- Pelvic pain
- Asymptomatic

Examination

- Papillomatous or ulcerative growth on the vaginal walls.
- Rectovaginal examination indicates the extent of spread.

Table 19.2. FIGO staging of carcinoma vagina	
STAGE	**DEFINITION**
St 0	Intraepithelial neoplasia
St I	Invasive carcinoma confined to the vaginal mucosa
St II	Sub-vaginal infiltration not extending to the pelvic wall
St III	Infiltration upto the pelvic wall
St IVa	Involvement mucosa of the bladder or rectum
St IVb	Spread beyond the pelvis

Investigations To know the extent of spread are colposcopy, cystoscopy, proctosigmoidoscopy, chest x-ray, trans-rectal ultrasound and MRI.

Treatment The options are:

1. *Radiotherapy*

    Interstitial with Iridium 192 for early cases i.e. stage I-IIa

    Teletherapy to the pelvis for cases with para-metrial involvement.

2. *Surgery*

    Radical hysterectomy, radical vaginectomy and pelvic lymphadenectomy for stage I lesions in the upper vagina.

    Pelvic exenteration for tumours involving the bladder or rectum.

20

Radiation Therapy in Gynaecological Cancer

Radiation therapy is a clinical modality dealing with the use of ionizing radiation in the treatment of a patient with malignant disease and occasionally benign diseases. The aim of radiation therapy is to deliver a precisely measured dose of radiation to a defined volume.

PRINCIPLES OF RADIOTHERAPY

In radiation therapy, X-rays and electron beams are directed at tumours which in turn interact with the subcellular constituents of the tumour and impart energy to them. Ionization is thereby produced, causing biological changes. All the basic particles which make up atoms are ionizing radiation and can be used to kill cells. Various kinds of radiation are emitted from radioactive nuclei. These may be α particles, β particles, protons, neutrons, γ rays etc.

Radiosensitivity

Radiosensitivity is the speed of regression of a tumour from radiation. Differences in radiosensitivity of various tumours are explained by four principles–

1. Hypoxia–hypoxic cells are relatively resistant to radiation.
2. Proportion of clonogenic cells–proliferating cells are more radiosensitive.
3. Inherent radiosensitivity of the tumour cells.
4. Repair of radiation damage–greater the repair of potentially lethal damage, less curable is the tumour.

Time dose factors

Fractionation allows for delivery of effective treatment to the tumour with minimum complications due to exposure of normal tissues. Radiation time dose factors are governed by the 4R's of ionizing radiation—

1. Repair of sublethal damage and potentially lethal damage to DNA in normal tissues

2. Repopulation of normal cells.

3. Redistribution of cells throughout the cell cycle so that more cells are in the radio sensitive phase.

4. Reoxygenation of hypoxic tumours.

The **cell cycle** (Fig. 20.1) is divided into four phases G_1, S, G_2 and M. The radiosensitivity of proliferating cells varies in the different phases of the cell cycle. The maximally affected are cells in G_2 and M phases of the cell cycle. Cells are most resistant in the late S phase.

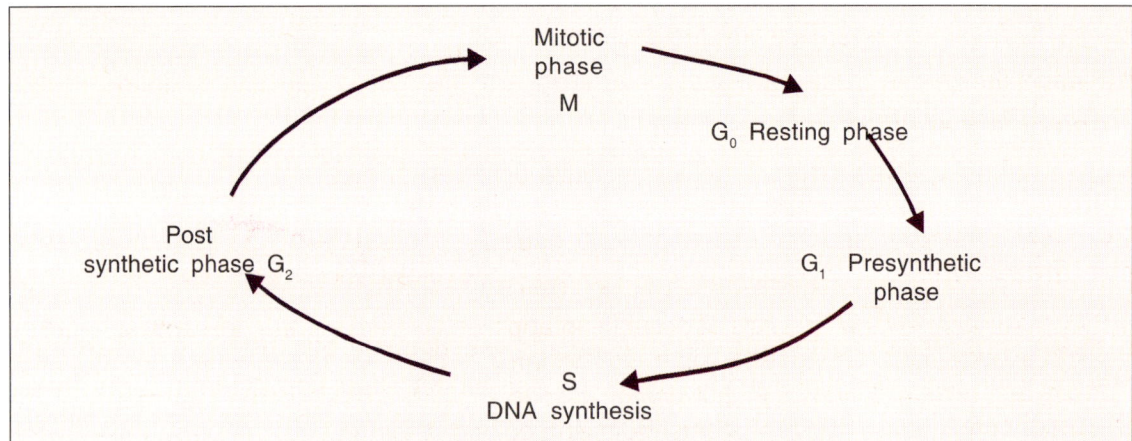

Fig. 20.1. The cell cycle

Radiation biology

DNA is the principal cellular target of ionizing radiation. Radiation effect may be *Direct* or *Indirect*. Radiation may *directly* interact causing ionization and excitation of the critical target molecule in the cells or it may produce biological damage through the generation of free radicals-known as the *indirect effect*.

Radiotherapy techniques

Teletherapy

Refers to application of radiation where radiation source is placed at a distance from the patient. Most commonly used teletherapy source is cobalt in our country. Linear accelerators which use x-rays or electrons are the preferred ones in developed countries. External beam pelvic radiation is delivered before intracavitary insertions in patients with

1. Bulky cervical lesions, to improve the geometry of the intracavitary application.

2. Exophytic, easily bleeding tumours

3. Tumours with necrosis or infection

4. Tumours with parametrial involvement

Brachytherapy

Refers to radiation therapy where radioactive sources are placed close to or within the tumour. Here dose to the healthy tissues is kept low while giving high radiation doses to the tumour. Several isotopes are available for brachytherapy eg. Radium, Cobalt, Cesium and Iridium. Cesium Cs^{137} is the most popular.

Of these radium is now obsolete because of–

* it's high photon energy (shielding problems)

* long half life

* possible leakage of radon gas and

* possible eruption of the source due to build up of helium gas

Two types of brachytherapy application are used in gynaecological cancers, *Interstitial* and *Intracavitary.*

i) *Intracavitary method* consists of positioning applications (bearing the radioactive sources) into a body cavity in close proximity to the target tissue. These are temporary implants and are removed after the delivery of a specified dose of radiation. The most widely used technique is insertion of a tandem and colpostat for treatment of carcinoma cervix (Fig. 20.2). A *Tandem* is a tube which is inserted through the external os of the cervix

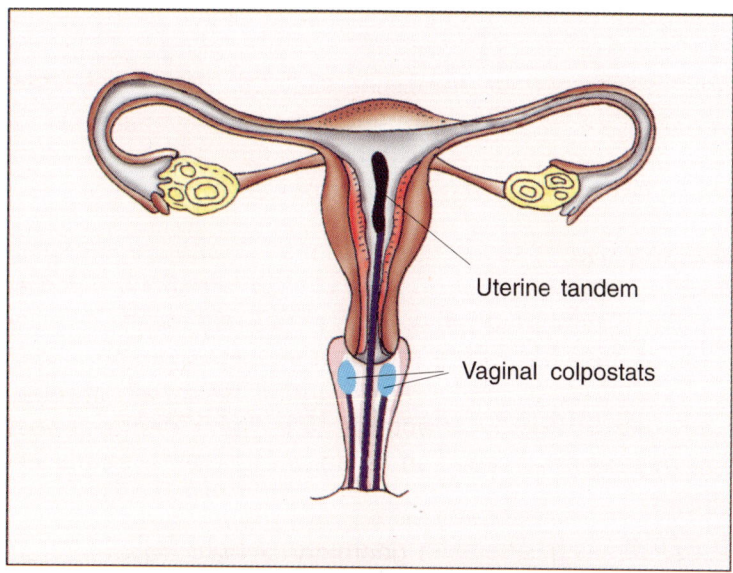

Uterine tandem

Vaginal colpostats

Fig. 20.2. Brachytherapy for cervical cancer

into the uterus and into which a source can be after loaded. *Ovoids or Colpostats* are devices which are placed in the fornices of the vagina. The doses delivered using these devices are calculated according to the maximum tolerable doses of surrounding tissues. The anatomical points used for cervical and uterine treatment are point A and point B. A is defined as 2 cm superior to the external cervical os and 2 cm lateral to the cervical canal. This is the point where the uterine artery crosses the ureter. Point B is defined as 3 cm lateral to point A in the same plane or 5 cm lateral to the uterine axes. This represents the lateral pelvic wall. The dose limiting normal structure here is the rectal and bladder mucosa.

With intracavitary therapy, there is a rapid dose fall off as a function of the distance, a high dose being given to the uterus and the paracervical tissues, but is inadequate to treat the pelvic lymph nodes. External irradiation is necessary to supplement the dose. The parametrium is therefore primarily treated with external irradiation.

Radiographs are always obtained using a dummy source; the active sources inserted after the films have been reviewed and the position of the applicators has been judged satisfactory. A vaginal pack soaked in 40% iodinated contrast material is used to identify it on radiographs.

In general, an intrauterine tandem with three or four Cs^{137} sources is inserted in the uterus, two colpostats are placed in the vaginal vault and packed with iodoform gauze to deliver 0.6 to 0.8 Gy/hr to pt. A.

ii) *Interstitial brachytherapy* consists of surgically implanting a small radioactive source directly into the target tissues. The implant procedures may be classified in terms of source loading techniques-preloaded, manually afterloaded or remotely afterloaded, the last one being the preferred as it provides protection to the health personnels.

Brachytherapy can also divided on the basis of dose rates delivered.

(Low Dose Rate)   LDR   0.4 to 2 Gy/hr

(High Dose Rate)   HDR   > 12 Gy/hr

Interstitial implants with Ra^{226}, Cs^{137} needles or Ir^{192} afterloading plastic catheters to limited tumour volumes are helpful in specific clinical situations, such as those patients with a localized residual tumour or with parametrial extension.

COMPLICATIONS OF RADIOTHERAPY

Early complications

- Transient nausea, vomiting, anorexia, diarrhoea, weight loss
- Bladder irritation causing frequency, dysuria or haematuria

- Rectal irritation leading to tenesmus and diarrhoea
- Malaise and irritability
- Flare up of sepsis, tubo-ovarian mass, pyometra, peritonitis and septicaemia
- Pyelitis, pyelonephritis and cystitis
- Pyrexia
- Skin reactions

Late complications

- Persistent anaemia
- Chronic pelvic pain due to fibrosis involving the nerve trunks
- Pyometra
- Proctitis followed later by radiation ulcers, rectal bleeding, rectal strictures, and rarely recto-vaginal fistula
- Post irradiation ulcers in the bladder causing dysuria, haematuria, or a vesico-vaginal fistula
- Small bowel strictures, obstruction, ulceration and gut perforation
- Colonic ulcer, telangiectasis, perforation, stricture or obstruction
- Atrophic vaginitis, fibrosis and vaginal stenosis
- Ureteric stricture and obstructive uropathy
- Osteoporosis, fracture neck of femur
- Psychological complications
- Ovarian destruction causing severe menopausal symptoms along with osteoporosis

INDICATIONS OF RADIOTHERAPY IN GYNAECOLOGICAL MALIGNANCIES

Radiotherapy can be used for curative or palliative treatment.

As palliative therapy it is useful for:

- Intractable bleeding in advanced cervical cancer
- Management of bone metastases
- Management of intractable pain
- Impending vertebral collapse/spinal cord compression
- Management of brain metastases
- Management of malignant pleural effusion

1. Carcinoma of the cervix

Carcinoma cervix is the commonest malignancy to affect the female population in developing countries. In countries where papanicolaou smear screening of masses is used, there is a marked decline in the number of invasive cervical cancers. Early stage cervical carcinoma is treatable and largely curable by radiotherapy. Patients should be treated with close collaboration between the gynaecologic oncologist and the radiation oncologist, and an integrated team approach should be vigorously pursued.

Carcinoma in situ

- Patients with carcinoma in situ, which may include those with severe dysplasia, are usually treated with a total abdominal hysterectomy with or without a small vaginal cuff.

- Occasionally, when the patient wishes to have more children, carcinoma in situ may be treated conservatively with a therapeutic conization, laser or cryotherapy.

- Indications of radiotherapy in in situ carcinoma—

    1. Patients with strong medical contraindications for surgery.

    2. Extension of the lesion to the vaginal wall.

    3. Multifocal carcinoma in situ in both the cervix and the vagina.

Stage Ia

Early invasive carcinoma of the cervix is usually treated with a total abdominal or a modified radical hysterectomy, but it can also be treated with intracavitary radioactive source alone (60 to 75 Gy to point A, in one or two insertions, respectively).

Stage Ib to IIa

Radical hysterectomy is used primarily because of the inability of the intracavitary sources to encompass all the tumour in a high dose volume, large doses of external irradiation to the whole pelvis are necessary.

Stage IIb, III and IVa

Patients with stage IIb and III tumours are treated with irradiation alone. Patients with stage IVa disease can be treated either with high doses of external irradiation to the whole pelvis, intracavitary insertions and additional parametrial irradiation or with pelvic exenteration.

Postoperative RT

Patients who have undergone radical hysterectomy with no preoperative radiation therapy are considered for postoperative radiation therapy if they have high-risk factors which are—

- Positive pelvic lymph nodes
- Microscopically positive tumour extending to <3mm of the margins
- Deep stromal invasion
- Vascular or lymphatic permeation

Extreme care should be exercised in designing postoperative irradiation treatment techniques, including intracavitary insertions. Because of the surgical extirpation of the uterus, the bladder and the recto-sigmoid may be closer to the radioactive sources than in patients with an intact uterus.

When metastatic pelvic lymph nodes are present, treatment consists of 50Gy to the whole pelvis delivered with a four field technique. Patients with positive common iliac or para-aortic nodes should receive 50Gy to the para-aortic region as well.

2. Carcinoma of the endometrium

Majority of patients of uterine corpus cancer present with early stage disease. Surgery is the conventional mode of therapy, the operation of choice is total abdominal hysterectomy and bilateral salpingo-oophorectomy. Adenocarcinoma of body of uterus is moderately radiosensitive. The postoperative adjuvant radiotherapy can be external irradiation, vaginal irradiation or both. The patients who should receive postoperative radiotherapy are—

1. Stage Ia or Ib with histologically grade 3 disease
2. Stage Ic G_1-G_3
3. Patients who have vaginal spread upto the margins, spread to the adnexa or pelvic lymph nodes.

Currently, post-op vaginal vault radiotherapy is recommended for all stage Ia-Ib (G_3) and Ic (all grades) patients. Additional pelvic RT is given to stage Ic patients.

Intravaginal radiotherapy is delivered by either vaginal ovoids or by the vaginal cylinder. Both low dose and high dose rates are used now-a-days, mostly with an afterloading system. The aim is to deliver between 50-60 Gy to vaginal epithelium, when given as intravaginal irradiation alone.

Patients with stage IV and recurrent disease with vaginal bleeding and pain can be relieved with a palliative radiotherapy course of 20Gy in 5 fractions.

Carcinoma of the ovary

The primary treatment is surgical. The indications of radiotherapy for carcinoma of ovary are—

1. In patients with bulky postoperative residual disease, Whole Abdomen Radiotherapy (WAR) is added as a consolidated treatment to decrease the risk of intra-abdominal recurrence.

2. Palliative radiotherapy is given in patients with metastatic disease to the bone, brain and liver.

Carcinoma of the fallopian tube

The primary treatment of adenocarcinoma of the fallopian tube is surgical resection at the time of initial diagnosis including total abdominal hysterectomy, omentectomy and bilateral salpingectomy as well as sampling of the ascitic fluid or peritoneal washings and peritoneal sampling of the diaphragm, bladder and bowel.

Postoperative radiation therapy has been a traditional form of therapy for fallopian tube carcinoma with dissemination or recurrence. The best results are with a total dose greater then 50 Gy in 5 to 6 weeks with megavoltage therapy.

Carcinoma of the vagina

The surgery involved is radical, involving exenteration of the pelvis and diversion of urine and to form a colostomy. If the tumour extends to the lower two thirds of the vagina, surgery involves removal of vagina along with total vulvectomy. As the surgery involved is extensive, radiotherapy is commonly selected as the primary treatment.

Paravaginal or parametrial interstitial implants or both should be considered if residual tumour is present after the planned external and intracavitary therapy has been completed.

Carcinoma of the vulva

The preferred method of treatment is surgery, which varies from wide local excision to partial vulvectomy; depending on the extent and multiplicity of intraepithelial lesions and the patients wish to preserve the vulva.

The indications of radiotherapy after radical vulvectomy and lymphadenectomy are:

1. Three or more positive groin nodes

2. Extracapsular extension of metastatic neck nodes

3. Extension of tumour to urethra, vagina and anal area

4. Primary tumour equal to or more than 4 cm

5. Positive surgical margins.

21

Chemotherapy in Gynaecological Cancer

Since the initiation of chemotherapy from the extended use of mustard gas in world war I many developments have taken place. A number of new drugs have been found, which are important in the treatment of gynaecological cancer.

THE BASICS OF CHEMOTHERAPY

The Cell Cycle: It is important to understand the cell-cycle kinetics for proper use of antineoplastic drugs. Many of the potent cytotoxic agents act by damaging the DNA during the various phases of cell division. Their toxicity is greater during the S, or DNA synthetic phase of the cell cycle; while vinca alkaloids and taxanes, block the formation of the mitotic spindle in the M-phase and hence are active only against rapidly dividing cells (Fig. 21.1).

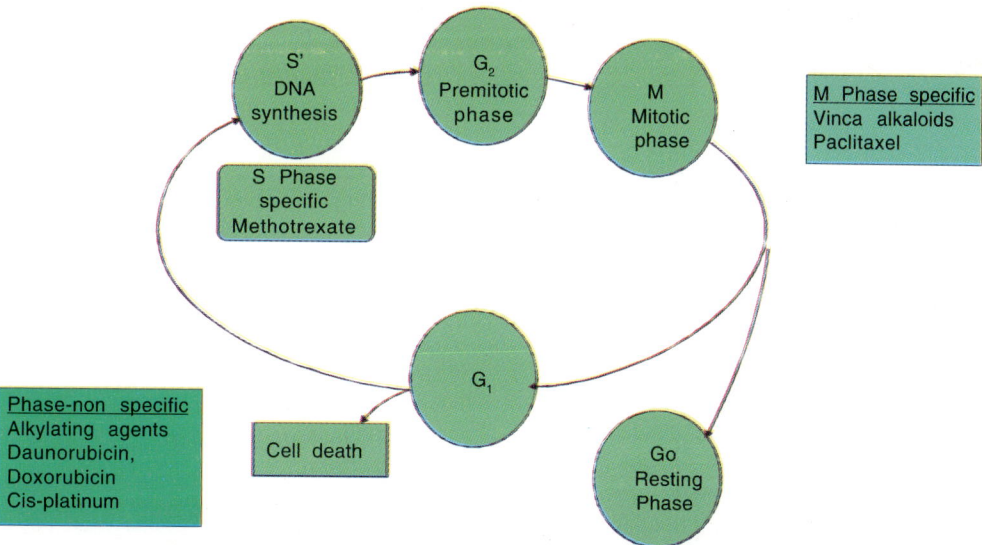

Fig. 21.1. The cell cycle and the site of action of anti-cancer drugs

263

The cell cycle may be characterized as follows:

1. Presynthetic (G_1) phase
2. Synthetic (S) phase: where DNA synthesis occurs
3. Premitotic phase (G_2)–termination of DNA synthesis
4. Mitotic (M) phase–DNA division occurs
5. Resting (G0) phase–taken up by some cells

Damaged cells that reach the G_1/S boundary undergo apoptosis, or programmed cell death; in the presence of a normal p53 gene as a checkpoint. If the checkpoint function fails, the damaged cells are not diverted to the apoptotic pathway. These cells will proceed through the S-phase and some will emerge as a drug-resistant population.

COMMONLY USED ANTI-CANCER DRUGS IN GYNAECOLOGICAL CANCER

The commonly used drugs, their mode of action and toxic effects are given in table 21.1.

Combination Chemotherapy: Combination of drugs acting at different inter-cellular targets are combined to have a synergistic effect. The advantages are a lower incidence of side-effects and development of resistance to individual drugs.

Multiple doses: These are needed as each cycle of therapy kills <99% of cells, it is necessary to repeat treatment in multiple cycles to kill all the tumour cells.

Table 21.1. Anti-cancer drugs: Mode of action and toxic effects

Class of drug	Mode of action	Toxicity
Alkylating agents: Cyclophosphamide Chlorambucil Ifosfamide Melphalan Treosulphan Platinum compounds (Cisplatin and Carboplatin) Gemcitabine	• Cross-link DNA strands by forming covalent bonds between highly reactive alkylating groups and nitrogen groups • Prevent division of the helix at mitosis> imperfect division > cell death	• Vomitings • Bone marrow suppression • Alopecia (Cyclophosphamide and Ifosfamide) • Chemical cystitis (Cyclophosphamide) • Nephrotoxicity (Cisplatin) • Myelotoxicity (Carboplatin) • Encephalopathy (Ifosfamide) • Peripheral neuropathy (Cisplatin)
Antimetabolites: Methotrexate 5-Flurouracil (5-FU)	Closely resemble metabolites essential for	• Oral ulceration (Methotrexate)

	synthesis of nucleic acids and proteins; get incorporated into natural metabolic pathways and enzyme systems and disrupt cell mechanism **Methotrexate**-Folic acid antagonist and inhibits dihydrofolate reductase in the synthesis of nitrogen bases of DNA **5-FU**-Pyramidine analogue which blocks thymidine synthesis and inhibits the incorporation of uracil into DNA	• Myelosuppression (5-FU)
Vinca alkaloids: (derivatives of the periwinkle plant, Vinca rosea) Vincristine Vinblastine Vindesine Vinorelbin	Metaphase arrest by acting on the micro-tubules of the mitotic spindle	Peripheral neuropathy (Vincristine)
Etoposide: Semi-synthetic derivative of podophyllotoxin	Acts on the cells in the G_2 phase in the cell cycle	• Myelosuppression • Alopecia
Antibiotics: Actinomycin D Doxorubicin (Adriamycin) Daunorubicin Bleomycin	Form irreversible complexes with DNA	• Alopecia • Myelosuppression • Cardiomyopathy (Epirubicin and Mitozantrone are less cardiotoxic) • Increased pigmentation • Pulmonary fibrosis
Taxanes: Paclitaxel (Taxol) Docitaxel (Taxotere)	Cytotoxic effects on the microtubules	• Total alopecia • Skin toxicity • Oedema • Bone marrow suppression
Hormones: Medroxyprogesterone acetate	Suppressive effect on endometrial cancer	• Fluid retention
Interferons:	Alter the host response to cancer	

Investigations necessary before starting chemotherapy

- Haemogram and platelet count as all the chemotherapeutic agents suppress the actively dividing cells in the bone marrow.
- Liver and renal function tests to know the renal and liver function as the drugs could be hepato/ nephro toxic.
- Urine routine and microscopy
- Chest X-ray PA view
- Details of operative findings (to know the extent and location of residual disease).
- Histopathology and grade of the tumour.
- CT scan of the abdomen and pelvis for staging and to know the amount of residual disease.
- Tumour markers: Serum CA 125 (in epithelial ovarian cancer), hCG (in gestational trophoblastic disease and teratomas), alphafetoprotein (in teratomas) LDH (in dysgerminomas).
- Echocardiography or MUGA scan (for women >45 yrs. or earlier if indicated).

CHEMOTHERAPY REGIMES IN GYNAECOLOGICAL MALIGNANCIES

Various combination chemotherapy regimes are used which have been found to be highly effective (table 21.2).

Table 21.2. Chemotherapy regimes in gynaecological cancers

1. Epithelial ovarian cancer
   - Cisplatin and Cyclophosphamide (CP)
   - Carboplatin and Cyclophosphamide
2. Dysgerminoma ovary–Bleomycin, Etoposide and Cisplatin (BEP)
3. Cervical cancer–Cisplatin, Ifosfamide and 5-FU
4. Gestational Trophoblastic Disease
   - Single agent Methotrexate
   - Etoposide, Methotrexate, Actinomycin-D, Cyclophosphamide and Vincristine (EMACO)

1. Epithelial ovarian cancer (EOC)

- ***Early stage (stage I and II)***
   - i) Stage Ia and Ib (grade I and II) do not need adjuvant chemotherapy
   - ii) Stage Ia, Ib (high grade), Ic and stage II-need adjuvant chemotherapy with 4-6 cycles of Paclitaxel and Platinum analogues

- *Advanced disease (stage III and IV)* Cytoreductive surgery is carried out primarily to reduce the tumour load followed by postoperative chemotherapy with Paclitaxel+ Platinum analogues (Cisplatin or Carboplatin).

- *Commonly used chemotherapy regimes are:*

  i) Inj Paclitaxel 135 mg/m^2 IV 24 hrs. infusion on D1

     Inj Cisplatin 75 mg/m^2 on D2

     The cycle is repeated 3 weekly for 6 cycles

  ii) Inj Paclitaxel 175 mg/m^2 IV infusion on D1

      Inj Carboplatin (dose calculated by area under curve) on D2

  The cycle is repeated 3 weekly for 6 cycles.

- *Neoadjuvant chemotherapy* In advanced ovarian cancer, initial chemotherapy is given in 3-4 cycles followed by surgery. This reduces the tumour volume, which facilitates surgery and reduces the postoperative morbidity. This form of chemo-therapy is undergoing trials at present.

2. Dysgerminoma ovary

- Initial surgery with bilateral salpingo-oophorectomy

- Stage Ia: no further treatment is needed.

- Bleomycin, Etoposide and Cisplatin (BEP) are given in combination for stage Ib-IV in 3-4 cycles.

- Radiotherapy which used to be given earlier has been given up in favour of chemotherapy due to the risk of ovarian failure and sterility with radiotherapy.

3. Cervical cancer

- Surgery and radiotherapy are the primary modalities of treatment.

- Chemotherapy given prior to radiotherapy or surgery (neoadjuvant or induction chemotherapy) or concurrently with radiotherapy (RT), helps in reducing tumour size, thus improving local control. It may also control micro-metastases at distant sites as well as in regional lymph nodes and improves the overall survival.

- The most effective drugs are Cisplatin, Ifosfamide and 5-Florouracil

4. Gestational trophoblastic disease

- Persistent Gestational Trophoblastic Disease (GTD) is diagnosed by the presence of persistently elevated beta hCG levels 9-11 weeks following evacuation or by a plateau in the level that persists for more than 3 weeks.

- *Prophylactic chemotherapy* The risk of persistent GTD is higher in older patients

(>39 yrs.), those with very high beta hCG levels, with excessive uterine enlargement at diagnosis; and in those with a history of multiple molar pregnancies. Studies have shown that prophylactic chemotherapy following evacuation of a complete molar pregnancy can reduce the risk of postmolar GTD by about 70%. At AIIMS, it is our policy to give prophylactic chemotherapy to all such patients following evacuation.

Chemotherapy regimes Chemotherapy is given as per the stage of the disease or by assessing the prognosis by prognostic scoring.

Prognostic Scoring

A modified FIGO scoring is given in chapter 9. Patients in low and medium risk category are given single agent chemotherapy with methotrexate and folinic acid. Those in the high risk group are given combination chemotherapy with EMA-CO regime.

Stage I (limited to the uterus)

- Methotrexate 1 mg/kg IV push on days 1, 3, 5, and 7
- Folinic acid 6 mg/m2 IV push on day 2, 4, 6 and 8

  The cycle is repeated every 2 weeks (calculating from day 1) till 3 consecutive weekly values of beta hCG are negative. Patients hypersensitive to methotrexate are given actinomycin-D.

  Hysterectomy is indicated in patients with placental site trophoblastic tumour (PSTT) who do not wish to remain fertile.

Stage II (vaginal metastases)

- Low or medium risk-single agent methotrexate and folinic acid.

Stage III (lung metastases)

- Combination chemotherapy with EMA-CO (Etoposide, Methotrexate, Actinomycin-D alternating with Cyclophosphamide and Vincristine) regimen.

Stage IV (cerebral metastases)

- Primary combination chemotherapy with EMA-CO regime
- Whole brain irradiation to reduce the risk of haemorrhage due to the tumour.

Section IV

Contraception and Medical Termination of Pregnancy

22

Contraception

On 11th May, 2000, India crossed a population of 1 billion with the birth of baby Astha. India's current annual increase in population of 15.5 million is large enough to neutralize efforts to conserve the resource endowment and environment. Hence, there is an urgent need to promote contraceptive practices.

A method or a system which allows intercourse and yet prevents conception is called a **contraceptive method**. A contraceptive could be used temporarily and be reversible (temporary method) or be permanent with no chance of reversibility.

Contraception is a reversible temporary prevention of fertility (active method) as opposed to **sterilization** which is both terminal and permanent. A contraceptive method should ideally be safe, long-acting, highly effective in preventing conception and be reversible.

METHODS OF CONTRACEPTION

The various methods available are given in the table 22.1.

Contraceptive failure rate Pregnancy rates with various types of contraceptives is expressed as the number of pregnancies per 100 women after 1 year of usage as the number per 100 woman years.

IUD event rates Incidence of an adverse events such as expulsion, removal for medical reasons, and pregnancy, at various times after the insertion of an IUD.

Method effectiveness The rate of effectiveness when the contraceptive method is always used correctly (also called *Perfect use*).

Pearl index A method used to determine the failure (pregnancy) rate of any contraceptive technique:

$$\text{Pregnancy rate} = \frac{\text{No. of pregnancies x 1200}}{\text{Women - months of use}}$$

Hence, Failure rate = Pregnancy rate per 100 woman years.

Use effectiveness used to the rate overall effectiveness in actual use for a specific contraceptive method (also called *Typical use*).

Table 22.1. Methods of contraception

I. Natural methods
- Abstinence
- Coitus Interruptus
- Lactational amenorrhoea method (LAM)

II. Barrier contraceptives
- Condoms
- Spermicidal agents
- Douching
- Occlusive devices
- Hormones altering cervical mucus

III. Intrauterine devices (IUD)
- Inert devices
- Copper containing devices
- Hormone containing devices

IV. Suppression of spermatogenesis
- Gossypol
- Testosterone enanthate
- GnRH analogues
- Medroxyprogesterone acetate

V. Hormonal contraceptives
- Short-acting–oral pills
- Long-acting–injectables, implants and vaginal rings

VI. Postcoital contraceptives/emergency contraceptives

VII. Surgical sterilization
- Male
- Female

NATURAL METHODS

1. Abstinence during the fertile phase

This depends upon the avoidance of sexual intercourse during the fertile period i.e., period of ovulation. Calculation of this period is as per the methods given below. It depends upon the individual woman's previous menstrual cycles and follows two assumptions;

i) Ovum is capable of being fertilized for only about 24 hrs. after ovulation

ii) A spermatozoon has the capacity to fertilize for only 72 hrs., though this rapidly diminishes after 24 hrs.

a) ***Calender / rhythm method*** Ovulation usually occurs 14 ± 2 days prior (12-16 days) to the onset of the subsequent menstrual cycle. Therefore, intercourse between the 9th and 17th day may result in pregnancy. Alternatively a woman may calculate her ***fertile period (or risk period)*** by subtracting 18 days from the length of her previous shortest cycle and 11 days from her pervious longest cycle. Rest of the days would be a *'safe period'.*

Pregnancy rates are high ranging from 14.4 to 47 per 100 woman years.

b) ***Mucus method (Billing's or Ovulation method)*** Oestrogen makes the cervical mucus copious, clear, slippery and elastic reaching a peak in the mid cycle 'peak mucus day'; thereafter it becomes thicker, opaque, scanty and dry due to progesterone effects. Intercourse is considered safe during 'dry days' with scanty mucus and 4 days after the peak day. In a WHO study, the failure rate calculated was 19.6%.

c) ***Temperature method*** A woman is required to note her basal body temperature (BBT) immediately on waking up. A rise in the BBT indicates progesterone influence, as progesterone is thermogenic. She is hence advised to abstain from coitus until the 3rd consecutive day of elevated BBT.

d) ***Symptothermal method*** A combination of the above three methods is the most effective natural method. Calender method and change in mucus method require the calculation of the beginning of risk period (fertile phase) with the end predicted by use of the basal body temperature.

2. Withdrawal method (Coitus interruptus)

Withdrawal of the penis just before ejaculation is a common method. It has a pregnancy rate of 25 per 100-woman years, since the prostatic fluid secreted prior to ejaculation frequently contains the active sperms.

3. Lactational amenorrhoea method (LAM)

Breast feeding provides more than 98% protection from pregnancy during the first six months postpartum if the mother is fully or nearly fully breast feeding and has not experienced vaginal bleeding after the 56th day postpartum.

BARRIER CONTRACEPTIVES

Barrier methods are effective for the motivated women with the advantage of reducing the rates of transmission of sexually transmitted diseases. However, the lack of bathroom facilities and privacy in the low socioeconomic groups deprives its wider use in India.

The types of barrier contraceptive available are given table 22.2.

Table 22.2. Types of barrier contraceptives
Condoms
Spermicidal agents
Douching
Cervical occlusive devices
– Dutch cap
– Cervical cap/vimule
– Dumas cap
– Contra-cap
Female condom (*Femshield*)
Sponge (*Today*)
Drugs altering cervical mucus

a) **Condoms** Condoms are made of very thin rubber and completely cover the penis.

   Advantages it is easily available, cheap, easy to carry, free from side effects, and requires no instructions. It emphasizes the male involvement and is the most effective means of preventing transmission of sexually transmitted diseases and HIV. It prevents sperm allergy and reduces the chances of cancer of cervix. Further, it has no adverse effects on the fetus, if the method fails.

   Disadvantages High failure rate of 10-14/100 woman years, partly due to bursting of the condom and partly due to non-compliance. The method is coitus dependant and some couples do not draw full sexual satisfaction.

b) **Spermicidal agents** These are chemicals that kill the sperms before the latter can gain access to the cervical canal. They usually contain surfactants such as nanoxynol 9(N9), octoxynon and enzyme inhibiting agents. These are available as foam tablets, soluble pessaries, creams, jellies, or film along with other barrier contraceptives.

   Used alone, the failure rate is high, approx. 30 per 100 woman years, but in conjunction with mechanical barriers they are an effective alternative. They are effective for 1-2 hrs. after application, and have no risk of congenital malformations. Some concerns have been expressed with N-9 causing higher HIV transmission due to local irrigation and breach of the vaginal epithelium.

ORF 13900, which agglutinates sperms, inhibits the sperm's acrosin and alters the mucus–sperm interaction. It is being evaluated as a spermicidal agent.

c) **Douching** Postcoital washing of the vagina with a spermicidal solution is effective if done immediately after intercourse, before the sperm gets the opportunity to reach the cervical canal. Apart from having a very higher failure rate of 40 per 100 woman years, it has obvious aesthetic disadvantages.

d) **Occlusive devices** These provide a barrier in the vagina preventing sperms from entering the cervical canal. However, sperms can gain access by passing around the edges. Use of spermicidal agents in conjunction increases the efficacy, A diaphragm needs to be left for 8 hrs. after coitus. Accurate fitting is essential as the size and type may vary due to weight, illness, delivery, prolapse or apprehension at the time of examination.

Type of occlusive devices

These are three main types and others are modifications of these with limited use.

1. *The Dutch cap or diaphragm* It is the most widely used and most comfortable cap. It consists of a dome shaped diaphragm of thin rubber with a rubber covered metal rim. It is available in 50 mm to 95 mm diameter sizes. It fits in the vagina from just behind the pubic ramus to the posterior fornix, covering the cervix.

   It is contraindicated in women with relaxed vaginal walls eg. prolapse, or if a woman is allergic to rubber and spermicidal agents.

2. *The Cervical cap / vimule* is made of rubber, with a solid rolled rubber rim, designed to the fit cervix. Available in four sizes, varying from 22 to 31 mm, it has the advantage that it can be left for 48 hrs. It can be used when a woman has prolapse of the uterus and vagina but, is contraindicated in diseases of the cervix.

3. *Dumas cap* is wider than the cervical cap, made of rubber, and fits well into the vault of the vagina and encloses the cervix.

4. *Contra cap* is a cervical cap with a one-way valve to permit egress of secretions and menstrual fluid but prevents the ascent of sperms.

5. *Femshield (female condom)* is a soft, loose fitting, 15-17 cm long sheath of polyurethane material having two flexible rings. One ring at the closed end of the sheath serves as an insertion and anchoring device while the other ring at the open end serves as the external edge, lying outside the vagina providing protection to the labia and the base of penis during intercourse. It combines the features of the diaphragm and a condom. It is pre-lubricated and designed for one time use.

   Advantages

   • Coital independent and can be worn well in advance

- Does not slip off easily
- Provides greater protection against STD/HIV and particularly herpes
- Less likely to rupture as polyurethane is stronger
- Failure rates are low

6. *Today* is a mushroom shaped polyurethane disposable sponge, 2 inch in diameter, 1.25 inches thick and contains 1 gm of nanoxynol-9. It is provided with a loop for easy removal. After insertion, it works as a mechanical barrier for upto 24 hrs. and needs to be replaced.

7. *Drugs altering cervical mucus* Low dose progestogen–only pill, called the 'Minipill', can make cervical mucus viscid and unconducive for sperm travel, thereby reducing fertility.

INTRAUTERINE DEVICES (IUD)

Intrauterine devices (IUD) are effective, safe and long-acting methods of contraception with no systemic side effects, and do not interfere with the act of coitus.

The device is commonly made of polyethylene, (incorporated with barium sulphate to render it radio-opaque) and impregnated with copper hormones. These plastic devices are flexible, can be straightened and fitted into an introducer by which they are pushed through the cervical canal into the uterine cavity. Each device has a nylon thread attached to its lower end, which protrudes through the cervical canal into the vagina. The types of IUDs are shown in Fig. 22.1.

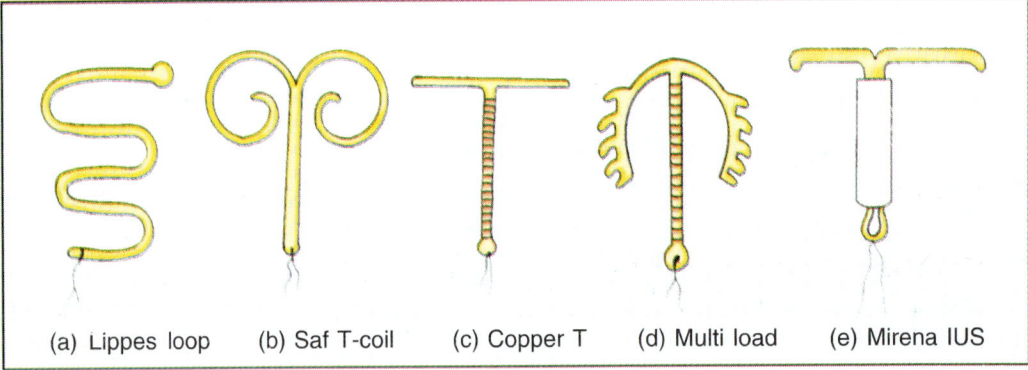

(a) Lippes loop　(b) Saf T-coil　(c) Copper T　(d) Multi load　(e) Mirena IUS

Fig. 22.1.　Types of intrauterine devices (IUD)

Classification of the common IUDs (table 22.3)

1. *INERT devices* The biologically inert devices include Lippes loop and Saf-T-coil. They exert their contraceptive effect by a local irritant inflammatory reaction. They are no longer in use.

2. **Copper containing devices** To decrease the side effects like uterine bleeding and pain, small devices covered with copper were developed in 1970's. A copper wire of surface area 200-250 mm is wrapped around the vertical stem of the polypropylene frame e.g. *Copper T 200, Copper 7.* In 1980s devices bearing a larger amount of copper, including sleeves on the horizontal arm, such as *Copper T 380*, and the *Copper T 220C* were developed as well as *multiload Cu 250 and Cu 375. NovaT* has silver added to the copper wire thereby increasing its life span to 5 yrs. Most of devices have a life-span of about 3 years, *Copper T 380* is effective for about 10 years.

   Gynefix is a frameless IUD comprising of six copper beads threaded on a nylon line, has recently been developed. The string has a knot at the proximal end, which is embedded, using a special introducer, into the myometrium, anchoring it in place. The device is 'free' to move in the uterine cavity, and has a lower incidence of dysmenorrhoea.

3. **Hormone containing devices** *Progestasert* is a T-shaped device carrying 35 mg of progesterone in a silicon oil reservoir in the vertical stem. It allows 65 mg of progesterone to diffuse into the endometrial cavity each day. It causes mucus plug thickening at the cervical os preventing entry of sperms. It needs to be changed every 18 months.

Table 22.3. Classification of IUDs

1. Inert devices–Lippes Loop and Saf-T coil
2. Copper containing devices
   * Copper T 200
   * Copper 7
   * Copper T 380
   * Copper 375
   * Nova T
   * CuT 380A
   * Multiload (ML 250 and ML 375)
   * Gynefix
3. Hormone containing devices
   * Progestasert
   * Levonova/Mirena

A levonorgestrel–releasing device (known as the intrauterine system IUS–to distinguish it from the copper IUD) has been developed. Known as **levonova/ mirena,** it contains a column of levonorgestrel (52-60 mg) within a rate-limiting membrane wrapped around the stem of the Nova-T frame. It releases a very low dose of the hormone (20μg/d) rendering it efficient for 5 years with a pregnancy rate of 0-3 (average 0.7) /100 woman years. Menstrual blood loss is markedly reduced and the device is recommended for management of menorrhagia.

Patient selection The intrauterine device is preferred in women who have

- A low risk of STD
- Are multiparous
- Are in a monogamous relationship
- Want a long term reversible method of contraception
- Unsatisfied with oral or barrier contraceptives

Contraindications (table 22.4)

- Suspected pregnancy
- PID, lower genital tract infection
- Genital bleeding of unknown origin
- Presence of fibroids or suspected malignancy
- Menorrhagia and dysmenorrhoea
- Severe anaemia
- Untreated acute cervicitis
- Postpartum endometritis or infected abortion in the past 3 months.

Relative contraindications are diabetes mellitus, past history of ectopic pregnancy (except progestasert), nulliparty, treated cervical dysplasia, steroid usage.

Table 22.4. Contraindications to IUD insertion
<ul><li>Suspected pregnancy</li><li>Lower genital tract infection</li><li>Genital bleeding of unknown origin</li><li>Associated fibroids</li><li>Suspected malignancy</li><li>Unmarried nullipara</li><li>Postpartum endometritis or infected abortion in the past 3 months</li></ul>

Insertion technique

A pelvic examination is carried out to determine the position and size of the uterus. The cervix is visualized and held with the vulsellum or allis forceps. The device is mounted into the pre-sterilised introducer as shown in Fig. 22.2.

The stopper is adjusted according to the length of the uterine cavity. The introducer with the plunger is pushed through the cervical canal, the plunger is pressed home, and the device uncoils within the uterine cavity. The introducer is then withdrawn, and the nylon

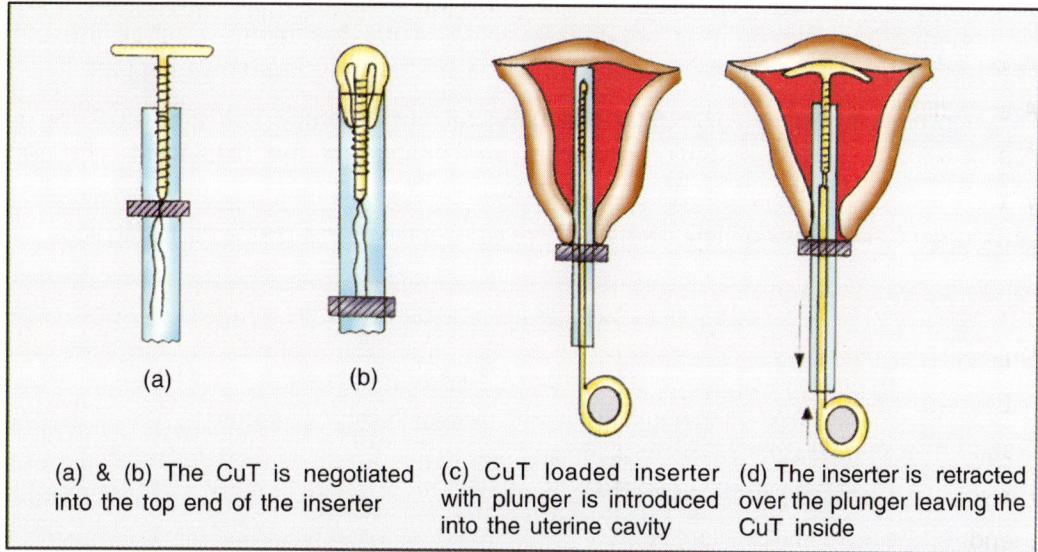

(a) & (b) The CuT is negotiated into the top end of the inserter

(c) CuT loaded inserter with plunger is introduced into the uterine cavity

(d) The inserter is retracted over the plunger leaving the CuT inside

Fig. 22.2a-d. IUD insertion technique

thread left in the vagina. The thread is cut to the desired length and rest of the instruments are removed. The woman is instructed to come for follow-up after the first cycle and every 6 months. She is asked to feel the thread herself once in 3 months.

Timing of insertion

- The optimal time for insertion of an IUD is during the menses or just after, through can be safely inserted on any day of the cycle provided the woman is not likely to be pregnant.

- It can also be inserted postpartum, preferably 2-3 months after delivery.

- Other suitable times are following an abortion or MTP.

Mechanism of action of IUDs

Several mechanisms have been postulated for the contraceptive effects of an IUD (table 22.5).

1. The main mechanism of the copper bearing IUD is spermicidal. This is caused by a local, sterile, inflammatory reaction produced by the presence of the foreign body in the uterine cavity. Copper markedly increases the extent of inflammatory reaction. There is an increase in leucocytes which cause phagocytosis of the spermatozoa; tissue break-down products of these leucocytes are toxic to all cells, including sperms and the blastocyst.

2. Copper also impedes sperm transport and viability in cervical mucus.

3. Increased uterine contractility due to a local irritant action with increased tubal peristalsis propells the fertilized egg faster than usual. Thus the ovum reaches the uterine cavity before the development of chorionic villi and is thus unable to implant.

4. Progesterone releasing IUDs alter the cervical mucus properties and slow the tubal transport of the embryo, thus preventing implantation of the blastocyst. This device however has a high ectopic pregnancy rate.

5. Levonorgestrel releasing IUD has a spermicidal action and prevents fertilization.

Table 22.5. Mechanism of action of IUDs
• Spermicidal due to a local sterile, inflammatory reaction • Alteration of sperm transport and viability in cervical mucus • Increased uterine contractility • Increased tubal peristalsis

Complications of IUDs

Immediate

• Vasovagal attack
• Uterine cramps

Early

• Expulsion
• Perforation
• Menorrhagia
• Dysmenorrhoea
• Actinomycosis

Late

• Pelvic inflammatory disease (PID)
• Pregnancy
• Ectopic pregnancy
• Perforation
• Menorrhagia
• Dysmenorrhoea

Long term follow up has shown no ill effects and has not shown any increase in either cervical or endometrial cancer.

1. *Uterine bleeding* Nearly all the medical reasons accounting for removal of IUDs (copper/inert) involve one or more types of abnormal bleeding which could be menorrhagia or inter-menstrual bleeding. Local release of prostaglandins may be responsible. There is 55% increase in menstrual blood flow compared to a significantly low (25 ml/cycle) blood loss with progesterone containing IUDs. Mefenemic acid ingestion (500 mg TDS) significantly reduces the menstrual blood flow. However, excessive bleeding requires removal of the device; 15% of patients get the IUD removed for bleeding and pain.

2. *Perforation* Uncommon but a potentially serious complication can occur in 0.3 to 1 per 1000 insertions. It can occur at the time of insertion specially in puerperal insertions. Nearly always asymptomatic, it should be suspected when the device has not been expelled and cannot be felt on vaginal examination.

3. *Expulsion* may occur in 3-10% of women in the first year of use; the rate of expulsion is higher in multiparous women, insertion during menses or insertion by an untrained doctor.

   The incidence of both expulsion and perforation is influenced by the skill of the person inserting the device, the incidence of both being increased with postpartum insertions.

4. *Pelvic infection* The risk is highest in young women with a maximum incidence in the first 3-4 weeks of use. If there is evidence of infection with pain, dyspareunia or discharge, the device should be removed and endocervical swabs sent for culture.

Misplaced IUD Is labelled when the tail of the IUD is not visualised through the Os. The causes could be

1. Perforation

2. Expulsion

3. Enlargement of the uterus due to pregnancy

4. Curling of the thread inside the uterus

An ultrasound scan is carried out to locate the IUCD, to find out if it is intrauterine or buried in the myometrium.

If intrauterine, a uterine sound is passed to feel for the IUD, If felt by the uterine sound, it is removed either by a Shirodkar's IUCD hook, an artery forceps or a curette. If it cannot be removed by these, a hysteroscopy is carried out to visualize the IUD embedded in the uterine wall.

Pregnancy with an IUD These devices do not exert a deleterious effect on fetal development and do not increase the risk of birth defects. The effect on the pregnancy could be—

1. **Spontaneous abortion** The incidence of spontaneous abortion is about 55%; approximately 3 times greater than would occur in pregnancies without an intrauterine IUD. This is reduced to 20%, if either the device is expelled spontaneously or removed.

2. **Septic abortion** Risk of septic abortion may be increased if the IUD remains in place specially in the multifilament variety.

3. **Ectopic pregnancy** Occurs in 1:30 pregnancies in women bearing a copper IUD though this risk is lower with copper T 380A and levonorgestrel releasing IUDs.

4. **Prematurity** The risk of prematurity is four times greater with an IUD in place than when it was removed.

The consequences should be explained to the patient. If the threads are seen easily, the IUD is removed. If the threads are not seen; the choice of removing it or not should be left for the patient to decide.

Advantages of IUD

• Coital independent

• One time insertion gives continuous protection for a long time.

• Highly effective, newer IUD with levonorgestrel (Mirena) is as effective as sterilization.

• No evidence of reduced fertility; 75% conceive within 6 months and about 90% in one year.

• No systemic side effects, unlike the oral contraceptive.

Other uses of IUD

Besides being used in family planning, IUD is inserted following division of adhesions in Asherman's syndrome and following excision of a uterine septum to prevent formation of fresh adhesions.

Copper T 380 A presently is inserted free of cost in government hospitals in India.

SUPPRESSION OF SPERMATOGENESIS

1. **Gossypol** is a yellow pigment isolated from cotton seed oil. Given in a dosage of 10-20mg daily for 3 months, followed by a maintenance dose of 20mg biweekly, it directly acts on seminiferous tubules inhibiting spermatogenesis. It does not alter FSH or LH levels. The side effects are weakness, hyponatremia and permanent sterility in 20% of cases.

2. **Testosterone enanthate** 200 mg once a week causes azoospermia in upto 58% of men; testosterone bucictate 600mg 3 monthly is undergoing trials.

3. **GnRHa** continuous administration of analogues of gonadotropin–releasing hormone

(GnRHa) causes a fall in sperm count and motility. The testosterone levels also fall, thus reducing the libido.

4. **Medroxy progesterone acetate** 250mg with 200 mg norethisterone given as weekly injections is reported to suppress spermatogenesis with 97% success.

HORMONAL CONTRACEPTIVE AGENTS

Discovered by Pincus in 1956, it is the most widely used method of reversible contraception among both married and unmarried women world-wide.

Initial combinations containing 150 mg of the oestrogenic component mestranol and 9.85 mg of the progestin component norethynodrel, resulted in side effects in a large number of patients and were soon replaced by low dose combinations. The various types of hormonal contraceptives are summarized in table 22.6.

Table 22.6. Hormonal Contraceptives

Short-acting		Long-acting	
1. *Combined pills* – Fixed dose combinations (Mala N/ Mala D) – Phasic pills (Triquilar) 2. *Progesterone* *only pills–* Minipill	*Injections* 1. Capronos 2. DMPA (3 monthly) 3. NET-EN (2 monthly) 4. Monthly Injections	*Implants* 1. Norplant I 2. Norplant II 3. Implanon	*Vaginal rings*

Mode of action (table 22.7)

1. Ovulation inhibition: Oestrogen and progesterones suppress the cyclical changes in LH and FSH thus suppressing ovulation

2. Decidualization of the endometrium

3. Thickening of cervical mucus by progesterone

The mode of action depends upon the hormones used, the mode of delivery and the time of administration. Three major types of OC formulations exist: fixed dose combination Mala N/Mala D, combination phasics with which have oestrogen and progesterone in varying combinations (Triquilar) and daily progestins (Minipill).

Table 22.7. Mode of action of hormonal contraceptives

1. Ovulation inhibition
2. Decidualization of the endometrium
3. Thickening of cervical mucus

Combined contraceptive pills

Chemistry

All current combinations contain synthetic oestrogen and progesterone. Two major types of synthetic progesterone exist, the progesterone component is a 19 Nor-testosterone derivative-nor-thrindrone, ethindrone acetate and ethinoidol di-acetate, desogesterol, norgestimate and gestodene.

Oestrogen on the other hand is either ethinyl estradiol (EE) or rarely ethinyl estradiol 3-methyl ether (mestranol).

Classification On the basis of development they can be as classified as

1st generation OC : > 50 µg of EE or mestranol with any progestin.

2nd generation OC : < 50 µg of EE with any progestin except lovonorgestrel (LNG) derivatives.

3rd generation OC : 20 µg or less of EE with a levonorgestrel (LNG) derivative (desogestrel/ norgestimate/gestodene). These three derivatives have greater progestogenic and lesser androgenic activity. They are more effective in preventing ovulation, the lower androgenic effect results in a lower incidence of adverse effects on the lipid profile.

Mala-D contains 0.5 mg of d-norgestrel, with 30 µg of ethinyl-estradiol.

Mala-N contains 1 mg norethisterone, with 30 µg of ethinyl-estradiol.

These are available free of cost in India and are supplied by the family planning association of India.

Mode of administration of combined pills

The pills supplied by the government are available in a 28 day pack (Fig. 22.3).

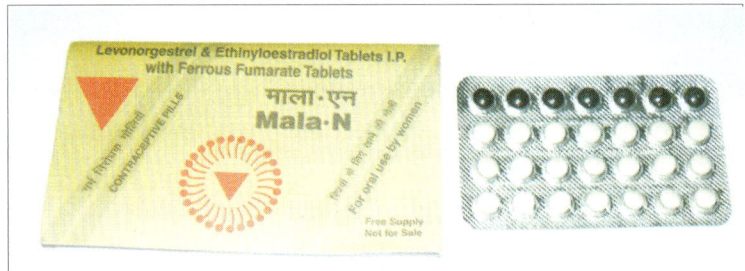

Fig. 22.3.   Combined contraceptive pill provided by govt. of India (Mala-N) (the black pills contain Iron only, the white pills contain the hormones)

The most important pill to remember is take – is the *first ONE OF EACH CYCLE.*

A new course should be commenced seven days after the cessation of the previous course with a 28 day pack, a second pack can be started without a break. During the first cycle of use, ovulation may not be suppressed. If can woman forgets to take a tablet, she should take two tablets the following day. If one pill in the first 7 days of the pack or 4 pills in the second half of the pack are missed, she is no longer protected and must use a barrier method during the rest of the cycle. The commonest cause of failure of OCs is failure to take the pill regularly. With regular usage pregnancy rate is 0.1 per 100 women years.

Benefits of combined pills

1. Relief of dysmenorrhoea and menorrhagia: By stopping ovulation, it relieves dysmenorrhoea and premenstrual tension. Decidualization of the endometrium results in reducing the menstrual blood loss and preventing anaemia.
2. Reduced incidence of ectopic pregnancy due to suppression of ovulation.
3. Reduction in the incidence of pelvic inflammatory disease due to thickening of the cervical mucus.
4. Suppression of ovulation results in a reduced incidence of endometrial hyperplasia and adenocarcinoma, ovarian cysts and ovarian cancer. There is also a reduction in the incidence of benign breast disease.
5. Risk of development of rheumatoid arthritis is reduced to half.

Contraindications of the combined pill are given in table 22.8.

Table 22.8. Contraindications of the combined pill	
ABSOLUTE	**RELATIVE**
Arterial or venous thrombosis	Age > 35yrs.
Ischaemic heart disease and cardiomyopathy	Factors increasing the risk of cardiovascular disease eg. obesity, smoking, hypertension
Most valvular heart diseases	Steroid dependant cancer eg. breast cancer present or past
Post cerebral haemorrhage	Severe depression
Hypercholesterolaemia	Chronic systemic disease eg. diabetes, chronic renal disease, sickle cell anaemia, chronic liver disease
Conditions predisposing to thrombosis eg. Polycythaemia	Long term partial immobilization
Migraine	Diseases requiring long term treatment with enzyme inducing drugs
Pulmonary hypertension	During or after definitive treatment of CIN
Porphyria	
History of a serious condition affected by sex steroids (trophoblastic disease)	
Suspected pregnancy	

Side effects of combined pills They could be major or minor

Major side effects

1. Venous thromboembolism:

    • The overall risk is 4-6 times more than non-users.

    • Related to the oestrogen component as they cause a reduction in anti-thrombin III and alter the platelet function.

    • Preparations containing Desogestrel and Gestodene have higher incidence of VTE (double that of second generation pills). Hence 3rd generation pills are contraindicated in a patient at high risk of thromboembolism i.e. obesity, varicose veins and a family history of thrombosis.

2. Cholestatic jaundice and an increased risk of gall-stones.

3. Arterial disease including myocardial infraction and cerebrovascular accidents resulting from the progesterone related alteration in lipid profile together with changes in blood coagulation i.e., oestrogens. Women with risk factors should be advised to stop the pill at 35 yrs. of age; those women with no risk factors can continue the low-dose pill till they reach the menopause.

4. Hypertension is seen in 2% of women on the pill.

5. Increased risk of glandular neoplasia of the cervix (relative risk is 2.1 and increasing to 4.4 after 12 yrs. of use).

Minor side effects

1. Nausea, vomitings, leg cramps, acne–these are transient

2. Weight gain–due to the anabolic effects of progestins

3. Menstrual irregularities–breakthrough bleeding, hypomenorrhoea

4. Diminished libido

5. Increased incidence of monilial vaginitis

Drug interactions of combined pills

• Rifampicin, an enzyme inducer can cause OC failure

• Drugs like barbiturates, sulphonamides, cyclophosphamides and rifampicin accelerate biotransformation of oestrogens and progesterones. Patients on these medications should be advised that the pill may fail and they will need to use additional contraception.

Checklist for prescription of oral contraceptives (to be used for screening by health workers) Table 22.9.

Table 22.9. Checklist for prescription of oral contraceptives
(to be used for screening by health workers)

Check the following by history and examination

Question	Yes	No
Age > 40 yrs.		
Age > 35 yrs.		
Heavy smoker		
Seizures		
Severe pain in the calves or thighs		
Symptomatic varicose veins in the legs		
Severe chest pain		
Unusual shortness of breath after examination		
Severe headaches or visual disturbances		
Lactating		
Intermenstrual bleeding or bleeding after sexual intercourse		
Amenorrhoea		
Abnormally yellow skin and eyes		
Blood pressure of > 140/90		
Mass in the breast		
Swollen legs (edema)		

If all the above are negative, the woman may be given the pill. If any are positive, she should be first seen by a doctor.

Triphasic combined pills (Triquilar)

They mimic the functioning pattern of steroid concentrations in the normal ovarian cycle, in an attempt to produce better cycle control. The triphasic preparations of ethinyl estradiol (EE) and levonorgestrel (LNG) are popular. However, there have been no published reports of comparative clinical trials which have shown a significantly lower adverse effects than fixed dose combinations.

Minipill / Progestogen-only pill (POP)

The low dose progestogen-only pills (norethisterone 350 µg, norgestrel 75µg or levonorgestrel 30 µg) have been introduced to avoid the side effects of oestrogen in the combined pills.

Mode of administration The tablet is taken daily without a pill free interval at the same time of the day.

Mode of action Alteration of cervical mucus preventing sperm penetration. It is well suited for lactating women and women with medical contraindications like migraine, headache etc.

Failure rate 2-3 per 100 woman years.

Indications

- During lactation
- Women >35 yrs. who wish to use a pill for contraception
- Women with migraine, hypertension, diabetes

Side effects

- Irregular bleeding
- Increased risk of ectopic pregnancy
- Increased incidence of functional ovarian cysts

Contraindications Ovarian cyst, breast and cervical cancers, abnormal vaginal bleeding, active liver disease, arterial disease and porphyria.

Long-acting contraceptive steroids

They overcome the inconvenience of daily administration and have better compliance. Types of long-acting steroids are–

1. Injectable suspensions
2. Implants
3. Vaginal rings

Mode of action

1. Continuous release of progesterone suppresses the LH surge and ovulation.
2. Thickening of cervical mucus prevents sperm penetration.

1. Injectable suspensions

(a) ***Depo medroxy progesterone acetate (DMPA or Depo-provera)*** in a dose of 150 mg 3 monthly (micro crystalline aqueous suspension) by deep intramuscular injection has been used with considerable efficacy.

Mode of action of DMPA

- Ovulation suppression
- Thickening of cervical mucus preventing sperm penetration

Timing of administration

- Day 1-2 of the cycle
- Postpartum 6 weeks after delivery
- Post MTP/miscarriage–can be given within the first 7 days.

Advantages

- Effective, convenient and reversible

- Lower incidence of PID and ectopic pregnancy

- Amenorrhoea often occurs with less anaemia, dysmenorrhoea and premenstrual tension.

Side effects

- weight gain

- delay in resumption of fertility of upto 1 year

- possible reduction in the bone mineral density.

(b) *Norethisterone enanthate (NET-EN)* 200 mg every 8 weeks (in castor oil solution)

After withdrawl, the contraceptive effect of DMPA lasts longer than NET-EN.

Pregnancy rate is 1 per 100 woman years for DMPA and 0.6 per 100 woman years for NET-EN.

(c) *Monthly depots* Several combined progestin – oestrogen injectables designed for once a month administration and production of regular withdrawal bleeding have been developed. Currently four of them are being used world wide.

(i) Combination of 17α hydroxyprogesterone caproate 250mg + estradiol valerate 5 mg

(ii) Dihydroxy progesterone acetophemide 150mg + estradiol oesmanthate 10mg

(iii) DMPA 25 mg + estradiol cypionate 5 mg (*cyclofem/cycloprovera/Lunelle*)

(iv) Norethisterone enanthate 50mg + estradiol valerate 5 mg (*mesigyna*)

2. Implants

These implants contain varying amounts of progesterone and are implanted subdermally. They ensure an even release of the hormone.

- *Norplant I* contains six silastic capsules each containing 36 mg crystalline levonorgestrel (total 2/6 mg) is inserted subdermally on the inner aspect of the upper arm. Contraceptive effect lasts for 5 years.

- *Norplant II* (Jadelle) consists of two rods each containing 70 mg of LNG the daily release of which is 50 µg and provides contraception of 3 to 5 years.

- *Implanon* is a single rod implant containing 68 mg of 3-keto-desogesterel and provides contraceptive efficacy for three years.

- *Capronos* is a bio-degradable capsule under trial, which does not require removal at the end of its tenure.

The **disadvantage** of long-acting steroid preparations is breakthrough bleeding and irregular cycles. The major reason for discontinuation of all progestin only long-acting steroids is menstrual irregularly. Pregnancy rate is 1.1 per 100 woman years.

3. Silastic vaginal ring (SVR)

Soft silastic or vinyl vaginal rings have been developed releasing progestogen either alone or in combination with oestrogen. The steroids are readily absorbed vaginally avoiding the first pass through the liver. Levonorgestrel ring has a daily release of 20mg and is designed to be worn for 3 weeks. A combination ring has been developed recently, which releases etonorgestrel and 15 mg of ethinyl-estradiol per day. This is used for 3 weeks in each cycle.

Centchroman

It is a synthetic non-steroidal contraceptive taken as a 30 mg tab, started on the 1st day of menses and taken twice weekly for 12 weeks, and weekly thereafter. It prevents implantation through endometrial changes. It exhibits a strong anti-oestrogenic and a weak oestrogenic action peripherally at the receptor level. The fertility returns usually within 6 months of stopping the drug. It is not teratogenic or carcinogenic, and exerts no pharmacological effect on other organs.

This drug has been developed by Central drug research Institute, Lucknow and is available in India as "Saheli". Clinical trials in the 1990's have shown a failure rate after perfect use of 4.2–6/100 woman years; however, post marketing surveillance has shown lower pregnancy rates of 1.83/100 woman years. There is also concern regarding development of ovarian cysts and delayed return of fertility due to its anti-oestrogenic effect. The drug has also been recommended as a "Post Coital Pill" in the dose of 60 mg, within 24 hrs. of unprotected coitus.

Contraindications are liver dysfunction, PCOD, cervical dysplasia and allergy to the drug.

Return of fertility

*   Contraceptive effect of oral pills is reversible within 6 months of withdrawal; about 70% of women are expected to conceive within a year.
*   Mini-pill suppresses ovulation in only 40% of cases, its reversible effect is faster than combined pills.
*   With DMPA ovulation returns, within 6 months and with NET-EN within 3 months of the last injection.

EMERGENCY (POST COITAL) CONTRACEPTION

High doses of oestrogen were first used by Morris and Van Wagenen in 1966 to prevent implantation of the embryo.

Indications

1. Contraceptive failure eg. ruptured or slipped condom, misplaced IUD, displaced diaphragm or a forgotten pill.

2. Failure to use a contraceptive (unprotected intercourse)

3. Incorrect or inconsistent use of a regular contraceptive.

4. Accidental intercourse due to rape, assault or sexual coercion.

Methods

The methods available are tabulated in table 22.10.

Table 22.10. Emergency contraceptives
• Oestrogen alone (5mg/day for 5 days)
• Yuzpe regime (two tabs of COC pill taken in two doses 12 hrs. apart)
• Levonorgestrel containing pill (Levonova) (0.75mg repeated after 12 hrs.)
• Antiprogestogens-Mifepristone (RU486)–(600mg single dose)
• Anti-oestrogens
– Danazol (400mg repeated after 12 hrs. for two doses)
– Centchroman/Saheli (50mg 12 hrly for 2 doses)
• Cu-T IUD
• GnRH agonist (daily injections)
• Prostaglandins (vaginal suppository)

1. ***Oestrogen alone*** Ethinyl estradiol 5 mg/day, or conjugated oestrogen, 30 mg per day. Treatment is continued for 5 days, beginning within 72 hrs. after an isolated act of coitus. Pregnancy rates are 0.7 to 1.6%. Side effects like nausea, vomiting, breast soreness and menstrual irregularities are common.

2. ***Combined pill*** Ethinyl estradiol 50 μg + d-norgestrel 500 mg (*Ovral*) given in doses of two tablets 12 hrs. apart was initially tested in Canada by Yuzpe in 1977 and is known after him as the *Yuzpe regime.* Effectiveness is 75%, if taken within 24 hrs.

3. ***Progestin only pills (POP)*** Levonorgestrel is the only progestin studied for emergency contraception, one tablet of 0.75 mg LNG is taken within 72 hrs. of coitus, and repeated after 12 hours. Available as *Plan-B* in US, Levonelle–2 (UK) and *Pill 72* (Cipla) in India, this regime is highly effective (95%) in preventing unwanted pregnancies. It is well tolerated with a lower incidence of side effects like nausea and vomiting.

4. ***Antiprogestogens*** These are anti-implantation agents and can be given as late as 24th-27th day of their cycle. RU 486 (*Mifepristone*) has been found effective in a dose of 600 mg, when used as an emergency contraceptive. It acts by blocking the action of progesterone on the endometrium, causing sloughing and shedding of the decidua.

5. ***Anti-oestrogens***
   A. Danazol: has a direct luteolytic effect with a 400 mg. dose repeated after 12 hrs. for two to three doses. It has lower incidence of side effects. It is contraindicated in undiagnosed abnormal vaginal bleeding, liver, kidney and cardiac dysfunction, porphyria, epilepsy, migraine and in lactation. In case of failure it has a virlizing effect on the female fetus. Pregnancy rate is 2.0%.
   B. Centchroman (Saheli) is used as two 50 mg. tablets given 12 hrs. apart within 72 hrs. of the act of coitus. It acts on the zygote, affecting ovum transport and blastocyst development.

6. ***CuT IUD*** Insertion of a CUT IUD upto 5 days of unprotected intercourse reduces the risk of pregnancy by 99%. Women at high-risk of harbouring sexually transmitted diseases should be given prophylactic antibiotics.

7. ***GnRH agonists*** Daily administration of gonadotropin releasing hormone agonist (*Buserelin*) prevents ovulation. The drug is undergoing trials for contraceptive effects. They cause initial ovarian stimulation followed by down regulation and luteolysis.

8. ***Prostaglandins*** Self administered vaginal suppository containing prostaglandin, by virtue of its proteolytic effect on the ovary, its effect on motility of the fallopian tubes and the uterus, can prevent implantation and bring about menstruation. Its specific role as a contraceptive is however yet to be established.

IMMUNOLOGICAL METHODS OF CONTRACEPTION

Immunological approach to family planning is in a developmental stage. The vaccines which are being experimented upon are:

1. An β sub-unit (300µg) of hCG which evokes specific antibodies and thereby prevents pregnancy for 6-12 months. It is also useful in hydatidiform mole and choriocarcinoma.

2. Vaccine against zona pellucida, develops antibodies which can either prevent penetration of the ovum by the sperm or prevents shedding of the zona after fertilization so that implantation is impossible. There vaccines can to lead irreversible interference with ovarian function, permanent sterility and premature menopause.

3. Antibodies to sperm antigens namely the enzyme lactate dehydrogenase, hydaluronidase and acrosin cause immobilization and destruction of the sperm.

4. Anti FSH vaccine (*Inhibin*) is also under trial.

STERILIZATION

A permanent act of contraception to prevent further pregnancies. It is suited for those couples who:

- Have completed their families.
- Do not want the inconvenience or cost of other methods of contraception.

Types

Male sterilization: Vasectomy

Female sterilization: Tubectomy

Male sterilization

Performed by vasectomy, a procedure of occlusion or division of the vas deferens to prevent the passage of sperms.

Procedure

- Outpatient procedure done under local anaesthesia.
- The vas is exposed through a small skin incision in the midline. It is separated from the surrounding tissues and approximately 1 cm is excised. It is ligated by silk, and the sheath of the vas interposed between the cut ends (Fig. 22.4).
- Vas is replaced back in the scrotal sac, the skin wound is closed with silk and a scrotal support given.
- Person can resume work after a rest of one or two days.

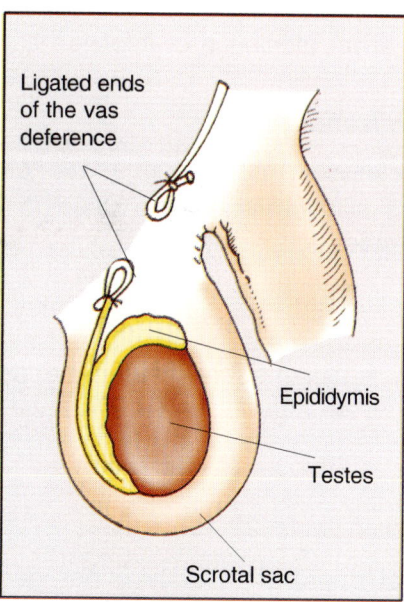

Fig. 22.4.   Technique of Vasectomy. The vas is exposed, approximately 1cm is excised and the ends ligated with silk.

Precautions Sterility is not immediate, since sperms are stored in the tract for upto 3 months. Usually 14-20 ejaculates are required to clear the semen of sperms. Abstinence or contraception should be observed till then.

Complications

- Local wound infection, scrotal bruising, post-op bleeding which can cause a scrotal haematoma.
- Sperm granuloma-inflammatory response to sperm leakage at the ends.
- Spontaneous re-anastomosis can occur even after years.
- Chronic intrascrotal pain and discomfort (*post-vasectomy syndrome*).
- Anti-sperm antibodies formation possibly due to leakage of sperms.
- Increased risk of prostatic cancer.

Reversal Restoration of fertility by anastomosing the cut ends is feasible in some cases and can be restored in upto 50-70% cases.

No-scalpel vasectomy (NSV)

- Developed in China in 1974.
- A specially designed instrument is used for isolating and delivering the vas through a small puncture in the skin.
- Quick and associated with lower incidence of infection and haematoma.

Newer advances in male sterilization

Percutaneous injection of sclerosing agents such as polyurethrane elastomers or occlusive substances such as silicone are being used in china. Silicon plug can be removed if required for restoration of fertility.

Female sterilization

Involves the blocking of both fallopian tubes. It can be performed in the postpartum period (*Postpartum sterilization*) or after 6 weeks (*Interval sterilization*).

Methods

The methods are summarized in table 22.11.

1. *Laparotomy*–Transperitoneal approach usually under general or spinal anaesthesia, may be combined with caesarean section or other gynae surgery.
2. *Mini-laparotomy (minilap)*–During the interval period or immediate postpartum; ligation

of the tube is performed by a mini-laparotomy. Absorbable or non-absorbable sutures are used to tie the oviducts by any of the following methods.

*   In *Pomeroy's technique* (Fig. 22.5) a loop of fallopian tube is tied at the base and the loop excised. Failure rate is 0.4%, due to recanalization.

*   In *Madlener's operation*, a loop of fallopian tube is crushed and ligated with non-absorbable suture i.e., silk. The failure rate is high (7%).

*   In *Modified Irving procedure* (Fig. 22.6) the middle portion of the tube is tied. The intervening portion is excised, the proximal end is buried in the uterus, whilst the distal end is buried in the broad ligament. A reliable and irreversible method.

*   In *Aldridge method* (Fig. 22.7), a hole is made in the anterior leaf of the broad ligament, and the fimbrial end buried into this.

*   In *Kroner's fimbriectomy* (Fig. 22.8), the fimbrial end of the tube is doubly ligated with silk sutures and excised.

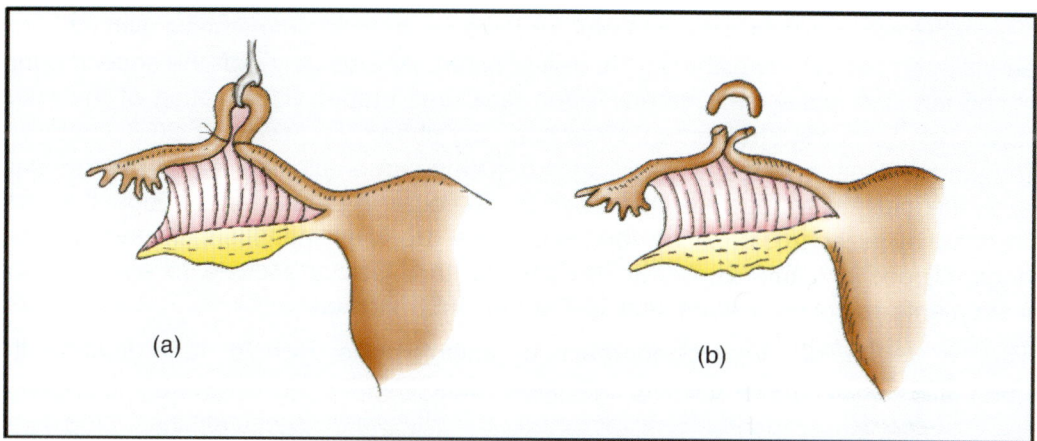

Fig. 22.5a-b. Pomeroy's technique

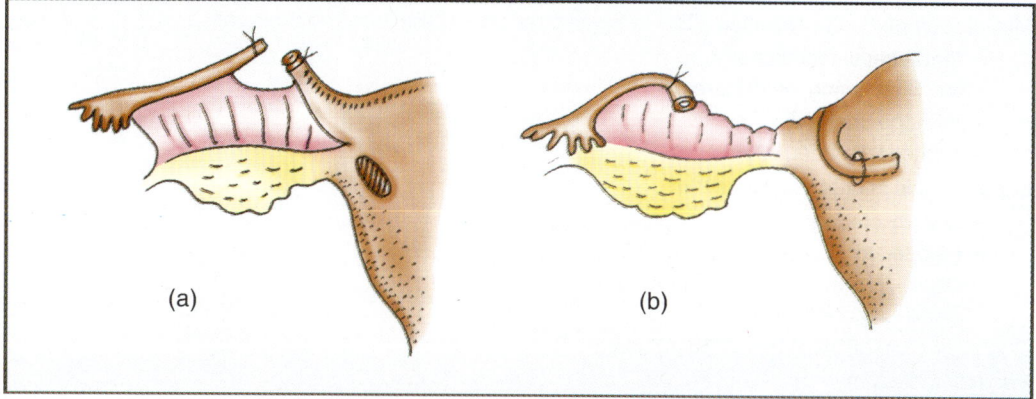

Fig. 22.6a-b. Modified Irving procedure

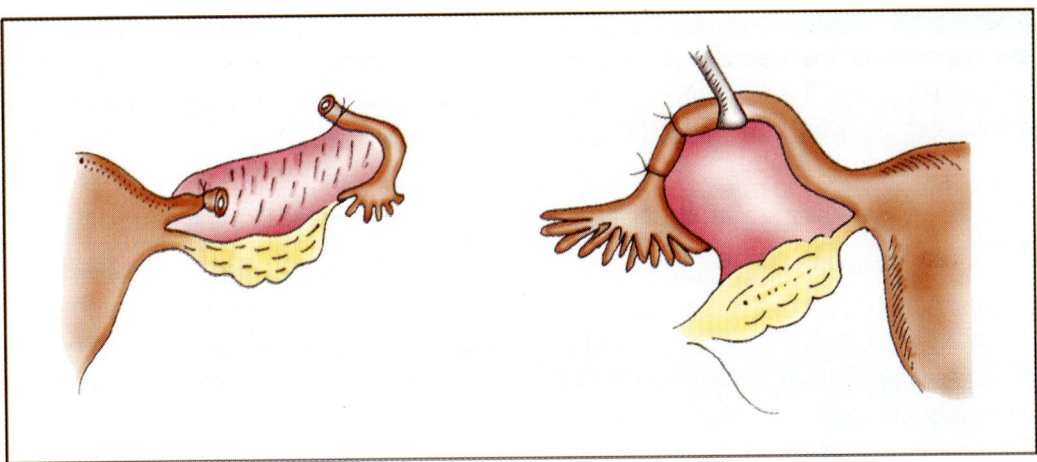

| **Fig. 22.7.** Aldridge method | **Fig. 22.8.** Kroner's fimbriectomy |

3. *Laparoscopic sterilization* Fibre-optic light source with laparoscopy allows access to the fallopian tubes with one sub-umbilical puncture under local anaesthesia with intravenous sedation or general anaesthesia. Double puncture laparoscopy with the second puncture in the left iliac fossa with camera vision facilitates proper visualization of the fallopian tube and occlusion. Instruments needed are shown in (*see* Fig 26.5 chapter 26). Pneumoperitoneum is first created by introducing carbon-dioxide using a verres needle. With the patient in head low the position, a trocar is pushed in through the incision followed by a laparocator. The fallopian tubes are then identified, ligated with falope rings, clipped or cauterized near the isthmic end. Gas is allowed to escape and the instruments removed. Failure rate is 0.2 per 1000 women.

4. *Vaginal sterilization* Vaginal approach by colpotomy is used for tubal ligation. It has been abandoned due to the high infection rates.

Table 22.11. Methods of female sterilization

1. Minilaparotomy – the fallopian tube is ligated by any of the three techniques
    – Madlener's technique
    – Modified Irving procedure
    – Aldridge method
    – Kroner's fimbriectomy
2. Laparoscopic method using either
    – Electro cautery
    – Falope rings
    – Clips - Hulka clemens/ Filshie clip
    – Laser vaporization
3. Chemical method with quinacrine pellets
4. Vaginal tubectomy
5. Hysteroscopic sterilization

5. *Chemical sterilization* New methods using quinacrine can be used to occlude the tube either directly or transcervically via the uterus. The quinacrine pellets are ready for use, are inserted into the uterus by a modified IUD inserter during the follicular phase. Usually two insertions, one month apart, are made.

6. *Hysteroscopic sterilization* Occlude of the utero-tubal junction through a hysteroscope. Now abandoned due to high failure rates (30%) and associated complications like uterine perforation, intestinal burns and infection.

Anaesthesia used

- Spinal anaesthesia is given for mini-laparotomies.
- Laparoscopic and hysteroscopic sterilizations–Local anaesthesia with intravenous sedation, or general anaesthesia is used.

Complications

Short term

1. Unipolar cautery can cause local burns.
2. Subcutaneous emphysema of the abdominal wall due to leakage of CO_2 gas into the abdominal wall.
3. Haemorrhage due to injury to the inferior epigastric vessels, mesosalpinx or uterus.
4. Uterine perforation.
5. Wrong placement of the falope ring eg. on the round ligament, ovarian ligament or the mesosalpinx.
6. Anaesthetic complications.
7. Gas embolism due to CO_2 embolism.
8. Post-op pain due to local tissue ischaemia and necrosis at the site of occlusion.
9. Wound infections.

Long term

1. Post-tubal sterilization syndrome–Symptoms include abdominal pain, dyspareunia, exacerbation of PMS or dysmenorrhoea, emotional and psychosexual problems. Younger women, may have manifestations of regret.
2. Psychological and psychosexual problems.
3. Ectopic pregnancies–15 to 17 pregnancies per 1000 procedures depending upon the type of procedure.
4. Failure–0.4% with modified Pomeroy's; 0.3-1.3% with laparoscopic method–The failure rate is higher with clips then with falope rings.

5. Dysfunctional uterine bleeding–thought to be due to altered blood supply to the tubes.

Contraindications

- Previous abdominal surgery is a relative contraindication as there could be extensive intra-abdominal adhesions.
- Cardiac/pulmonary disease where head low position is not possible.
- In puerperal cases, the uterus is not involuted and insertion of trocar can injure the uterus.
- Extreme obesity, diaphragmatic or umbilical hernia.
- Previous pelvic inflammatory disease (PID) where omental adhesions may mask the tubes.

23

Medical Termination of Pregnancy

Medical termination of pregnancy (MTP) is intentional medical or surgical termination of pregnancy before 20 weeks of gestation.

MTP ACT

The MTP act was passed in India by the Parliament in 1971, and came into force on 1st April, 1972. Any abortion performed outside the conditions of the act is called an illegal abortion. It identifies the persons performing the MTP and the indications for the same.

The following persons can perform an MTP under the MTP act:

- A registered medical pracfitioner with a degree / diploma in gynaecology and obstetrics
- Any registered medical practitioner if

  a) He/she has completed a 6 months of house job in obstetrics and gynaecology

  b) He/she has experience of not less than one year in the practice of obstetrics and gynaecology

  c) He/she has assisted in the performance of 25 cases of MTP in an established hospital or at a recognised training centre

Place The places where it can be performed are:

a) In a hospital established and maintained by the government

b) In a place recognised and approved by the government under this act

Gestation If the pregnancy is <12 weeks, opinion of one medical practitioner is sufficient. If the pregnancy is >12 weeks, opinion of two medical practitioners is essential.

INDICATIONS FOR MEDICAL TERMINATION OF PREGNANCY

A pregnancy could be terminated on the following grounds:

1. **Medical**

   – When the continuation of pregnancy is likely to endanger the life of a pregnant woman.

   – When pregnancy causes serious injury to her physical or mental health as in severe hypertension, NYHA Class III or IV heart disease, uncontrolled diabetes, serious psychiatric illness, advanced genital or breast cancer.

2. **Eugenic** When there is a substantial risk of the child being born with serious physical or mental abnormalities eg. hereditary disorders, congenital malformations in a previous offspring with a high risk of recurrence in subsequent childbirth, severe degree of Rh isoimmunization, active maternal rubella infection posing a risk of anomalies in the fetus. Chorion villus sampling (CVS), cordocentesis and sonographic evaluation of the fetus have contributed significantly in identifying the fetus at risk.

3. **Humanitarian** When the pregnancy is caused by rape or incest.

4. **Contraceptive failure** When pregnancy results from failure of a contraceptive device or method. India is one of the few countries in the world where women have this option in case of failed contraception.

EVALUATION OF A PATIENT FOR MEDICAL TERMINATION OF PREGNANCY

History

A detailed history should include the following points:

– *Gynaecological:* period of amenorrhoea, previous menstrual history, obstetric history including the mode of deliveries, and reasons for any prior interruption of pregnancy should be inquired.

– *Medical and surgical:* history of medical problems and any surgical procedure undertaken should be enquired.

• **Examination** A complete general examination to look for icterus, anaemia, any cardiac murmur should be carried out. Blood pressure should be checked. A pelvic examination is then carried out to note any local infection, the size of the uterus and any adnexal mass.

• **Investigations**

– *Haemoglobin percentage:* As per the guidelines issued by the govt. of India, procedure should be deferred if the haemoglobin is < 8 g%.

- *Urine routine and microscopy*

- *Blood group and Rh type:* If the patient is Rh negative, her husband's blood group should also be performed. If the husband is Rh positive, inj anti-D needs to be given following the MTP to prevent isoimmunization (50µg if the pregnancy is <12 wks and 300µg if >12 wks).

- *Ultrasound pelvis:* is indicated if the size of the uterus cannot be made out due to obesity, a retroverted uterus or an uncooperative patient.

Prerequisites

1. Consent: An informed consent should be obtained from the patient herself. She should be informed of the risks due to the procedure and the various methods of contraception available. Parents' or guardians' consent is required if she is <18 yrs. of age (minor) or >18 yrs. and mentally deranged. Husband's consent is not mandatory though desirable in cases of dispute.

2. A responsible person, preferably the spouse should accompany when under-going the procedure. The procedure is to be kept confidential and the patient's identity should be treated as a personal matter.

3. If the pregnancy is <12 wks, certification by one registered medical practitioner is sufficient. If the pregnancy is advanced to >12 wks, certification by two registered medical practitioners is essential.

4. Blood should be booked in case of second trimester termination as the incidence of postpartum haemorrhage is increased.

METHODS OF MTP

The methods of MTP in the first and second trimester are summarized in table 23.1.

First Trimester MTP

Medical methods These regimes are safe, effective and offer a new range of choices for patients. Pregnancy is terminated spontaneously with the help of pharmacologic methods. It has a well documented failure rate and may require a surgical method for completion. An ultrasound scan needs to be carried out after one week to check for completeness of the abortion. The drugs which are used are RU 486 (mifepristone), methotrexate and danazol. Mifepristone is the most popular.

RU 486 (Mifepristone) is an anti-progestational compound, which acts by binding to progesterone receptors inhibitng it's action, leading to increased uterine contractility and expulsion of the fetus. In a dose of 200mg orally followed by misoprostol 800 µg vaginally 48 hrs. later, a complete abortion rate of 98% can be achieved at <9 wks of gestation.

Table 23.1. Methods of MTP	
I Trimester	**II Trimester**
Medical	**Medical**
• Antiprogesterones (RU 486)+ Misoprostol	• Antiprogesterones (RU 486)+Misoprostol
• Methotrexate+Misoprostol	• Misoprostol only
	• Extra-amniotic solutions (saline, ethacridine lactate)
	• Prostodin injections
Surgical	**Surgical**
• Menstrual regulation	• Dilatation and evacuation
• Manual vacuum aspiration	• Hysterotomy
• Dilatation and evacuation	

Methotrexate, an antimetabolite acts by blocking dihydrofolate reductase, thus inhibiting folate production and DNA synthesis. In a dose of 50mg/sqm given intramuscularly followed by misoprostol 3-5 days later, a complete abortion rate of 92-93% can be achieved at <9 wks of gestation.

Surgical methods

1. *Menstrual regulation*

   • Method of aspiration of the contents of uterine cavity within 42 days of the last menstrual period.

   • Performed with the help of a special plastic cannula (Karman's cannula) and a plastic 50cc syringe capable of creating vacuum of over 60 mm of Hg.

   • Preoperative sedation or local paracervical block is sufficient.

   • The procedure is easy, safe, inexpensive, efficient and can be performed on an outpatient basis.

   • Complication rate is low and includes haemorrhage, incomplete evacuation, cervical laceration, perforation and sepsis.

2. *Manual Vacuum Aspiration (MVA)*

   • A variation of menstrual regulation

   • The MVA syringe is a double syringe of 60 cc capacity, capable of adapting to cannulae ranging from 4-12 mm. It is easily sterilised, tough, resilient long lasting, and cost effective (Fig. 23.1).

- It does not require the use of electricity and is suitable for performance in the rural setup.

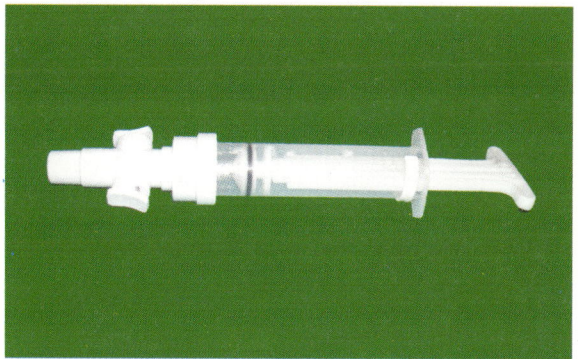

Fig. 23.1. The MVA syringe

3. *Dilatation and suction evacuation*

- Involves dilatation of the cervix and evacuation of its contents using a karman's cannula and an electric suction device.

- Pre-op sedation with paracervical block (using 1% xylocaine injected into the lateral fornices avoiding the blood vessels) is usually sufficient.

- Pre-operatively the patient is given misoprostol 400 µg orally or vaginally to soften the cervix and facilitate cervical dilatation. Laminaria tents were used earlier which were hygroscopic and expanded to dilate the cervix when introduced intra-cervically.

- The cervix is held with a vulsellum and dilated with metallic Hegar's dilators, or silastic dilators.

- Karman's cannula of size corresponding to the period of gestation is introduced through the cervical canal, the suction machine is turned on and the products of conception sucked out. The instruments used are shown in Fig. 23.2.

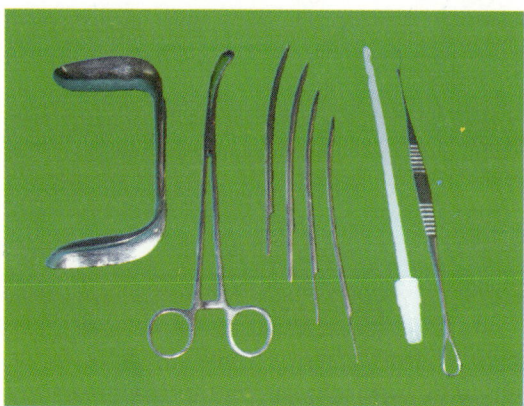

Fig. 23.2. Instruments used for suction evacuation. From left to right: Sims speculum, vulsellum, cervical dilators, Karman's cannula and endometrial curette

- Emptiness of the uterine cavity is indicated when a grating sensation is felt in the walls, no further tissue is aspirated, the internal os begins to grip the cannula and blood stained froth is seen coming through the cannula.
- Inj ergometrine (methergin) is given to contract the uterus.
- The contents aspirated are checked for products of conception.
- The procedure is usually followed by IUCD insertion, or sterilization if the patient desires.
- Post-operatively, the patient is discharged after 4-6 hrs. and asked to report if she has excessive pain or bleeding per vaginum. Antibiotics are given for a week and abstinence till the next period is advised.
- Complications:
  a) Uterine perforation: can occur during cervical dilatation or due to the suction and can cause injury to the bowel and omentum. It should be suspected when there is sudden loss of resistance of the uterine musculature. The procedure should be stopped immediately, a laparoscope introduced to know the size of the perforation and extent of injury. A laparotomy may or may not be needed subsequently.
  b) Incomplete evacuation: can lead to excessive bleeding.
  c) Infection: Introduction of infection in the uterus can lead to endometritis, pelvic inflammatory disease and can cause infertility at a later stage.

4. *Dilatation and curettage:*
   - Evacuation and curettage is done with an ovum forceps and curette.
   - Bleeding is more as compared to vacuum aspiration.
   - Risk of perforation and cervical injury is six fold higher than vacuum aspiration.

Second trimester methods

The incidence of such abortions is only 10% in the present times.

1. **Medical methods** Use of abortifacient drugs to accomplish pregnancy termination. The methods available are:
   - *Intra-amniotic instillation of hypertonic saline or urea* This method was used extensively in the past but given up due to electrolyte imbalance, fluid imbalance and renal complications.
   - *Extra-amniotic ethacridine lactate, hypertonic saline and prostaglandins* have been successfully tried. Ethacridine lactate (acenol lactate or lacto acridine) is a yellow dye with antiseptic properties. This is used as a 0.1% solution, is injected extra-amniotically via a foley catheter introduced intra-cervically in a dose of 10 ml/wk of gestation. It causes stimulation of the uterus by detachment of the membranes leading to uterine contractions. It also damages the decidual lysosomes leading to

release of prostaglandins. Side-effects include retained placenta, pelvic infection, nausea and vomiting, epigastric pain, haemorrhage and fever. It is used only is the other methods fail.

- *Prostaglandins* are a group of poly-unsaturated 20 carbon fatty acids which are subdivided into several groups according to the number of double bonds. Prostaglandin analogues are longer lasting compared to the natural prostaglandins. The commonly used prostaglandins are:

  a) PG E1 analogue (*Misoprostol*): This is being commonly used either alone or in combination with Mifepristone. Mifepristone 200mg is given orally followed 36-48 hrs. later by misoprostol 800 mg vaginally and 400 mg orally 3 hourly to a maximum of four oral doses. Misoprostol alone as 200 mg orally or vaginally four hourly upto a maximum of 10 doses, is commonly used though has not got FDA approval.

  b) 15 Methyl PG F2 alpha is available as inj Prostodin is given to a maximum of ten doses. This causes myometrial contractions of increased tone and amplitude with expulsion of the uterine contents, with an abortion rate of 95%. However it can cause bronchospasm.

2. Surgical methods

There are not very popular but may be resorted to if other medical methods fail.

- *Dilatation and evacuation* is the method of choice in the USA; but not practised routinely in India. However, some surgeons perform it between 13-15 wks. The cervix needs to be dilated upto 20mm before the fetal parts are extracted. This can result in cervical tears, bleeding and uterine perforation.

- *Hysterotomy* This involves is a mini-caesarean section which can be carried out in parous women who need concurrent sterilization. However, it has a higher incidence of haemorrhage, anaesthetic problems and used only if medical methods fail.

The advantages and disadvantages of medical and surgical abortion are summarized in table 23.2.

Table 23.2. Medical vs surgical abortion			
Medical abortion		**Surgical abortion**	
Advantages	*Disadvantages*	*Advantages*	*Disadvantages*
Avoids surgical and anaesthetic risk	Longer waiting period for completion	Shorter time to completion	Greater risk involved
Increases choice	Requires multiple visits	Fewer visits	Limited access
Less painful than surgical methods	Available upto 9 wks only	Can be performed at later gestations	Requires more equipment and investment
Offered earlier in pregnancy	Expensive	Pathologic confirmation possible	Providers more vulnerable to risk
More patient control over the procedure	Slightly less effective	Shorter bleeding duration	Less patient control over the procedure

Section V

Disorders of Pelvic Floor & Urinary Tract

24

Genital Prolapse

The normal position of the uterus is of ante-version and ante-flexion. It thus lies almost horizontally, when the woman stands erect. In a woman a natural hiatus is present in the pelvic floor through which increased intra-abdominal pressure acts. Prolapse is herniation or protrusion of an organ or structure outside it's anatomical boundaries.

Prevalence It is found in 50% of parous women, but symptomatic in only 20%.

THE NORMAL SUPPORTS OF THE UTERUS

The uterus is held in position by the muscular pelvic floor, the pelvic ligaments and the endopelvic fascia.

The pelvic floor This includes

1. The levator ani with it's parts, the pubo-coccygeus, ilio and ischio-coccygeus
2. The obturator internus muscles
3. Superficial and deep perineal muscles

The pelvic ligaments These are condensations of pelvic fascia that form a sling for the cervix, uterus and upper part of the vagina. They comprise:

1. The *pubo-cervical ligament* (Fig. 24.1a)–which extends from the anterior aspect of the cervix to the back of the body of the pubis.

2. The *lateral cervical ligament* (Fig. 24.1b)–extends from the lateral aspect of the cervix and the upper vagina to the pelvic side walls. It contains the uterine vessels and nerves running from the pelvic side walls to the uterus. The ureter passes underneath it to the ureterovesical junction.

3. The *uterosacral ligaments* (Fig. 24.1c)–extend form the back of the uterus to the front of the sacrum.

4. The *posterior pubo-urethral ligament*–extends from the postero-inferior aspect of the symphysis pubis to the anterior aspect of the middle third of the urethra and on to the bladder.

5. The *round ligament*–is not a true ligament but passes from the uterine cornu through the inguinal canal to the labium majus (see Fig. 1.1 in chapter on anatomy).

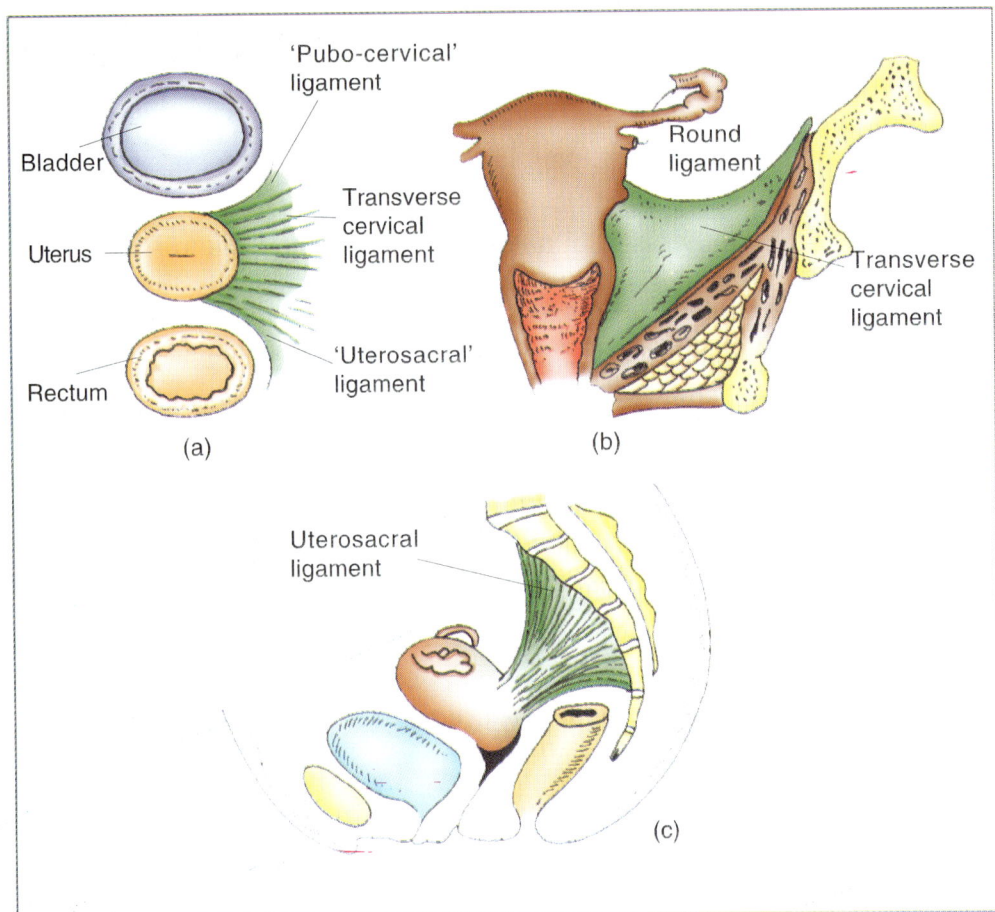

Fig. 24.1a-c. Supports of the uterus

The endopelvic fascia is composed of fibrous tissue and smooth muscle supported by blood vessels and nerves and is continuous with the uterus, cervix and vaginal walls. It envelops these structures and attaches them to the pelvic side-walls.

AETIOLOGY OF PROLAPSE

1. **Postmenopausal atrophy** Oestrogen is important for maintenance of the structural integrity of many tissues. Lack of oestrogens slackens tissues as a process of aging, hence prolapse is more often seen in the menopausal age group.

2. **Injury due to childbirth** Undue stretching of pelvic floor during childbirth is one of the aetiological factors implicated in prolapse. An episiotomy is better than excessive stretching of the pelvic floor. A woman with complete perineal tear rarely develops prolapse as she continuously exercises her sphincters to control her faeces. Prolonged bearing down, ventouse extraction from an incompletely dilated cervix, delivery of a big baby, pregnancies in rapid succession before full recovery cause weakening of the pelvic tissues and may cause prolapse in later life (Fig. 24.2).

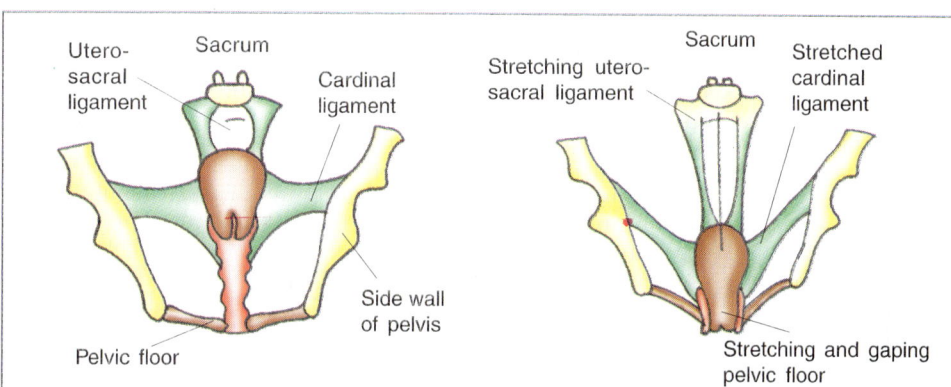

Fig. 24.2. Pathophysiology of genital prolapse

3. **Congenital prolapse** is seen in nulliparous females due to congenital weakness of pelvic tissues. It is usually not associated with a cystocele or rectocele. It may be associated with spina-bifida or a split pelvis. Prolapse may be seen in a new born, though it may be reduced, and usually recurs later on in life. These patients may also have a family history of prolapse.

4. **Pulsion type of prolapse** is seen in conditions of raised intra-abdominal pressure as in ascites, intra-abdominal tumours or in patients with chronic cough or constipation.

5. **Iatrogenic prolapse** is seen after abdomino-perineal resection of the rectum or in cases of radical vulvectomy due to extensive tissue excision.

6. **Traction type** is seen in cases of large fibroid polyp which drags on to the uterus.

7. **Traumatic type** is seen in bony injuries to pelvis as in fracture pelvis and diastases of pubic symphysis.

CLASSIFICATION OF PROLAPSE

According to the anatomical location, the pelvic structures are divided into three compartments and prolapse termed accordingly (Fig. 24.3a-d).

Anterior compartment

- Lower 1/3–Prolapse of the urethra–Urethrocele

- Upper 2/3–Prolapse of the bladder–Cystocele

Middle compartment

- Uterovaginal prolapse–Prolapse of the uterus and vaginal vault.

Posterior compartment

- Upper 1/3–Prolapse of peritoneum of pouch of douglas along with the small bowel or omentum into the vagina–Enterocele
- Mid 1/3–Prolapse of the rectum–Rectocele
- Lower 1/3–Prolapse of the perineal body–Perineal hernia

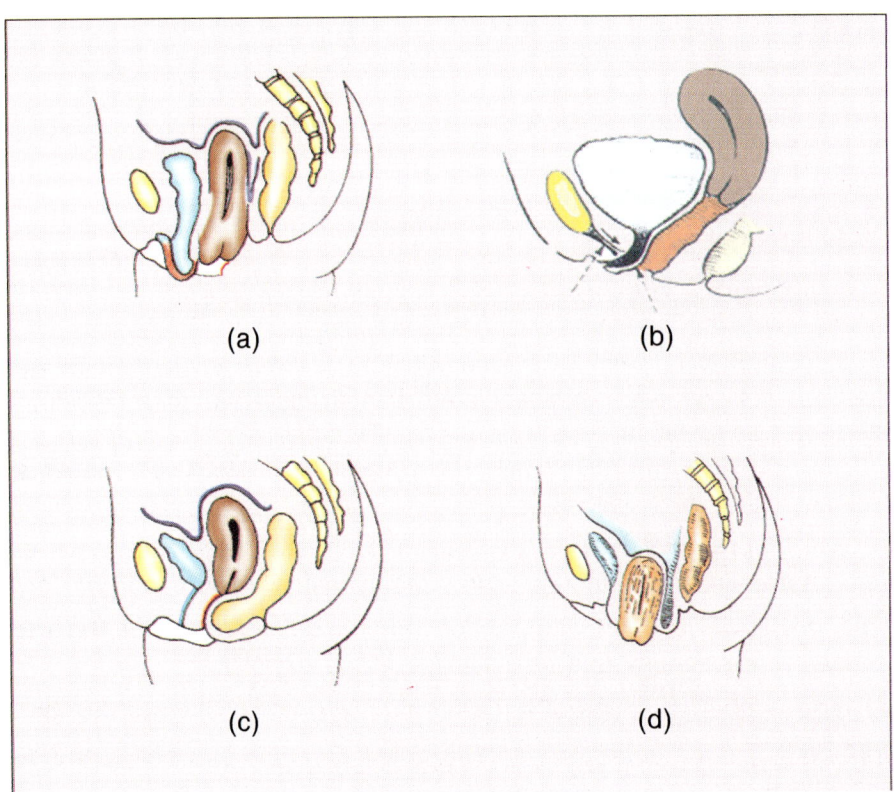

Fig. 24.3a-d. Types of prolapse (a) Cystocele, (b) Urethrocele, (c) Rectocele and (d) Enterocele

Grading of prolapse (Shaw's method) (Fig. 24.4) This is the most popular method where uterine prolapse is graded depending on it's relationship to the ischial spines.

- First degree–the cervix is below the level of ischial spines.
- Second degree–the cervix is at the level of introitus.
- Third degree–the cervix lies outside the introitus.

- Procidentia–in this the whole uterus lies outside the introitus with eversion of vaginal walls.

POP Classification standardized by the International continence society

0 – No descent of pelvic organs during staining.

I – Leading surface of he prolapse does not descend below 1 cm above the hymenal ring.

II – Leading edge of he prolapse extends from 1cm above to 1 cm below the hymenal ring.

III – From 1 cm beyond the hymenal ring belt without complete vaginal eversion.

IV – The vaginal is completely eversted.

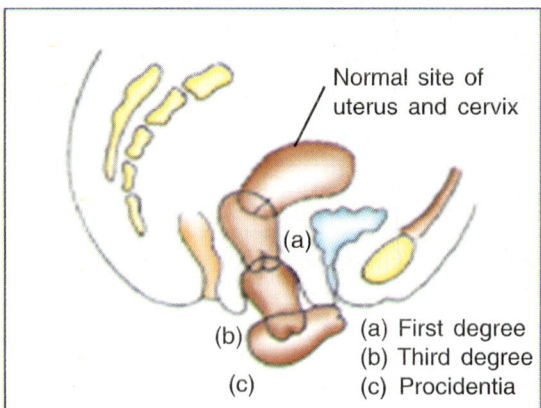

Fig. 24.4. Degrees of uterine prolapse–Note the position of uterus

- *Vault prolapse*–Following a hysterectomy, commonly a vaginal hysterectomy, the entire vault prolapses, if the defect has not been repaired properly.

COMPLICATIONS OF PROLAPSE

- **Keratinization**–due to prolonged rubbing of the prolapsed part.
- **Decubitus ulcer**–is caused by venous congestion due to prolonged venous engorgement and blockage of venous return.
- **Stress urinary incontinence (SUI)**–the urethrovesical angle descends with formation of cystocele and rectocele and stress urinary incontinence can be seen.
- **Incarceration of prolapse**–prolonged prolapse without reposition may cause incarceration.
- **Obstructive uropathy**–in long standing prolapse, especially in procidentia, the ureters

get kinked leading to obstructive uropathy and hydronephrosis. Prolonged retention of urine in the cystocele causes infection and hypertrophy of the bladder.

EVALUATION OF A PATIENT WITH GENITAL PROLAPSE

Symptoms

- *Mass per vaginum*–The patient complains of something coming out, with a bearing down feeling. This increases in the evenings especially after prolonged standing and squatting.

- *Urinary symptoms*–Initially there are symptoms of increased frequency, later on this is followed by difficulty in initiation of micturition and a feeling of incomplete evacuation, due to retention of urine in the cystocele pouch. Cystitis may occur due to residual urine collection in the bladder. Symptoms of stress urinary incontinence can occur.

- *Bowel complaints*–A feeling of incomplete evacuation after having passed stools occurs as stool collects in a pouch formed by the rectocele.

- *Discharge and spotting*–Due to laxity of the introitus, there is an increased chance of infection leading to vaginal discharge. Descent of the cervix and vagina causes congestion, which leads to decubitus ulcer formation and therefore spotting. Treatment of decubitus ulcer is by reduction of the prolapse. As venous stasis decreases, the ulcer heals. Biopsy should be taken if the decubitus ulcer does not heal by 2 weeks.

- *Coital difficulties*–Laxity of the introitus leads to coital problems, which is usually not revealed by the patient. In procidentia and third degree prolapse, laxity of the introitus and the prolapsed uterus prevents penetration.

EXAMINATION

General examination

- The general build, nutritional status and gait are noted.
- Her spine and hernial sites are checked.
- The chest is examined for any evidence of chronic bronchitis or bronchial asthma which could be the cause of intra-raised intra-abdominal pressure.
- The blood pressure should be checked as any hypertension needs to be controlled prior to surgery.
- The abdomen is examined for any mass which could be the reason for the prolapse.

Local examination

- Condition of vulva and laxity of the introitus are noted.

- The presence or absence of stress incontinence is assessed by the presence or absence of leakage on straining with a full bladder.

- The patient is then asked to strain and the part prolapsing first is noted. This is the leading part of prolapse. Repair would depend on this. The degree of prolapse, presence and degree of cystocele, rectocele, enterocele, urethrocele, the rugosity of vagina and status of cervix are noted on per speculum examination.

Per-vaginal examination is carried out to note the position and size of the uterus, and to look for any adnexal pathology.

Rectal examination

A low rectocele can easily be identified by a finger in the rectum, as the rectovaginal septum is unusually thin.

Diagnosis of enterocele

- Keeping one finger in the rectum and one in the vagina, the patient is asked to strain. If an enterocele is present it will bulge into the space between the cervix and the upper posterior vaginal wall.

- Intra-vaginal USG can be done to identify loops of small intestine in the enterocele sac. The distance between the anal orifice and rectum should also be noted.

Thickness of the perineum and tone of the levator-ani muscles is noted by keeping a finger in the rectum and the thumb over the perineum and asking the patient to contract the perineal muscles. Strong contraction with thickening of the perineal muscles indicates good perineal tone.

Cervical length is assessed by palpation and sounding the cavity. Uterovaginal prolapse is associated with supravaginal elongation of the cervix and an increase in length of the utero-cervical canal.

DIFFERENTIAL DIAGNOSIS

All the following conditions cause the patient to present with a mass per vaginum.

1. Vulval cyst–The vaginal orifice can be identified separately.
2. Urethral diverticulum arises anterior to the vaginal hiatus.
3. Cervical fibroid polyp–The vaginal wall can be felt all around the polyp.
4. Chronic inversion of the uterus–the fundus of the uterus is not palpable abdominally and the cervix can be palpated as a ring all around the inverted uterus.
5. Rectal prolapse–occurs posterior to the vagina.
6. Cyst of the anterior vaginal wall.
7. Varicocele of the vagina.

MANAGEMENT OF PROLAPSE

This includes Investigations and Treatment:

Investigations These include

General Investigations to know the patient's fitness for surgery and specific investigations related to the prolapse.

General Investigations as for any routine surgical procedure like a complete haemogram, urine routine and microscopy, blood urea, serum creatinine, random blood sugar, P A P smear, a chest x-ray and ECG are carried out.

Specific Investigations These are indicated in specific circumstances

- Intravenous urography (IVU)–is indicated in procidentia of long standing as it could be associated with bilateral hydronephrosis.
- Urine culture and sensitivity–indicated if urinary symptoms are present.
- Urodynamic studies–are indicated if the patient has stress incontinence or voiding difficulty.
- Ultrasound–Perineal and transvesical ultrasound can be used to visualize the pelvic floor and measure the bladder pressure simultaneously.
- Pelvic floor fluoroscopy–specially useful for the detection of an enterocele.
- Dynamic MRI–offers superior anatomical imaging and detail but is expensive.
- Isotope defecography–involves the use of technitium 99m labelled 'porridge' into the rectum and visualization with a gamma camera to note the descent of the pelvic floor and rectum. This is specially useful to demonstrate an enterocele.

Treatment of prolapse

Prophylaxis of prolapse Tissue damage starts at the time of childbirth. Multiparity, macrosomia, prolonged second stage of labour, home delivery by a dai with premature bearing down efforts increases the risk. A timely episiotomy, avoidance of prolonged second stage and good postnatal nutrition and exercises decrease the risk.

Conservative management This is advocated in case of

1. Old debilitated patients
2. Pregnancy
3. Any patient refusing surgery
4. Patient medically unfit for surgery
5. Postponement of surgery till the next childbirth

The options are

1. Pelvic floor exercises: There is no evidence to prove that they prevent or treat minor grades of prolapse.

2. Vaginal pessary: Pessary treatment can be recommended provided the patient is compliant. They are indicated in a woman who is unfit or refuses to have surgery. A pessary forms a shelf and prevents descent of the uterus and vagina (Fig. 24.5).

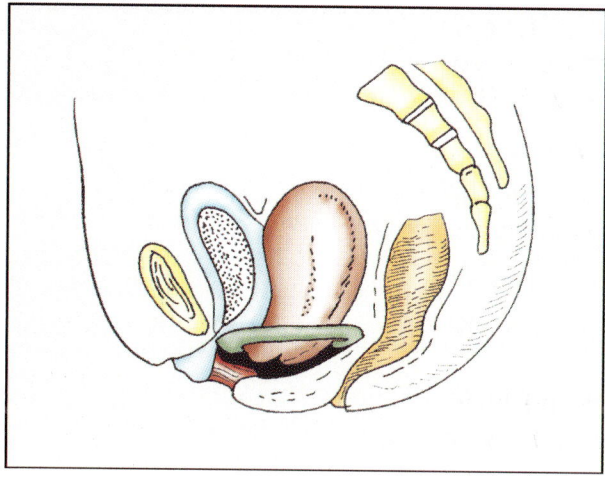

Fig. 24.5. Vaginal pessary for prolapse

Limitations of pessary usage

• It should be changed every 6 months

• Follow-up is needed as prolonged usage can cause vaginitis, ulcers, fistulas and carcinoma of the vagina.

• Failure of retention can occur in case of a patulous vaginal orifice.

• A pessary is only palliative and cannot correct the associated problems of stress-incontinence

Surgery for prolapse

The *principles of prolapse surgery* are to:

1. Restore anatomy

2. Restore vaginal function

3. Correct urinary and faecal incontinence

4. Prevent de-novo prolapse and incontinence

Prerequisites to be fulfilled before surgical treatment is undertaken:

- Symptoms should be caused by the prolapse and not by other pelvic or spinal conditions.
- Child bearing should preferably be completed before surgery is undertaken as vaginal delivery causes recurrence of prolapse.
- Marital life and coital activity should be noted to avoid overzealous shortening and narrowing of the vagina.
- Chronic cough and constipation should be corrected to prevent recurrence. Obese women should be advised weight reduction.
- Any urinary infection should be treated prior to surgery as symptoms can recur in the post-op period.
- Decubitus ulcer should be treated by an acriflavine-glycerine pack before surgery.
- Topical oestrogen creams are used 6-8 weeks preoperatively to improve the vaginal rugosity. They should be stopped 2 weeks before surgery.

Types of surgery

Surgery is chosen depending on

- The age of the patient
- Degree of prolapse
- The type of prolapse
- Associated menstrual problems
- Her desires regarding childbearing and menstrual functions
- Her fitness for surgery

1. *Vaginal hysterectomy with pelvic floor repair*–this the preferred operation in a woman with second or greater degree of prolapse with cervical elongation, age more than 45 yrs. or <45 yrs. whose family is complete or she has associated menstrual problems. A hysterectomy is done with posterior and anterior repair, if cytocele and rectocele are associated. The steps of vaginal hysterectomy are detailed in chapter 27 and shown in Fig. 27.3.

2. *Anterior colporrhaphy*–this procedure is used to correct an isolated cystourethrocele. The principles are reduction of the prolapsed bladder and vagina using interrupted absorbable sutures placed in the pubo-cervical fascia, excision of excess vaginal skin and approximation of the vagina with continuous locking sutures (Fig. 24.6a-e). Nowadays a prolene mesh is inserted if the prolapse is recurrent.

3. *Manchester repair*–is carried out in women of less than 40 yrs. age with a second

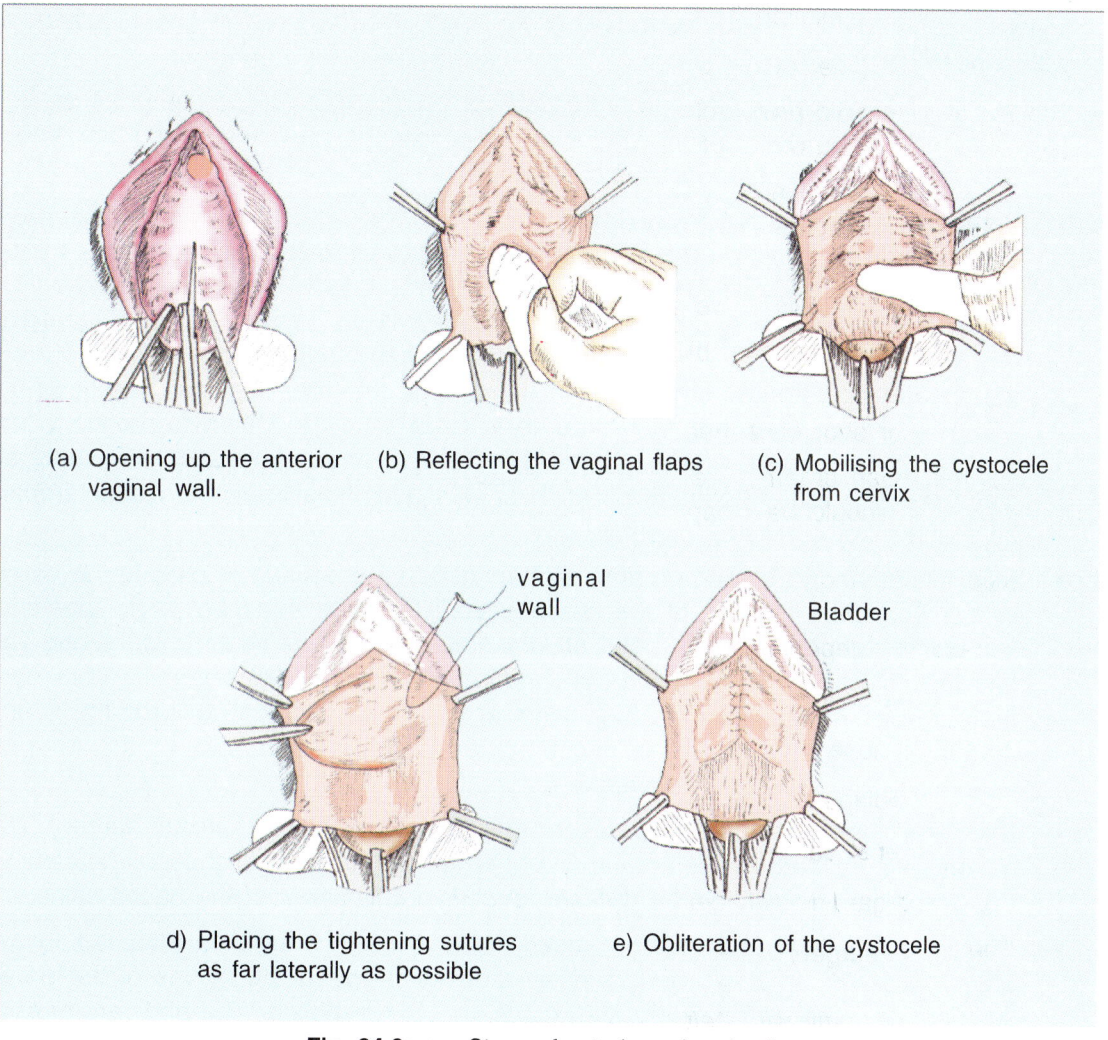

(a) Opening up the anterior vaginal wall.

(b) Reflecting the vaginal flaps

(c) Mobilising the cystocele from cervix

vaginal wall

Bladder

d) Placing the tightening sutures as far laterally as possible

e) Obliteration of the cystocele

Fig. 24.6a-e. Steps of anterior colporrhaphy

degree uterovaginal prolapse along with cervical elongation, who is keen to retain her uterus for menstrual functions or child bearing. It consists of cervical dilatation with anterior colporrhaphy, cervical amputation and posterior colpoperinorrhaphy. The mackendrodt ligaments are shortened and brought anteriorly in front of the cervix and held with Fothergill's sutures. Postoperative complications are secondary haemorrhage, habitual abortion, repetitive preterm deliveries, cervical stenosis and dystocia during labour in the long term.

4. *Shirodkar's repair*–this is preferably done with a second or third degree prolapse when cervical elongation is not present, the patient is less than 40 years of age and is keen on maintaining her menstrual functions and fertility. Following an anterior colporrhaphy, the pouch of douglas is opened, bilateral uterosacral ligaments are clamped, shortened,

ligated and brought in front of the cervix. A high closure of the pouch of douglas is done with a posterior repair.

5. *Abdominal sling operations*–these are carried out in case of a nulliparous prolapse in a young woman. The types of sling operation which can be performed are Purandare's, Shirodkar's and Khanna's abdominal sling operations.

- Purandare's sling operation: A rectus sheath sling is used to elevate the cervix. A low transverse incision is made in the abdominal wall to expose the rectus sheath and 1/2 an inch thick fascial sheaths are fashioned from it. These are elevated from the underlying muscle and divided in the middle with its base at the lateral margins of the rectus abdominis. After entering the abdomen the UV fold is opened up and the sheaths are brought intra-abdominally through the deep inguinal ring along the round ligaments. They are then sutured to each other and then anchored to the isthmus of the uterus. Anteriorly, the UV fold is then sutured back. This may be combined with round ligament plication or with abdominal repair of the enterocele by a purse string suture.

- Modified Purandare's sling: A sling of merselene tape is used to elevate the cervix in this procedure instead of fascial sheaths. These are attached to the posterior surface of the cervix at the point of attachment of the uterosacral ligaments. The tape is brought forward between the uterine vessels and the isthmus. From here they are passed between the two layers of the broad ligament towards the lateral margin of rectus muscle and anchored on to the aponeurosis of the anterior abdominal wall with non-absorbable sutures.

- Shirodkar's abdominal sling operation: It is technically a very difficult surgery. The abdomen is opened, merselene tape is attached to the isthmus of cervix posteriorly, the other end attached to the anterior longitudinal ligament of the sacral spine.

- Khanna's sling surgery: In this procedure, a merselene tape is attached to the uterine isthmus, the two ends are brought out between the leaves of the broad ligament near the lateral side of the rectus abdominis muscle. The ends are passed below the external oblique aponeurosis on either side and attached to the anterior superior iliac spine.

6. *Le Fort's partial colpocleisis*–is indicated in a patient who has her uterus, is not sexually active and is medically unfit to undergo major reconstructive surgery. A raw area is made on the anterior and posterior vaginal wall by sharp dissection; the cut edges are sutured together with interrupted delayed absorbable sutures to obliterate the vagina. An aggressive perinenorrhaphy is performed to narrow the introitus.

25

Urogynaecology

Urogynaecology, which deals with urological problems in gynaecology is a newly emerging sub-speciality. In the last decade, a lot of advances have taken place in this sub-speciality particularly after better understanding of female urogynaecological problems like over-active bladder, stress urinary incontinence, urinary tract infection during pregnancy, female sexual dysfunction and female urethral syndrome.

Recent advances in video urodynamic studies and better imaging modalities have greatly helped both urologists and gynaecologists in managing these problems.

The following are the common urogynaecological problems encountered by the gynaecologist:

A. Stress urinary incontinence (SUI)

B. Urogynaecological fistulae

C. Female urethral syndrome

D. Urinary tract infection (UTI)

E. Overactive bladder (OAB)

F. Female urethral disorders

ANATOMY OF THE FEMALE GENITO URINARY SYSTEM (GUS)

Female urethra

The female urethra is 4 cm long with its opening just superior to the introitus. The lining epithelium gradually changes from transitional to non-keratinized stratified squamous epithelium from above downwards. Many small mucus glands open into the urethra and can give rise to urethral diverticula. Distally these glands group together on either side of urethra and are known as the Skene's glands and empty on either side of the external urethral meatus. The submucosa of the female urethra is thick, richly vascular and supports the urethral epithelium and glands. The mucosa and submucosa together form a cushion that contributes significantly to urethral closure pressure. These layers are oestrogen dependent. At menopause they atrophy resulting in a decrease in the urethral closure pressure which further decreases during any increase in the intra-abdominal pressure resulting in stress incontinence. In contrast to the male proximal urethra, no circular muscle sphincter can be identified in the females.

The striated urethral sphincter invests the distal two thirds of the female urethra. Proximally it forms a complete ring around the urethra that corresponding to the zone of highest urethral closure pressure. The suspensory ligament of the clitoris and the pubo-urethral ligaments form a sling that suspends the urethra beneath the pubis.

Blood supply

*   The *arterial supply* to the female urethra is derived from the inferior vesical, vaginal and internal pudendal arteries.
*   *Venous drainage* drains into the internal pudendal veins.
*   *Lymphatic drainage* from the external portion of the urethra is to the inguinal and sub-inguinal lymphnodes. Drainage from the deep urethra is into the internal iliac lymphnodes (hypogastric).

Female urogenital triangle

The vestibule of the vagina runs vertically throughout the length of the urogenital triangle (see Fig. 1.1 in chapter 1). The labia majora form its lateral sides and fuse anteriorly as the hood of the clitoris. The subcutaneous fat pad of the mons pubis continues posteriorly in the labia majora to form the vestibule. The urethra enters the vestibule between the clitoris and the vagina. The perineal membrane is pierced in its centre by the vagina and is less well developed than that of the male.

Blood supply to the urogenital triangle is derived from the internal pudenal vessels. The internal pudendal veins communicate freely with the dorsal vein complex by piercing the levator ani muscles.

Nerve supply By the pudendal nerve which follows the vessels.

Mechanism of voiding The bladder adapts to increased urinary volume by maintaining the pressure below 10cm of H_2O until it is filled upto 500 mls of urine. The intraurethral pressure is normally higher than the intravesical pressure. The urethrovesical anatomy during rest and voiding is given in Fig. 25.1.

A. STRESS URINARY INCONTINENCE (SUI)

Definition Involuntary loss of urine during any increase in the intra-abdominal pressure like coughing, sneezing or physical exertion and sudden changes in position.

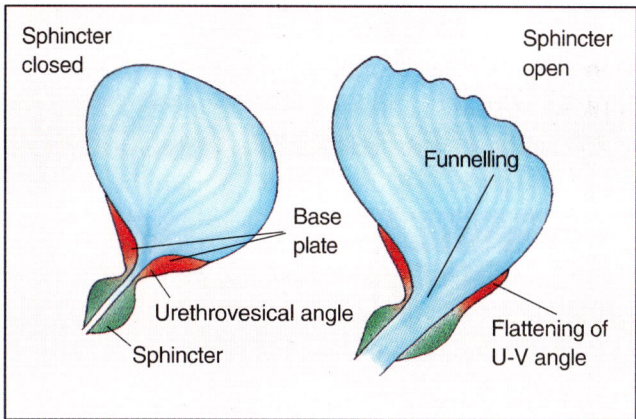

Fig. 25.1. Mechanism of micturition (a) During rest, the urethra and bladder neck are maintained in the closed state by the trigonal condensation of muscle and the urethral sphincter (b) During micturition, the detrusor contracts, the bladder neck relaxes causing funnelling and flattening of the U-V angle

Pathophysiology of SUI

SUI is strictly an anatomic problem. In the normal continent woman, in the standing position, the bladder neck and proximal urethra are intra-abdominal and lie parallel to the pelvic floor. Any increase in the intra-abdominal pressure causes compression of the urethra and the urethral pressure exceeds the intra-vesical pressure.

Urethral sphincter incontinence is principally due to two factors

1. Distortion of the normal urethrovesical anatomy with descent of the bladder neck and proximal urethra, the intra-urethral pressure then fails to rise during straining (Fig. 25.2).

2. Lowered urethral pressure–lowered intra-urethral pressure at rest below the intra-vesical pressure.

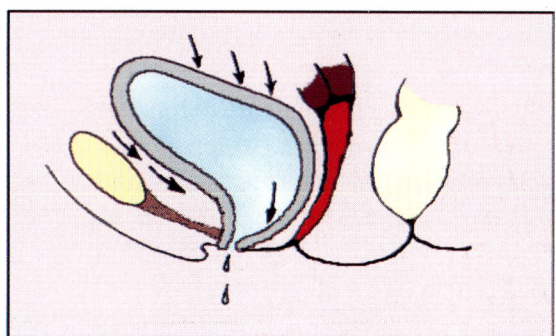

Fig. 25.2. SUI–Involuntary leakage in the absence of detrusor contraction due to displacement of the bladder neck

Causes of SUI

The components of the nervous system and bladder wall remain structurally intact; however, there is failure of urethral closure. The risk factors identified are:

1. Urethral hypermobility and loss of sub-urethral support as seen in pelvic organ prolapse.

2. Intrinsic sphincter deficiency
   - oestrogen deficiency after due to menopause resulting in a decrease in the functional urethral length and urethral closure pressure.
   - previous surgery on the urethra

3. Labour and delivery as vaginal delivery is associated with direct injury to the pelvic soft tissues as well as partial denervation of the pelvic floor, may play a role in the aetiology of SUI.

Diagnosis

1. *History* A detailed history is taken regarding the severity of incontinence as well as its impact on the quality of life. Details regarding any treatment received are also elicited.

2. *Physical examination*
   a) Bonney's test–

   The patient should be examined with a full bladder. Light forward pressure is applied using two fingers inserted along each side of the upper urethra. The patient is then asked to cough. If there is no escape of urine, it confirms the diagnosis and also predicts the success of local repair.

   b) A pelvic examination is then carried out to look for a cysto-urethrocele.

3. *Micturition diary* Frequency-volume chart–the patient keeps a record of the time of voiding, the volume of urine voided and any episodes of leakage.

4. *Pad test* A one-hour extended pad test is recommended in cases when the clinical stress test is negative.

   The patient wears a pre-weighed sanitary pad, drinks about 500 ml of water and rests for 15 min. She then performs exercises like walking or climbing stairs for 30 min.; followed by provocative exercises like bending, jumping, coughing etc. for another 15 min. After a period of one hour, the sanitary pad is removed and weighed. An increase in weight by 1 gm is considered as a significant loss.

5. *Cysto-urethroscopy* Optical visualization of the bladder and urethra is not indicated routinely but can exclude a urethro-vaginal or vesicovaginal fistula.

6. *Urodynamic evaluation* clinches the diagnosis.

a) *Cystometry:* This involves the measurement of pressure/volume relationship of the bladder during filling and voiding and is the most useful test of bladder function. The woman is first asked to void and is then catheterized to measure the residual volume. The bladder is filled using a 12F catheter with a continuous infusion of normal saline at room temperature, the intra-vesical and intra-abdominal pressure are measured. During filling, the woman is asked to indicate her first desire to void, the maximal desire to void, the volumes at which these events occur are noted. Once the bladder is filled, the patient is asked to stand and cough and any leakage is noted. The woman is then asked to void in the commode with the pressure lines in place.

Normal Cystometry: The parameters of normal bladder function are:

 – Residual urine of < 50 ml

 – First desire to void between 150 and 200 ml

 – Bladder capacity of > 400 ml

 – No detrusor pressure rise on filling with no detrusor contractions.

 – No leakage on coughing.

Abnormal Cystometry:

 – Leakage on coughing without a rise in the detrusor pressure suggests *Genuine Stress Incontinence (GSI).*

 – Spontaneous detrusor contractions while the woman is attempting to inhibit micturition is called *Detrusor Instability.*

b) *Uroflowmetry:* This is a simple non-invasive test and easily performed in an outpatient setting to know the flow rate of urine during voiding. The normal flow rate is 15 mls/sec, the voided volume should be above 150 ml. A low peak flow rate and a prolonged voiding time suggests a voiding disorder.

c) *Urethral pressure and urethral closure pressure profiles.*

7. **Lateral cystourethrogram** The procedure is the same as cystometry except that the filling medium is urografin 35% and the test is performed with x-ray screening. The woman is tilted upright and asked to cough and strain, any leakage, bladder neck opening and bladder base descent are noted with x-ray diagrams. Ureteric reflux can be demonstrated but this test is not necessary in a routine evaluation.

8. **Ultrasound** is useful to assess the bladder neck and volume of residual urine, the advantage being that it is non-invasive.

The investigations in a patient with urinary incontinence are summarized in table 25.1.

Table 25.1. Investigations in a patient with incontinence

History
Physical examination with Bonney's test
Pelvic examination
Micturition diary
Pad test
Cysto and urethroscopy
Urodynamic evaluation
    – Cystometry
    – Uroflowmetry
    – Urethral pressure and closure profiles
Lateral cytourethrogram
Pelvic ultrasound

Treatment of SUI

Medical management

a) *Anticholinergic drugs* improve the urethral tone, thereby preventing leakage. Alpha-agonists eg. ephedrine, phenylpropanolamine are given to increase the urethral tone.

b) *Electrical stimulation* is used to strengthen the pelvic muscle tone.

c) *Bio-feedback* is useful in patients who cannot perform pelvic floor exercises. In this, a signal, auditory or visual tells the patient that she is contracting the right muscles.

d) *Periurethral injections* with collagen polymers is indicated in recurrent GSI.

e) *Pelvic floor exercises* were introduced by Kegel in the 1950s, the subjective cure rate varies from 17-75%.

Surgical management

Aims of surgery are: To correct the anatomic defects i.e.,

1. Descent of the bladder neck

2. Correct intrinsic sphincter weakness

3. Correct loss of urethral support

Surgical procedures suspend and support the vesicourethral segment in a normal position. The various procedures are:

a) *Marshall-Marchetti-Krantz* and *Burch's Colposuspension*

There are the two most commonly performed surgeries for SUI. They are performed by the retropubic approach. The purpose is to bring the bladder neck back to an intra-abdominal location. In this procedure catgut or vicryl sutures are used to suture the peri-urethral tissues to the pubic bone. In *Burch's* procedure, a permanent suture is placed on both sides of the bladder neck and the ipsilateral ilio-pectineal ligament (Fig. 25.3).

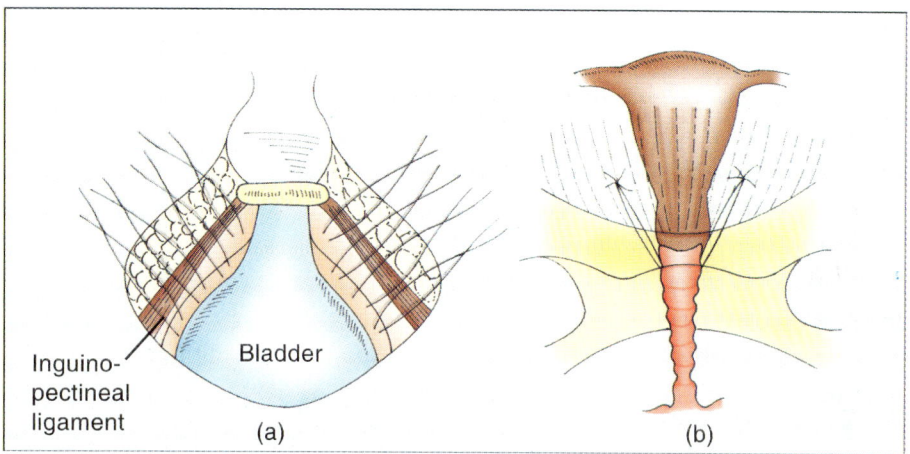

Inguino-
pectineal
ligament

Bladder

(a)

(b)

Fig. 25.3ab a) Burch's colposuspension–The paravaginal fascia is sutured on each side to the ilio-pectineal ligaments   b) Stamey colposuspension–A nylon suture attaches the vaginal wall to the rectus sheath, to elevate the vagina and bladder base.

b) *Kelly's procedure*–cystourethroplasty usually combined with a cystocele repair, however the success rate is low.

c) *Needle suspension procedures*–Stamey, Pareyra are not very effective.

d) *Tension free vaginal tape (TVT)*–This is a latest technique in which a prolene tape is used at the level of the mid-vagina to form a sub-urethral sling.

e) *Pubo-vaginal slings* (Fig. 25.4)–A sling of synthetic material, fascia of the rectus sheath or fascia lata is used to form a sub-urethral sling.

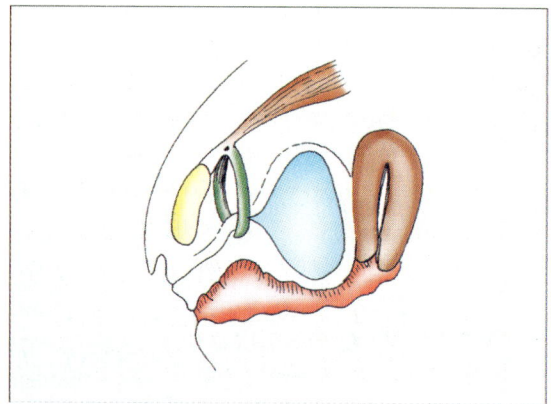

Fig. 25.4. Principle of the pubo-vaginal sling

f) *Peri-urethral injections* are used in recurrent GSI. A bulking agent (Collagen, Macoplastique) is injected transurethrally via an operative cysto-urethroscope into the urethral submucosa of the bladder neck.

g) *Artificial sphincter* is an implantable device that occludes the urethra but can be voluntarily opened by the patient when she desires to empty her bladder.

B. UROGYNAECOLOGICAL FISTULAE

Definition A fistula is defined as an abnormal communication between two or more epithelial surfaces.

Types of urinary fistulae

1. Vesicovaginal fistula

2. Urethrovaginal fistula

3. Ureterovaginal fistula

1. Vesicovaginal fistula (VVF)

Causes of VVF

A. *Obstetric trauma* – The obstetric causes include obstructed labour, accidental injury at caesarean section, forceps delivery, craniotomy, symphysiotomy or criminal abortion. In developing countries birth trauma still accounts for the majority of fistulae. In obstructed labour, the anterior vaginal wall, bladder base and urethra are compressed between the fetal head and the posterior surface of the pubis and get devitalized by ischaemia. The devitalized area separates as slough between the 3rd and 10th day postpartum resulting in incontinence. The bladder may also be injured with difficult operative deliveries eg. forceps, rotation of the fetal head with Kielland's forceps, symphysiotomy or rupture uterus.

B. *Surgical trauma* – In industrialized nations the most common cause of vesicovaginal fistula is routine abdominal or vaginal hysterectomy. Factors which increase the risk are prior caesarean section, intrinsic uterine disease or prior radiotherapy for malignancy. Uretero-vaginal fistulas can occur after abdominal hysterectomy following ligation of the ureters.

C. *Malignancies* – Carcinoma of the cervix, vagina or rectum. Development of a fistula indicates a late stage of the disease.

D. *Iatrogenic* – Rarely foreign bodies, vaginal pessaries, diaphragms and intra-uterine devices may lead to fistula formation. Iatrogenic CO_2 laser therapy for cervical disease has also resulted in bladder fistulas. Autoimmune diseases such as Behcet's disease have also been implicated as causative for vesicovaginal fistulas.

E. *Infections* – Inflammatory bowel disease, tuberculosis, lymphogranuloma venereum can rarely cause a VVF.

Prevalence

The exact prevalence of obstetric fistulas is unknown, but is estimated as 1-2/1000 deliveries. Post-hysterectomy fistulas are seen in about 1 in 1300 operations.

Clinical features

Continuous urinary drainage from the vagina in cases of vesicovaginal fistula and intermittent in case of urethrovaginal fistula. Pain in the loin area is observed in case of ureterovaginal fistulae.

Evaluation

- Physical examination with a sims speculum.

- Dye test–when the diagnosis and the site of fistula is in doubt. Methylene blue dye is instilled into the bladder via a catheter and the site of leakage noted. The traditional three swab test has it's limitations and is not recommended. If leakage of clear fluid occurs after instilling the dye, a ureterovaginal fistula is likely.

- Examination under anaesthesia (EUA)–may be necessary to determine the presence of a fistula and the access for vaginal repair.

- Cystourethroscopy–is essential to know the site, size of fistula and it's relation to the ureteric orifices.

- IVP–is carried out to know the renal function and to diagnose a ureterovaginal fistula.

- Retrograde pyelogram may need to be carried out if IVP is not helpful.

- Voiding cystourethrogram–is essential to diagnose a urethrovaginal fistula.

- Cystography and fistulography–dye test is used to identify the fistulous tract and is useful in small complex fistulas.

Treatment

Surgery

Timing of surgical repair is most important. Fistulas identified within the first 24 to 48 hours post-operatively can safely be repaired immediately. If identified later continuous bladder drainage should be carried out for 6-8 weeks to allow for spontaneous closure of the fistula. If the fistula persists, at least twelve weeks should be given before repairing the fistula as time is required to soften the tissues to obtain a better surgical plane. In radiation fistulas, one should wait for 12 months or more.

Preoperative preparation of the patient is of paramount importance in fistula surgery.

- Proper and appropriate antibiotic cover is to be given to ensure a sterile environment.
- Vaginal douches with antiseptic agents prior to surgery should be undertaken.
- Oestrogen replacement therapy is also used in these patients with poor quality of vaginal tissue.
- Silicone barrier cream is used to reduce the ammoniacal dermatitis.
- The nutrition of patients with long standing obstetric fistulas needs to be improved.

Selection of suture materials is very important. Long acting polyglycolic acid or polydioxone material is used.

Surgical Options: The repair can be performed by either of the three approaches:

- Vaginal
- Abdominal
- Combined vaginal and abdominal

Criteria for selection of the right type of surgical approach depend on several factors like the location of fistula, quality of tissue, size of the fistula and age of the patient.

Vaginal repair is best suited for

- small fistulas
- fistulas low in the anterior vaginal wall
- fistulae not close to the ureteric orifices
- there is good vaginal access
- the vaginal tissues are sufficiently mobile

    Principles

    – Sharp dissection and mobilization to separate the tissues and closure without tension.
    – The vaginal approach uses the creation of an anterior vaginal wall mucosal flap.

- **Sims technique** (Fig. 25.5) involves saucerization of the fistulous tract into a crater which is then closed without dissection using a single row of interrupted sutures. This technique is applicable for small fistulae and residual fistulae after closure of a large defect.
- A suprapubic catheter should be placed for urinary drainage.

Abdominal repair: It is best suited for

- large fistulas
- fistulas involving the trigone and near ureteric orifices
- recurrent fistulas and
- those with poor vaginal access

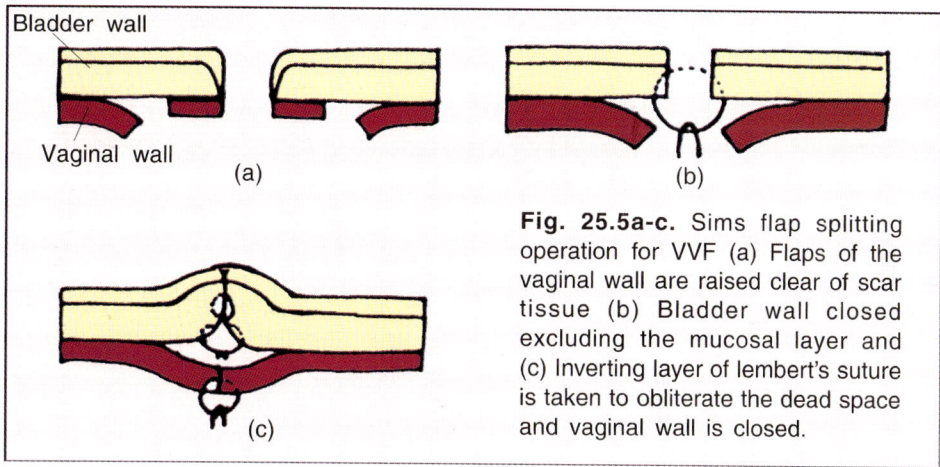

Bladder wall

Vaginal wall

(a)

(b)

(c)

Fig. 25.5a-c. Sims flap splitting operation for VVF (a) Flaps of the vaginal wall are raised clear of scar tissue (b) Bladder wall closed excluding the mucosal layer and (c) Inverting layer of lembert's suture is taken to obliterate the dead space and vaginal wall is closed.

Post-op care: Continuous bladder drainage is the key to success. A bladder neck fistula should be drained by a suprapubic catheter. The urethral catheter is removed first, the suprapubic catheter is removed once the residual urine volume is < 50mls and the patient is voiding normally. A laxative is given to prevent excessive straining at stool, enemas and suppositories are avoided.

Duration of bladder drainage: Post-surgical fistulas-12 days, obstetric fistulas-21 days and radiation fistulas-21-42 days.

2. Urethrovaginal fistulas

Causes: mainly birth trauma

Treatment

• Vaginal approach is the most suitable. Urethrovaginal fistula should not be completely excised but rather circumcised and oversewn.

• Flaps may be taken from the anterior vaginal wall and the urethra reconstructed. Muscle or fat may be interposed between the flaps.

3. Ureterovaginal fistula

Causes: Ligation of the ureter while performing an abdominal hysterectomy.

Treatment

1. If diagnosed intra-operatively the ligature should be released.

2. If diagnosed late then urinary diversion by PCN (percutaneous nephrostomy) followed by a planned uretero-neocystostomy should be performed with an anti-reflux procedure with DJ stenting.

C. FEMALE URETHRAL SYNDROME (FUS)

The female urethral syndrome whether acute or chronic usually refers to any symptoms or combination of symptoms suggestive of UTI occurring in patients considered to be uninfected.

Clinical features

Female urethral syndrome is a very non specific constellation of symptoms including urinary frequency, urgency, dysuria and suprapubic discomfort without any objective finding.

Types

- Acute
- Chronic

Pure urethral syndrome includes patients who have neither a microbial cause nor interstitial cystitis. Many of these patients have an emotional basis for their discomfort. Dysfunctional voiding may contribute to the symptoms. It is in this group that urodynamic studies may be useful.

Treatment

If associated infection is ruled out and interstitial cystitis is excluded then the treatment is mainly symptomatic.

D.   URINARY TRACT INFECTION DURING PREGNANCY

Although the prevalence of bacteruria does not change with the occurrence of pregnancy, certain anatomic and physiologic alterations associated with this state probably do change the course of bacteriuria during pregnancy. These changes may cause the pregnant woman to be more susceptible to pyelonephritis and may require alteration of therapy. These changes are as follows:

1. Increase in renal size.

2. Smooth muscle atony of the collecting system and bladder–There is decreased peristalsis during pregnancy and most women in their third trimester show significant ureteric dilatation. This hydroureter has been attributed to muscle relaxing effect of progesterone during pregnancy and also due to the mechanical obstruction of the ureters by the enlarged uterus.

3. Bladder changes–The enlarging uterus displaces the bladder superiorly and anteriorly and the bladder becomes hyperaemic and congested.

4. Augmented renal function–The GFR and the renal plasma flow increases. The urinary protein excretion also increases.

5. The prevalence of bacteriuria found in females of childbearing age is 4 to 6%. Whether treated or not, pregnant females with bacteriuria are at a high risk of suffering from recurrent urinary tract infection. The incidence of acute clinical pyelonephritis in pregnant women with bacteriuria is significantly increased over that of non-pregnant women. Of the 1-4% of women who develop pyelonephritis during pregnancy, 60% to 75% acquire it during the third trimester.

Complications associated with UTI during pregnancy

1. An increase in the incidence of preterm labour with an increase in perinatal mortality.
2. Maternal anaemia
3. Maternal hypertension and pre-eclampsia

Treatment of UTI during pregnancy

- Selection of an antimicrobial agent to treat the bacteriuria must be made, however, special consideration should be given to maternal and fetal toxicity.

Drugs considered safe during pregnancy

- Penicillin
- Amoxicillin
- Ampicillin
- Cephalosporin
- Nitrofurantoin – safe in 1st and 2nd trimester but contraindicated in the 3rd trimester as it may cause haemolytic anaemia.

Drugs to be avoided during pregnancy

- Fluroquinolones–can cause damage to the immature cartilage of the fetus.
- Chloramphenicol–may result in "grey baby syndrome".
- Trimethoprim–may cause megaloblastic anaemia since it is a folate antagonist.
- Erythromycin–associated with maternal cholestatic jaundice.
- Tetracycline–may cause acute liver decompensation and inhibition of new bone growth in the fetus.

E. OVERACTIVE BLADDER (OAB) / DETRUSOR INSTABILITY

Overactive bladder is a form of urinary leakage due to involuntary bladder contraction characterized by an increased frequency of micturition, a strong and sudden desire to void, which may or may not be associated with urge incontinence.

- The risk of developing OAB increases with age. The incidence is 12-22% in females between 40 to 60 years of age and rises to 30 to 40% at 70 years of age.

- The condition is characterized by an uncontrolled contraction of the bladder muscle during bladder filling phase resulting in increased frequency, urgency and urge incontinence.

- In majority of cases the cause of OAB is unknown. In some patients there may be neurological causes like parkinsonism, spina bifida, multiple sclerosis and spinal cord damage.

- Other factors increasing the risk are increasing parity and a positive family history.

Diagnosis of OAB

- Clinical history with a frequency volume chart to evaluate their fluid intake and voiding pattern.
- Bonney's test: no leakage is seen on coughing.
- Urine analysis by MSU as urinary tract infection can cause similar symptoms.
- Urodynamic evaluation–Detrusor contractions are seen on bladder filling.

Treatment of OAB

- *General measures:* Limit fluid intake to 1-1.5 l / day, avoid tea, coffee and alcohol, incontinence pads.

- *Medical treatment*

    a) Anticholinergic drugs: The detrusor is innervated mainly by para-sympathetic nerves, hence anti-cholinergic drugs need to be used to stop detrusor contractions. However, they can all cause anti-muscarinic side-effects eg. dry mouth, blurred vision, tachycardia, drowsiness and constipation. The drugs used are

        – Oxybutynin
        – Tolterodine–has a more selective action on bladder receptors.

    b) Bladder training and behavioural therapy

- *Surgical treatment*

    a) Bladder augmentation cystoplasty to increase the capacity of the bladder.

F. FEMALE URETHRAL DISORDERS

i) Congenital

- – Distal urethral stenosis
- – Labial fusion

ii) Acquired

- – Urethritis-acute / chronic / senile
- – Urethral caruncle
- – Urethral mucosal prolapse
- – Urethral diverticulum
- – Urethral strictures

Distal urethral stenosis

There is spasm of the external urinary sphincter due to an external striated muscle ring. After puberty the ring disappears. Treatment of such a condition is periodic overdilatation of the urethra with urethral dilators.

If symptoms persist, urethrotomy is indicated to split the ring at 12 O'clock position.

Labial fusion (*Synechiae-vulvae*)

Fusion of the labial folds may be seen in children. Local application of oestrogen cream thrice daily results in spontaneous separation. Surgical separation is rarely indicated.

Urethritis

- Acute urethritis frequently occurs with gonorrhoeal infection in females. Immediate antimicrobial drugs are to be given.

- Chronic urethritis is one of the most common urological problems in females. The distal urethra normally harbours pathogens. The risk of infection may be increased by wearing contaminated diapers, catheterization, sexual intercourse with infected partners. On local examination the external urethral meatus looks red, edematous and tender on touch. Patients will have features of dysuria, frequency and urgency.

  Urine for c/s and urethral smears are recommended to identify the causative organism. Appropriate antimicrobial agents are to be started immediately with maintenance of personal hygiene.

- Senile urethritis occurs in post-menopausal women due to oestrogen deficiency resulting in atrophy of the urethral mucosa. Such patients present with stress incontinence, vaginal and vulval itching and discharge.

- The diagnosis is confirmed by Papanicolaou smear which reveals hypoestrogenic cells which appear yellow in colour in comparison to normal mucosa cells which are brown.
- Senile urethritis responds well to diethylstilbestrol vaginal suppositories, 0.1 mg daily for 3 weeks. Oestrogen cream locally applied is also effective.

Urethral caruncle

Urethral caruncle is a benign, red, raspberry like vascular tumour involving the posterior lip of the external urinary meatus. It is rarely seen before the menopause. Microscopically it consists of connective tissue containing inflammatory cells and blood vessels covered with an epithelial layer.

Local excision is the treatment of choice.

Urethral mucosal prolapse

It is an uncommon condition, usually seen in children or paraplegic patients suffering from lower motor neuron lesion resulting in urinary obstruction. The mucosal prolapse should be reduced or fixed after indwelling catheterization.

Urethral diverticulum

In females urethral diverticula are not very common. Most of these diverticulae are secondary to obstetric urethral trauma or secondary to urethral infection. Diagnosis is made by feeling a round cystic mass in the anterior wall of the vagina. Post-voiding film on excretory urographic series may demonstrate the lesion. Treatment consists of removal of the sac though an incision in the anterior vaginal wall. Care should be taken not to injure the urethral sphincter musculature.

Urethral stricture

True urethral stricture of adult female urethra is not common. It may be congenital or acquired. Trauma at intercourse and especially after childbirth may lead to periurethral fibrosis with contraction or stricture. Treatment includes gradual urethral dilatation or urethrotomy under anaesthesia.

Section VI

Operative Gynaecology

26

Minor Operative Procedures

Operative procedures performed in gynaecology can be broadly divided into minor and major procedures. The commonly performed procedures are described in this chapter. The most common major procedure is hysterectomy and is described in chapter 27. The other commonly performed major procedures are laparotomy (see chapter on ovarian tumours), pelvic floor repair (see chapter on genital prolapse).

The procedures described in this chapter are:

1. Dilatation and curettage
2. Endometrial biopsy
3. Cervical biopsy
4. Cryocauterization of the cervix
5. Endoscopic Procedures
   - Hysteroscopy
   - Laparoscopy

DILATATION AND CURETTAGE (D&C)

It is a technique involving dilatation of the cervix and curettage of the endometrial cavity.

Procedure

- It can be done on an outpatient or inpatient basis in patients with medical problems.
- The patient is preferably asked to come fasting for 6-8 hours.
- IV sedation (using pentazocine and promethazine) or general anaesthesia are given.
- Perineum and vagina are cleaned and draped. Pelvic examination is done to note the size of uterus and position of the cervix.

The instruments needed are shown in Fig. 26.1.

- Posterior vaginal wall is retracted with a Sims speculum
- Anterior lip of the cervix held with an allis tissue forceps or vulsellum
- A uterine sound is introduced to confirm the position and to note the length of the uterocervical canal
- Cervical canal is dilated with graduated dilators (Hawkin Ambler's or Hegar). The tip should be directed anteriorly in an anteverted uterus or posteriorly in a retroverted uterus. When the dilator is introduced, the cervix is made steady by pulling on the vulsellum.
- After desired dilatation, uterine cavity is curetted. The sharp end is used in a non-pregnant uterus and the blunt end in a pregnant uterus. Curettage should be gentle but thorough, scraping along the walls of the uterus. Vigorous curettage may damage the basal layer of the endometrium and uterine muscle.
- The curetted material is taken on a gauze piece, examined microscopically and sent for histopathology in 10% formalin saline solution. Another sample is sent in normal saline if endometrial tuberculosis is suspected.

Discharge

- The patient can be allowed to go after a short period of stay.
- She is prescribed a course of antibiotics and analgesics.

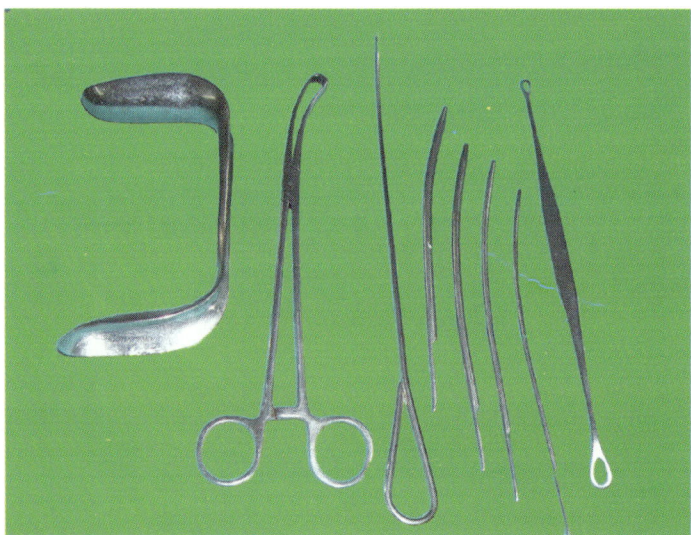

Fig. 26.1.   Instruments for D & C (from left to right) Sims speculum, vulsellum, uterine sound, cervical dilators, double sided curette (double sided with a sharp and blunt end)

- If the patient has been pregnant, blood group and rhesus type is checked and anti-D given, if necessary.

The **indications** for D&C could be diagnostic or therapeutic as shown in table 26.1.

Table 26.1. Indications for D&C	
Diagnostic	**Therapeutic**
• Menorrhagia in a patients >40 yrs. • Any patient with postmenopausal bleeding • Suspected choriocarcinoma	• DUB • Endometrial polyp • Incomplete abortion

Complications

Immediate

1. Vasovagal attack–sudden bradycardia and hypotension can occur during cervical dilatation. This can be avoided by proper pre-medication.

2. Cervical tears can occur due to forceful traction on the cervix with the tenaculum or, during cervical dilatation.

3. Uterine perforation can occur either during dilatation, or during curettage. It is diagnosed by a sudden loss of resistance at the uterine fundus and passage of the curette for more than the length of the uterine cavity. The principle dangers are bleeding due to injury to the uterine vessels and trauma to the abdominal viscera. The procedure should be immediately stopped, laparoscopy is carried out to know the extent of damage. If the perforation is large or there is a suspicion of bowel injury, laparotomy is carried out.

Late

1. Asherman's syndrome or intrauterine synechiae formation can occur if the curettage has been rigorous, or is performed in the puerperium.

2. Cervical incompetence in subsequent pregnancy due to injury to the internal os. This is more common if dilatation is continued after 8 mm.

Dilatation of the cervix alone is carried out–

1. Prior to drainage of pyometra.

2. Prior to insertion of an IUCD if the cervix is stenosed, this is commonly necessary with the newer IUCD, Mirena coil.

3. Prior to introduction of intracervical and intrauterine radium or cesium.

Fractional curettage

Endocervical curettings are also taken with uterine curettage, this is indicated in a patient with perimenopausal or postmenopausal bleeding when endocervical or endometrial carcinoma is suspected.

• The cervical canal is curetted before dilatation of the cervical canal and curettage of the endometrial cavity.

• A small curette is used for this purpose.

ENDOMETRIAL BIOPSY (EB) / ASPIRATION (EA)

It is a method of sampling the endometrium. The sample obtained is smaller than in D & C.

Indications

1. Patients with infertility to check if ovulation is occurring (secretory endometrium indicates ovulation).

2. Patients with menorrhagia who are > 40 yrs. of age to exclude endometrial cancer, a small sample by EA is taken for rapid diagnosis prior to a formal dilatation and curettage.

3. Patients with postmenopausal bleeding.

Procedure

The instruments used are shown in (Fig. 26.2). The patient is placed in a lithotomy position, perineum is cleaned and draped.

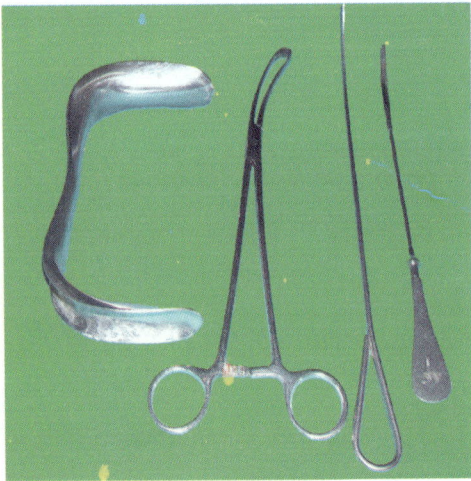

Fig. 26.2.   Instruments for endometrial biopsy (L–R). Sims speculum, vulsellum, uterine sound, endometrial biopsy curette (Karmann's cannula is used in place of EB curette in endometrial aspirations)

- A Sims speculum is introduced into the vagina and the posterior vaginal wall retracted.

- The anterior cervical lip is held with a vulsellum.

- Endometrial biopsy curette or 4mm Karman's cannula is introduced into the cervix.

- A 20 cc syringe is used to create suction and aspirate the curettings which are usually inspected and sent for HPE and AFB culture in patients with infertility.

Advantages of endometrial biopsy Dilatation of cervix with the resulting complications can be avoided. Curettage with a plastic cannula decreases the risk of perforation.

CERVICAL BIOPSY

The types of cervical biopsies performed are:

1. Punch biopsy
2. Cone biopsy

1. Punch biopsy

A small bit of the ectocervix is taken with a punch biopsy forceps. The area to be biopsied is initially visualized with 3% acetic acid or Schiller's iodine. The instruments used for cervical biopsy are shown in Fig. 26.3.

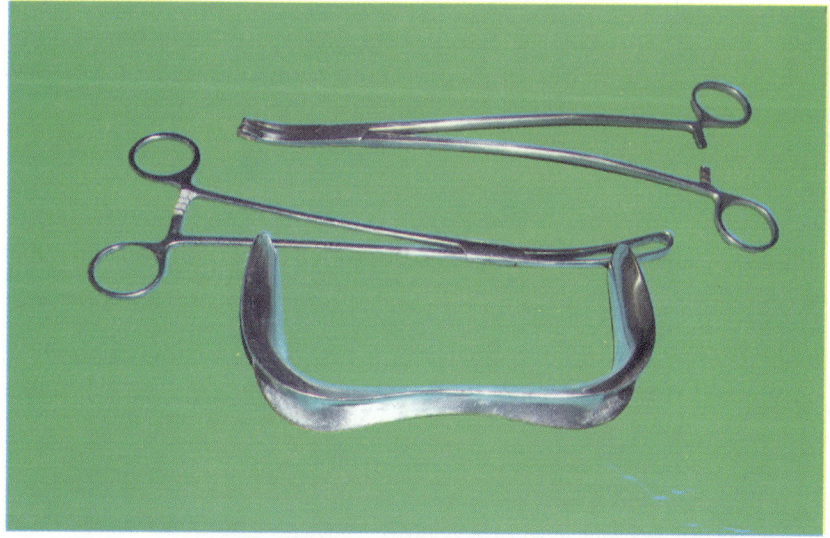

Fig. 26.3. Instruments for cervical biopsy (from above downwards) (1) Punch biopsy forceps, (2) Toothed vulsellum and (3) Sims speculum

2. Cone biopsy

This involves removal of a cone of the cervix including the squamocolumnar junction. The cone can be removed with a Knife-Cold-Knife Conization (CKC) or using an electrocautery.

Indications

1. In the presence of an abnormal smear when colposcopy is unsatisfactory.
2. When the lesion on colposcopy is inconsistent with the cytology report.
3. Presence of severe dyskaryosis on paps smear.
4. Presence of neoplastic glandular cells on the smear–i.e. when endocervical neoplasia is suspected.

Procedure

Cold-Knife Conization (CKC)

General anaesthesia is to be given and blood is to be arranged preoperatively. Haemostatic sutures are taken at 3 & 9 O'clock positions by ligating the descending cervical branches of the uterine artery. Schiller's iodine is used to mark out the abnormal area. A cold-knife (*Beevor's knife*) is used to remove a cone of the cervix with the apex below the level of the internal os. Haemostasis is secured by a continuous locking suture. A silk suture is placed at 12 O' clock position of the cone for identification of the margins.

Conization with electrocautery

A diathermy loop of adequate size to incorporate the entire transformation zone is used (LLETZ–Large loop excising of the transformation zone) instead of the Beevor's knife. A ball diathermy is used to cauterize the bleeding points (Fig. 26.4).

Complications of cone biopsy

1. Secondary haemorrhage
2. Cervical stenosis leading to non-progress of labour in subsequent pregnancies
3. Cervical incompetence leading to mid-trimester abortions and preterm labour.

These complications can be reduced by limiting the depth of the cone to <2.5cm. The cone of the cervix is extensively sectioned and examined by histopathologists.

CRYOCAUTERIZATION

Cryotherapy is a destructive technique using nitrous oxide or carbon dioxide as a refrigerant to lower the temperature of the tissues below–22°C to produce cell death by intracellular and extracellular water crystallization.

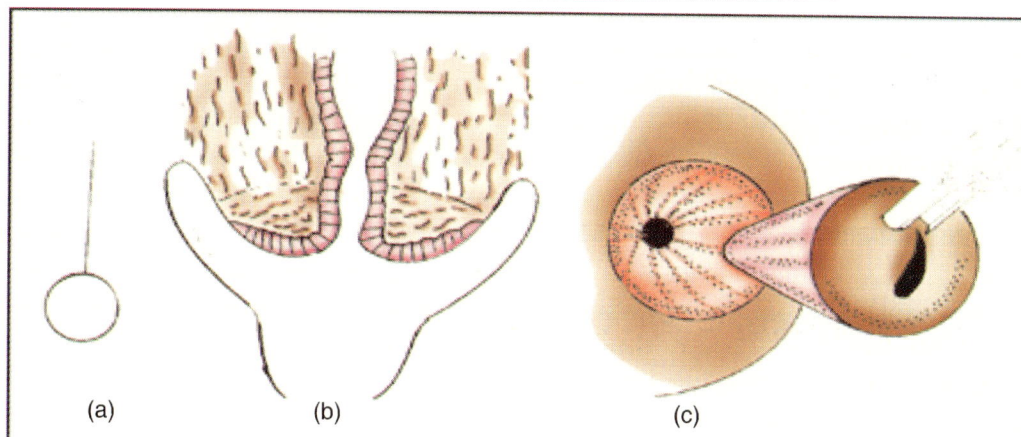

Fig. 26.4a-c. Large loop excision of the transformation zone (LLETZ) (a) Wire loop used for taking a cone, (b) The part below the dotted line shows the part of cervix taken for biopsy and (c) A cone of the cervix with the transformation zone is sent for histopathology

Indications

1. Benign cervical lesions–such as CIN, condyloma acuminata, leukoplakia etc.

2. Condyloma acuminata of the vulva and VIN diagnosed colposcopically and not more than 2 cms in size.

3. VAIN, condyloma acuminata or vault granulation tissue following hysterectomy.

Methods

This is done as an out patient procedure. The vulva and vagina and cleaned, the cryoprobe is applied to the cervix and the gas is switched on to activate freezing. When a good ice ball is found 4-5m beyond the edge of the probe, the freezing is carried out for further 3 min. and then stopped; the probe is kept applied to the cervix until it can be easily released.

Post-op

The patient is advised that she will have a profuse watery discharge per vaginum for about 2 weeks and that she should abstain from having intercourse.

Cryocauterization has been largely replaced by electrocautery in the western countries. However, it still has a place in India with limited resources as the complication rate is low.

Advantages over thermal cauterization

• Anaesthesia is not required

- Precise destruction of tissue.
- There is no secondary haemorrhage.
- Cervical stenosis is rare.

Drawbacks

- Excessive discharge for 2-3 weeks as healing is complete by 6-10 weeks.

ENDOSCOPIC PROCEDURES–(I) HYSTEROSCOPY

Endoscopic visualization of the uterine cavity.

Indications

1. *Abnormal uterine bleeding* in the form of meno-metrorrhagia, inter-menstrual bleeding or postmenopausal bleeding is an indication for hysteroscopy as submucous fibroids and endometrial polyps can be diagnosed.
2. *Infertility* Hysteroscopy is useful to diagnose submucous fibroids, septate, sub-septate, bicornuate uterus or intrauterine synechiae (Asherman's syndrome) which may be the cause of infertility.
3. *Missing IUCD* An IUCD embedded in the uterus can be visualized and removed under hysteroscopic guidance.

Contraindications

1. Infection–acute PID, vaginitis or cervicitis.
2. Suspected pregnancy–uterine perforation can occur.
3. Cervical cancer–malignant cells may disseminate during introduction of the hysteroscope.
4. Cardiopulmonary disorders–as CO_2 gas embolism and fluid overload can be fatal.

Technique

- *Anaesthesia* general for operative procedures, local anaesthesia with a paracervical block is sufficient for diagnostic procedures.
- Distension media–normal saline, 1.5% glycine or CO_2 gas.
- *Procedure of diagnostic hysteroscopy* In lithotomy position, the vulva and vagina are cleaned and draped. A pelvic examination is performed to know the size and direction of the uterus. The telescope is assembled, connected to the bag of distending medium. A sims speculum is introduced in the vagina, the cervix is held with a vulsellum, dilated if necessary and the hysteroscope introduced into the cervical canal under vision. The camera system gives a magnified view of the endocervical canal and

uterine cavity. Any endometrial hyperplasia is noted, the tubal ostia are visualized; a guided biopsy is then taken from the side-channel provided for biopsy.

Operative hysteroscope A wide bore hysteroscope with a port for operative instruments is used. The procedures which can be performed are:

- – Resection of an intrauterine septum
- – Resection of intrauterine adhesions
- – Removal of a pedunculated fibroid or a large polyp
- – Endometrial resection or ablation as treatment for menorrhagia.

Complications

1. Uterine perforation, cervical injury.
2. Fluid overload, hyponatremia due to excessive absorption of the distending medium.
3. Carbon-dioxide absorption can lead to gas embolism which can be fatal.
4. Haemorrhage and infection.

ENDOSCOPIC PROCEDURES–(II) LAPAROSCOPY

Visualization of the peritoneal cavity using an endoscope.

Equipment

The instruments essential to perform laparoscopy are: (Fig. 26.5)

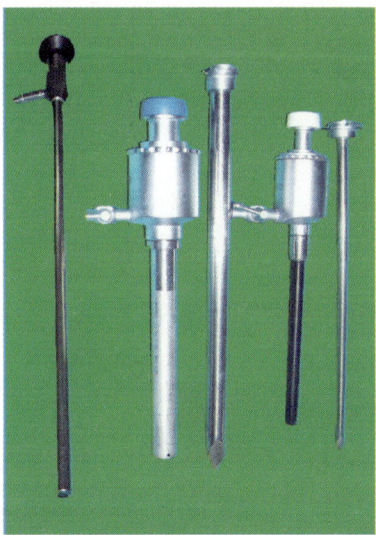

Fig. 26.5. Instruments for laparoscopy (a) laparoscope, (b) 10mm trocar and (c) 7mm trocar

1. ***Trocars*** of diameters 7mm, 10mm & 12mm. They have a conical tip and an outer sleeve and make a defect in the rectus sheath for introduction of the telescope and ancillary instruments.

2. ***Laparoscope*** is a high-precision engineered instrument which contains a fibre-optic bundle for light transmission and a series of lenses for transfer of the image back to the eye piece. The commonly used laparoscopes are 10mm & 5mm is diameter.

3. ***Light source*** and lead is made of a xenon cold light source and a fiberoptic cable to transmit the light to the laparoscope.

4. ***Camera system*** is used to project the image on to a television screen to provide a magnified view visible to all the members of the surgical team. The image seen through the eye piece is converted into electrical signals by a charge-coupled drive (CCD) bound in the camera lead. These signals are then processed by the camera control facility which is in turn connected to the television monitor.

5. ***Insufflator*** fills CO_2 gas to create a pneumoperiloneum so that the bowel loops fall away from the pelvis to provide a clear view of the pelvis.

Procedure

The patient is placed in a lithotomy position with a Trendelenburg tilt after ensuring that the bladder is empty. A small incision is given in the infraumbilical or subumbilical region for introduction of a verres needle. Pneumoperiloneum is created using approximately 3.5 litres of CO_2 gas to allow the intestines to fall away from the pelvis. The incision is widened, the trocar with the trocar sleeve is introduced with its tip directed towards the pelvis, The trocar is then taken out, leaving the trocar sheath in the abdominal wall. The laparoscope is then introduced and the abdominal contents visualized. The assistant at the foot end elevates and anteverts the uterus to bring the pelvic structures in view. Accessory ports are used for introducing laparoscopic grasping forceps, scissors etc. through a smaller 5 mm diameter port.

Indications of laparoscopy

- ***Diagnostic*** for investigation of infertility, chronic pelvic pain and assessment of pelvic masses.

- ***Therapeutic*** The procedures which can be performed laparoscopically are laparoscopic sterilization, aspiration of simple cysts, adhesiolysis, diathermy of endometriosis, myomectomy, ovarian cystectomy, salpingectomy or salpingotomy for ectopic pregnancy and also complicated procedures like laparoscopic hysterectomy, lymphadenectomy and incontinence procedures.

Complications of laparoscopy

1. Bowel injury–commonly the transverse colon or small bowel either during trocar insertion or while performing the laparoscopic procedures.

2. Vessel injury–to the inferior epigastric vessels, common iliac arteries, aorta or inferior venacava.

3. Omental, bladder injury during insertion of the trocar or while performing the laparoscopic procedures.

4. Surgical emphysema due to extravasation of CO_2 gas.

27

Hysterectomy

Hysterectomy is the operation of removal of the uterus and the cervix.

TYPES OF HYSTERECTOMY

Depending on the extent of removal of the uterus and the adjacent structures, the following types of hysterectomy are described:

- **Total** – removal of the entire uterus

- **Subtotal or supracervical** – removal of only the body or corpus of the uterus leaving the cervix behind

- **Hysterectomy with bilateral salpingo-oophorectomy** – earlier known as 'panhysterectomy', involves removal of the uterus with both fallopian tubes and ovaries

- **Extended hysterectomy** – removal of uterus, both fallopian tubes and ovaries with a cuff of vagina

- **Radical hysterectomy** – removal of uterus, both fallopian tubes and ovaries, upper one third of vagina, adjacent parametrium and pelvic nodes.

INCIDENCE AND HISTORICAL ASPECTS

The estimated extrapolated incidence rate of hysterectomy in the population of India is approximately 2,310,263 annually. Approximately 590,000 hysterectomies are performed annually in the United States and 130,734 in the UK. By the age of 60, over one third of U.S. women would have undergone a hysterectomy.

Hysterectomy rates vary with geographic, patient-related and physician-related factors. Newer alternative treatments to hysterectomy have affected the hysterectomy rates especially in the developed countries where more women are opting for conservative methods.

The history of hysterectomy

- The first hysterectomy was performed by Soranus in Greece in 120 A.D.

- The first authenticated vaginal hysterectomy was performed by Berengario da Capri of Bologna in 1507.

- The first subtotal abdominal hysterectomy was performed by Charles Clay in 1843 in Manchester, England, for a large uterine fibroid. The patient died soon after of massive haemorrhage.

- The first successful abdominal hysterectomy with a surviving patient was performed in Massachusetts, USA by Ellis Burnham in 1853.

- In 1929, Richardson in the USA performed the first total abdominal hysterectomy.

- Kurt Semm in 1984 first described the use of laparoscopic assistance in vaginal hysterectomy. The first laparoscopic vaginal hysterectomy was performed by Harry Reich in 1988.

The mortality rate after a hysterectomy was considerably high in the 19th century. With the development of instruments, revolutionary improvement in anaesthesia and antisepsis, a considerable reduction in the mortality rate was observed by the beginning of the 20th century.

INDICATIONS

Indications of performing a hysterectomy have been described in a very simplified and simplistic manner by Dr. D.C. Dutta.

Benign lesions

- Fibroid uterus
- Dysfunctional uterine bleeding unresponsive to medical treatment
- Uterovaginal prolapse
- Endometriosis
- Adenomyosis
- Chronic pelvic pain
- Chronic pelvic inflammatory disease with persistent symptoms
- Cervical intraepithelial neoplasia (CIN) of high grade in a woman who has completed her family and cannot come for follow-up
- Complex endometrial hyperplasia

Malignant lesions

- Carcinoma cervix
- Carcinoma endometrium
- Carcinoma ovary and fallopian tube
- Uterine sarcoma
- Choriocarcinoma in rare specified circumstances

Traumatic as a last resort for uncontrolled haemorrhage when dealing with

- Extensive cervical tears which cannot be repaired vaginally.
- Large uterine perforation in which uterus cannot be repaired.
- Rupture uterus (in a parous woman).
- Incorrectable uterine inversion.

Obstetric

- Massive atonic postpartum haemorrhage unresponsive to medical and other surgical interventions.
- Morbidly adherent placenta–placenta accreta/increta/percreta
- Septic abortion (selected cases)
- Cervical ectopic pregnancy

ROUTES OF PERFORMING A HYSTERECTOMY

- Abdominal
- Total vaginal
- Laparoscopic assisted vaginal
- Total laparoscopic

Currently there are no specific criteria and guidelines to determine the route of hysterectomy. The ideal surgical approach should be cost-effective, meet the standard of quality care, be best suited to that particular patient with her presenting pathology, and, comfortable for the surgeon.

- The vaginal route is the least traumatic and utilizes a "natural access" i.e., the vagina. It is much like a vaginal delivery with rapid patient recovery. This route should be the first line approach, even in the absence of uterine descent.
- The laparoscopic approach is a "minimal access" approach since only small cuts/ punctures in the abdomen are used to perform the procedure.

- The abdominal approach was more popular amongst the gynaecologists in the past. A transverse muscle splitting (Pfanensteil) or muscle cutting incision (Maylard) is used. In patients with large uteri, multiple fibroids or malignancy a midline or paramedian vertical abdominal incision is used. Abdominal hysterectomy has a higher incidence of complications, a longer length of hospital stay and convalescence. It is more expensive for the patient and the hospital when compared to unassisted vaginal hysterectomy.

Vaginal hysterectomy

Gynaecological surgeons have long considered an enlarged uterus a contraindication to vaginal hysterectomy. A normal sized uterus weighs approximately 70 to 125 grams. The American College of Obstetricians and Gynaecologists (ACOG) advocates that vaginal hysterectomy is best performed in women with mobile uteri no larger than 12 weeks gestational size (approximately 280 grams). Other authors suggest that a uterus as large as 16 weeks gestational size (approximately 400 grams) or even larger can be safely approached vaginally.

The two factors limiting vaginal accessibility are an undescended and immobile uterus, and a vagina narrower than two finger-breadths, especially at the apex.

Laparoscopic hysterectomy

If it is suspected that the patient's pathologic condition is severe enough for an intra-abdominal operative intervention, a laparoscopic examination can help in assessment of the extent of disease, help determine the mobility of the uterus, and exclude conditions which might contraindicate a hysterectomy.

Although the American College of Obstetricians and Gynaecologists recommends laparoscopically assisted vaginal hysterectomy as an acceptable alternative to abdominal hysterectomy, it is debated by many skilled gynaecologists as addition of laparoscopy only increases the time taken and the cost of the procedure.

Subtotal hysterectomy (Fig. 27.1)

The potential indications for performing a subtotal or supracervical hysterectomy are—

- Endometriosis with the obliteration of the anterior and posterior cul-de-sac.
- Caesarean hysterectomy when the cervix is fully dilated and difficult to identify.
- Concern that sexual function may be compromised by the loss of cervical stimulation during sexual intercourse.

The possible advantages of leaving the cervix behind are a lower incidence of operative and postoperative morbidity, vault prolapse, vaginal shortening, abnormal cuff granulations and fallopian tube prolapse.

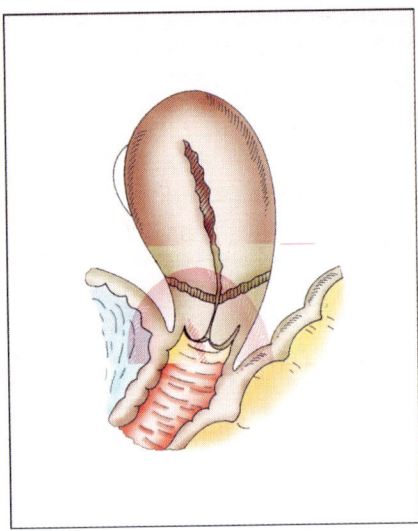

Fig. 27.1.   Subtotal hysterectomy—area above the line indicates the part of uterus removed in subtotal hysterectomy

However, in India, there is a high incidence of carcinoma cervix and regular follow-up of patients is unlikely. Leaving behind the cervix at the time of hysterectomy, regardless of the reason, is not practical. Subtotal hysterectomy should only be performed if the pre-operative pap smear is normal, she is prepared to have regular long term cervical screening and an informed consent has been taken.

COUNSELLING AND CONSENTING

An informed consent must be obtained prior to performing a hysterectomy. The discussion should include

- Issues pertaining to surgery, nature and extent of the disease process, extent of the proposed surgery, the potential modifications of the operation depending on the intraoperative findings, the anticipated benefits of the operation, and the potential complications of surgery.

- Alternative methods of therapy available, the risks and results of the same.

- The likely outcome if the patient is not treated at all.

- The need for hormone replacement therapy in the postoperative period after a bilateral oophorectomy along with its risks and benefits.

- The anaesthesiologist responsible for the surgical procedure should also assess the patient, review laboratory findings and discuss the proposed anaesthetic method with the patient.

Pre-operative assessment and workup

- *History and examination*

- *Investigations as appropriate*

    - Paps smear

    - USS abdomen and pelvis with colour doppler (in specific condition)

    - Pre-anaesthetic investigations

    - Endometrial biopsy / D&C

    - Hysteroscopy

- **Thrombophylaxis**

    - Thromboembolic deterrent (TED) stockings molecular weight

    - Low heparin 12 hrs. before surgery

    - Pneumatic intermittent compression device

- **Antibiotic prophylaxis**

    - All antibiotics are given preoperatively, ideally within 30 minutes of induction of anaesthesia as a single dose (roughly 30 minutes before operation if given intravenously or 1 hour before if administered intramuscularly), unless otherwise stated. This achieves maximum tissue concentrations at the time of surgery. A single dose of antibiotic at therapeutic concentrations is sufficient for prophylaxis under most circumstances unless there is blood loss of over 1500ml during surgery, haemodilution occurs of up to 15ml/kg or when surgery lasts for over 4 hours. In these cases, a repeat dose is given.

    - For abdominal hysterectomy, co-amoxyclav 1.2 grams (if penicillin allergic gentamicin 5mg/kg) with metronidazole 500mg are recommended.

    - For vaginal hysterectomy, co-amoxyclav 1.2 grams iv with gentamicin 160mg iv (if penicillin allergic or known to be MRSA colonized clindamycin 600mg iv with gentamicin 160mg iv) are recommended.

- **Bowel preparation** is needed in surgery for malignancies.

- **Blood** should be cross-matched and blood components should be arranged if massive blood loss is anticipated.

- **Pre-operative pharmacological interventions** (GnRH analogues) can be used to decrease the blood loss or reduce the size of fibroids.

Hysteroscopy, dilatation and curettage before hysterectomy–Is it mandatory?

It is indicated

- In women over 40 yrs. with menorrhagia.

- Women with postmenopausal bleeding or where there is a possibility of an intrauterine polyp or a submucosal fibroid.

Hysteroscopy and endometrial biopsy is taken to exclude endometrial hyperplasia or neoplasia. It may change the type of hysterectomy performed if malignancy is detected or in patients with polyps, the need for a hysterectomy may be avoided altogether once the polyps are removed.

STEPS OF THE OPERATION

The uterus is a pelvic organ attached to the pelvic cavity by ligamentous attachments (i.e. the round, infundibulopelvic, cardinal and uterosacral ligaments) and endopelvic fascia. In order to remove the uterus, it must be detached from its attachments.

In an **abdominal hysterectomy**, the steps of performing a hysterectomy after the abdomen has been opened are detaching the uterus from its attachments in a cranio-caudal sequence as shown in Fig. 27.2a-e.

- Detachment from round ligaments

- Detachment of the utero-ovarian or infundibulopelvic ligaments after identification of the ureter crossing the common iliac artery

- Mobilization of the urinary bladder after detaching the uterus from the uterovesical fold of peritoneum

- Separation of anterior and posterior leaves of the broad ligament

- Ligation and detachment of uterine vessels at the junction of cervix and the body of the uterus

- Detachment after incision of the posterior peritoneum to free the uterus from its rectovaginal fold of peritoneum (pouch of douglas)

- Detachment of cardinal ligaments

- Detachment of cervix from its vaginal wall attachments

- Removal of uterus and cervix (with a cuff of vagina in radical hysterectomy)

- Closure of the vaginal vault

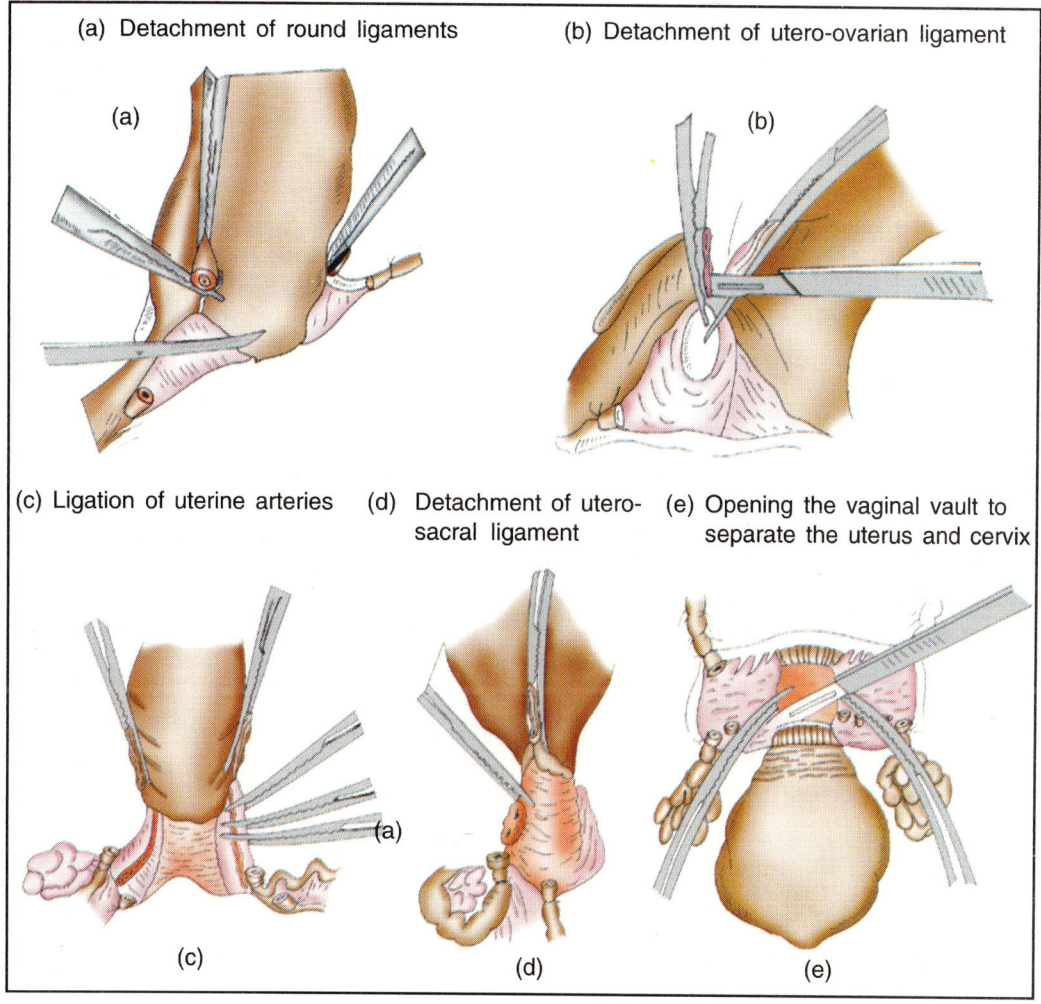

(a) Detachment of round ligaments

(b) Detachment of utero-ovarian ligament

(c) Ligation of uterine arteries

(d) Detachment of utero-sacral ligament

(e) Opening the vaginal vault to separate the uterus and cervix

Fig. 27. 2a-e. Steps of abdominal hysterectomy

- Re-approximation of the pelvic peritoneum (optional)
- Closure of the abdomen

In *vaginal hysterectomy*, the ligaments are detached in a caudo-cranial manner as shown in (Fig. 27.3a-f).

- Examination under anaesthesia to confirm feasibility of a vaginal approach
- Incising the vagina circumscribing the cervix
- Dissection of the vaginal wall off the cervix
- Opening the posterior cul-de-sac to detach the rectovaginal peritoneum

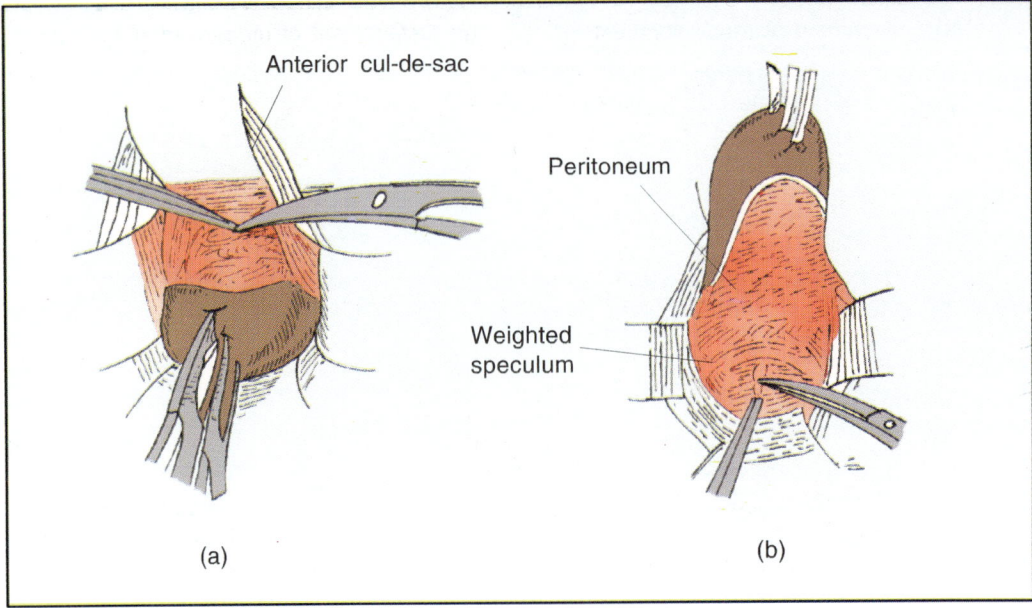

Fig. 27.3ab.   Steps of vaginal hysterectomy (a) Opening the utero-vesical fold of peritoneum after giving a circular incision in the vagina, (b) Opening the pouch of douglas

- Detachment of the uterus from it's attachment to the uterosacral ligaments
- Entry into vesicovaginal space to detach the vesicouterine fold of peritoneum
- Detachment of the uterus from the attachment of the cardinal ligaments
- Advancement of bladder with any adhesiolysis if bladder is adherent to the lower uterine segment
- Detachment of the uterine artery as it approaches the uterus
- Uteroovarian and round ligament ligation
- Ligation of infundibulopelvic ligaments if adnexa are removed
- Removal of the uterus and cervix
- Ensuring haemostasis
- Peritoneal closure
- Vaginal mucosal closure
- Anchoring the vault–If vaginal hysterectomy is being performed for prolapse, the uterosacral ligaments are anchored to the vaginal vault to prevent subsequent vault prolapse. Pelvic floor repair is done concomitantly (details given in the chapter on genital prolapse).

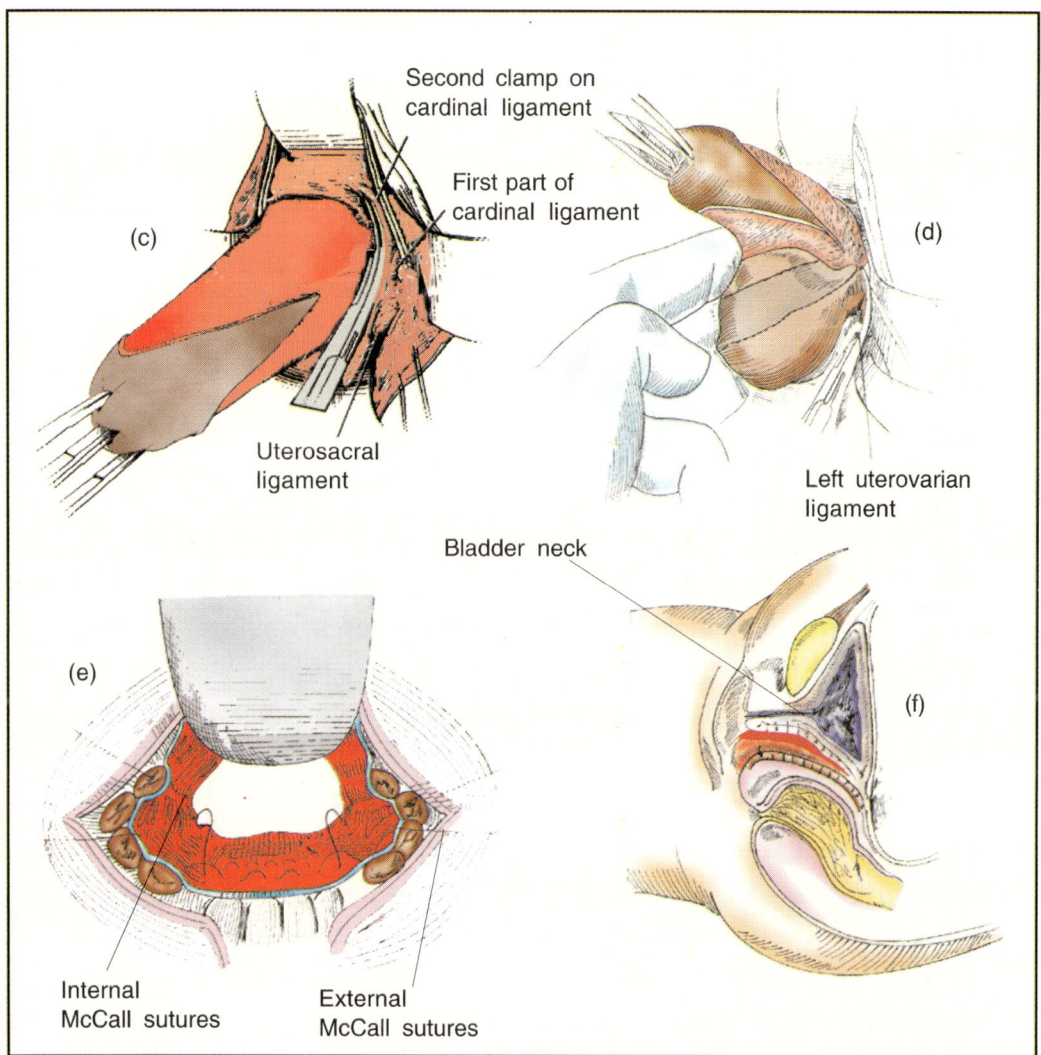

Fig. 27.3.c-f. Steps of vaginal hysterectomy (c) Clamping and detachment of the uterosacral and cardinal ligaments, (d) Clamping and detachment of the uteroovarian ligaments, (e) Closing the peritoneal sac and anchoring the uterosacral ligaments and (f) Cross-section of the pelvis shows the position of the vagina following anterior and posterior repair of the pelvic floor.

In a ***laparoscopic assisted vaginal hysterectomy (LAVH)***, the laparoscopic part of the operation begins with the mobilization of the uterus and adnexa from the pelvic side walls by its attachments to the round ligament and the infundibulo-pelvic ligament. The extent of the procedure performed laparoscopically can vary depending on the individual patient and the surgeon. The uterine vessels may be divided laparoscopically or vaginally. Usually the uterosacral and the cardinal ligaments are clamped and cut vaginally and the uterus and cervix delivered per vaginum.

In a *total laparoscopic hysterectomy*, the entire procedure is performed laparoscopically including closure of the vaginal vault.

Concomitant procedures

Numerous concomitant procedures that can be performed with hysterectomy are:

- Adnexectomy – removal of fallopian tubes and ovaries
- Bilateral salpingectomy with conservation of both ovaries
- Vault suspension
- Pelvic floor repair – repair of pelvic floor defects
- Adhesiolysis – lysis of intra-abdominal adhesions
- Stress incontinence procedures
- Lymphadenectomy – removal of the draining lymph glands performed in cases of malignancies
- Omentectomy – removal of the omentum performed in cases of carcinoma ovary, carcinoma fallopian tube, papillary serous or clear cell carcinoma of the endometrium.

Prophylactic oophorectomy is the most common surgical procedure performed concurrently with hysterectomy. It is performed to prevent ovarian cancer and eliminate the need for further surgery for either benign or malignant ovarian disease. In women with prior or family history of ovarian tumours, 0.14% can subsequently develop ovarian cancer, if the ovaries appear normal at hysterectomy. The only concern with prophylactic oophorectomy is the need for earlier hormone replacement.

Additional procedures performed

The following additional procedures can be performed along with hysterectomy with no increase in intra-operative or postoperative morbidity.

1. Appendicectomy may be performed under the same anaesthetic with hysterectomy to prevent appendicitis and to remove disease that may be present on the appendix.
2. Gall stone disease is common in women in the age group of 45-65 years. This is also the time when a hysterectomy is most often performed. Cholecystectomy when performed with hysterectomy does not increase febrile morbidity or the length of hospital stay.
3. Abdominoplasty when performed with hysterectomy has a shorter hospital stay, shorter operating time and lower intraoperative blood loss than when the two operations are performed separately.
4. Liposuction can also be safely performed at the time of vaginal hysterectomy.

Postoperative monitoring, care and recovery

- Monitoring of vital signs and vaginal bleeding
- Provision of adequate analgesia
- Provide bladder drainage and urinary catheterization
- Ensure mobilization and activity
- Ensure adequate calorie and fluid intake
- Watch bowel movement for return of bowel activity
- Continue thromboprophylaxis
- Provide chest and leg physiotherapy
- Assess requirement of transfusion of blood or blood products
- Continue antibiotic cover in patients with infection

COMPLICATIONS OF HYSTERECTOMY

Intraoperative complications

- Haemorrhage
- Urinary tract injuries
- Gastrointestinal injuries
- Other visceral injuries
- Nerve injuries
- Vascular injuries
- Those related to the laparoscopic route
  - Laparoscopic entry related injuries
  - Complications due to pneumoperitoneum

Immediate postoperative complications

- Reactionary haemorrhage
- Pyrexia
- Acute pelvic infection and abscess
- Thrombophlebitis
- Paralytic ileus
- Urinary tract infection
- Lung complications from aspiration and infection

- Pharyngitis
- Laryngitis
- Deep vein thrombosis
- Pulmonary embolism
- Depression and psychological problems

Long term complications

- Intestinal obstruction
- Urinary tract infection
- Urogenital fistula
- Fallopian tube prolapse
- Bowel dysfunction
- Persistence of chronic pelvic pain
- Sexual dysfunction
- Patient dissatisfaction
- Depression and psychological problems

Pregnancy after hysterectomy

Pregnancy after hysterectomy is the most unusual form of ectopic pregnancy reported in literature. Intraperitoneal access is provided by the cervical canal after a subtotal hysterectomy, or a vaginal mucosal defect after a total hysterectomy. Pregnancy may occur in the perioperative period with implantation of the fertilized ovum in the fallopian tube.

QUALITY OF LIFE ISSUES

Some women feel relieved as they no longer have to use contraception or worry about their periods. However, the quality of life after a hysterectomy can be impaired due to a feeling of loss of femininity

Symptoms of acute oestrogen deficiency can be distressing; they can be relieved by oestrogen replacement in the postoperative period which can be gradually withdrawn.

HRT "to give or not to give"

In those women who have had a concomitant oophorectomy during their reproductive years, it is necessary to offer HRT until they reach the average age of menopause (i.e., 50 years). In women over 50 years who develop symptoms of acute oestrogen deficiency, HRT is given to provide symptom relief in the immediate postoperative period. It should then be gradually weaned off.

Section VII

Frequently Asked Questions (FAQ)

28

Frequently Asked Questions (FAQs)

There questions are taken from the past papers of various medical colleges in India are listed topic wise (LQ indicates long questions/essay and SN indicates short notes).

MAKING A GYNAECOLOGICAL DIAGNOSIS

LQ

1. Discuss the differential diagnosis of an abdomino-pelvic mass of about 16 weeks gestational size in a 35 year old woman.

SN

– Cervical cytology, Pap smear

PUBERTY AND MENOPAUSE

LQ

1. Enumerate the different menstrual problems observed in an adolescent girl. Describe the management of pubertal menorrhagia.

2. Describe the normal menstrual cycle. Write the management of a case of pubertal menorrhagia.

SN

– Hormonal therapy for menopausal symptoms

AMENORRHOEA

LQ

1. Amenorrhoea

SN

– Asherman's Syndrome

- Haematocolpos
- Turner's Syndrome

MENSTRUAL DISORDERS

LQ

1. Enumerate the causes of menorrhagia at 40 yrs. of age and discuss the management of cystic glandular hyperplasia in this age group.

2. Discuss the physiology of menstruation. How will you treat anovulatory DUB?

3. What are the causes of menorrhagia? How will you manage a case of dysfunctional uterine bleeding (DUB)?

4. Define DUB. Discuss the causes of perimenopausal bleeding.

5. Mention the causes of menorrhagia in a 35 year old woman.

6. What is spasmodic dysmenorrhoea. Briefly outline its management.

7. What are the cause of irregular bleeding per vaginum in a 45 year old lady? How will you investigate such a case?

8. Define dysfunctional uterine bleeding (DUB). How will you investigate menorrhagia in a 40 year old lady.

SN

- Cystic glandular hyperplasia
- Transcervical resection of the endometrium (TCRE)
- Metropathia haemorrhagica
- Dysmenorrhoea
- Adenomyosis
- Endometrial hyperplasia

PROBLEMS OF EARLY PREGNANCY

LQ

1. Classify trophoblastic diseases.

2. Describe the differential diagnosis of a patient with 8 weeks amenorrhoea and acute pain in the lower abdomen?

3. How will you classify trophoblastic disease. Give the treatment of a diagnosed case of molar pregnancy with a uterus of 20 weeks size.

4. A 25 year old patient prevents with two months amenorrhoea and acute pain in the

lower abdomen. Enumerate the causes for such pain. How will you manage a care of ruptured ectopic pregnancy?

5. Discuss the diagnosis and management of ectopic pregnancy?
6. How will you manage a care of acute abdomen brought to the emergency with history of seven weeks amenorrhoea?
7. Describe the symptoms, signs, diagnosis and differential diagnosis of acute ectopic pregnancy.

SN

– Diagnosis of ectopic gestation
– Diagnosis of molar pregnancy
– Choriocarcinoma
– H. Mole
– Missed abortion
– Carneous mole
– Diagnosis of ectopic pregnancy
– Carneous Mole
– Pelvic haematocele

SEXUALLY TRANSMITTED DISEASE IN THE FEMALE

LQ

1. Enumerate the sexual transmitted diseases. How will you treat a case of a Bartholin's abscess?

SN

– Candida albicans
– Bartholin's abscess
– Bartholin's cyst
– Gonorrhoea
– Syphilis

PELVIC INFLAMMATORY DISEASES (PID) AND GENITAL TUBERCULOSIS

LQ

1. An 18 year old married girl is admitted with acute pain in the lower abdomen. Discuss the differential diagnosis.

2. How will you proceed to diagnose a case of genital tuberculosis?

SN

- Trichromonal vaginitis
- Endometrial Tuberculosis
- Pathology of TB of genital tract
- Diagnosis of TB of genital tract
- Clinical signs and investigation of TB of genital tract
- TB endometrium

INFERTILITY

LQ

1. How will you investigate a care of Primary Infertility?
2. Describe the clinical features of fibroid uterus. Enumerate the possible complications in the tumour.
3. Tests for detection of ovulation.
4. Investigation of an infertile couple.
5. Drug therapy for anovulation.
6. Common causes of female infertility in India? Discuss the management of a case of tubercular endometritis.
7. How would you investigate and manage a case of Infertility due to Tubal factor? Discuss the management of isthmic tubal block.
8. Discuss the various investigations done in an infertile female.
9. Causes of tubal factor infertility and methods of diagnosis.
10. Enumerate the cervical factors responsible for infertility. How do you assess them?
11. How will you investigate the tubal factor in an infertile female?
12. What are the causes of female infertility? How will you investigate such a case?

SN

- Test for Ovulation
- Seminogram
- Clomiphene Citrate
- Fern test

- Secretory endometrium
- Semen analysis
- PCOD
- HSG
- Basal body temperature
- Drug therapy for anovulation
- Secretory endometrium
- Tests for ovulation
- Diagnostic laparoscopy
- Basal body temperature (BBT)

BENIGN DISEASES OF THE VULVA AND VAGINA

LQ

1. What are the causes of vaginitis in an adult female. How will you diagnose and treat a case of monilial vaginitis.
2. How will you manage a patient aged 35yr. with complaints of Leucorrhoea.

SN

- Monilial vaginitis
- Trichomoniasis

ENDOMETRIOSIS

LQ

1. What are the clinical features of endometriosis. Briefly mention the treatment?

SN

- Chocolate cyst of the ovary

CARCINOMA CERVIX

LQ

1. Give the classification of carcinoma cervix. Discuss the management stage I cancer.
2. How will you diagnose a case of early carcinoma of cervix? Discuss the treatment of carcinoma in-situ of cervix.

3. How will you evaluate a case of carcinoma of the cervix? Briefly outline various forms of treatment.

4. Discuss the various roles of PAP smear study in modern gynaecological practice.

SN

– Paps smear

– FIGO's classification of cancer cervix

– Cervical erosion

– Staging of cancer cervix

– Cone biopsy

– Pyometra

– Shiller's test

– Carcinoma in-situ of the cervix

– Cervical intraepithelial neoplasia (CIN)

FIBROID

LQ

1. Enumerate the degenerative changes in a leiomyoma and describe the management of a case with an 8×8 cm fibroid in an 80 year old lady.

2. Enumerate the various degenerations possible in a fibroid uterus. Describe the clinical features and management of any one of them.

3. Describe the clinical featues of fibroid uterus. Enumerate the possible complications in the tumour.

4. Signs of fibromyoma, indications and contraindications of myomectomy.

5. Enumerate the cause of menorrhagia. How with you mange a case of fibroid uterus in a woman of 35 years?

6. Write the clinical features and management of a fibroid uterus.

SN

– Fibroid polyp

– Cystocele repair

– Red degeneration

TUMOURS OF THE OVARY

LQ

1. Discuss the differential diagnosis of a lump in the lower abdomen in a 35 year old woman.

2. Give the differential diagnosis of a lower abdominal mass. How will you manage a case of benign ovarian tumour in a 60 year old woman?

3. A 35 year old female is diagnosed to have a lump in the supra-pubic region, Discuss the differential diagnosis and outline the management.

4. Enumerate various cysts arising from the surface epithelium of the ovary. Write a note on any one of them.

5. Discuss the differential diagnosis of a lump in the hypogastric region.

6. Describe the clinical picture, diagnosis and management of a twisted ovarian cyst.

7. Describe the different modalities of treatment of malignant ovarian tumours.

SN

- Dermoid cyst
- Functional cyst of the ovary
- Krukenberg's tumour
- Complications of ovarian tumours
- FIGO staging of ovarian tumours
- Meig's syndrome
- Granulosa cell tumour
- Ovarian cyst
- Brenner tumour
- Dysgerminoma
- Malignant ovarian tumours

MALIGNANT TUMOURS OF THE UTERINE BODY

LQ

1. What are the cause of postmenopausal bleeding? Write in detail the investigations in such a case.

2. Enumerate the differential diagnosis of postmenopausal bleeding and describe the management of a case of carcinoma of endometrium.

3. Define DUB, discuss the causes of perimenopausal bleeding.

SN

- Fractional curettage
- Grading and investigations of carcinoma endometrium and Genital TB

DISEASES OF THE VULVA

LQ

1. Enumerate the causes of pruritus vulvae

BENIGN DISEASES OF THE VULVA AND VAGINA

LQ

1. What are the causes of vaginitis in an adult female. How will you diagnose and treat a case of monilial vaginitis?
2. How will you manage a patient aged 35year with complaints of Leucorrhoea?

SN

- Monilial vaginitis
- Trichomoniasis

CONTRACEPTION AND STERILIZATION

LQ

1. What are oral contraceptives?
2. Discuss the indications, contraindications and advantages of oral pills.
3. What are the various methods of contraception? Discuss briefly the advantages and disadvantages of each method.
4. Discuss different techniques of female sterilization.
5. Oral contraception
6. Methods, advantages and disadvantages of contraception
7. Female sterilization techniques

SN

- Techniques of female sterilization

– Conventional contraceptives

– Misplaced Cu T

– Methods of female sterilization

– Laparoscopic sterilization

– Benefits of OC pills

– Post-coital contraception/ Interceptives

– Triphasic pill

– Complications of IUCD

– Postpartum sterilization

– Injectable contraceptives

– Barrier methods of contraception

– Vasectomy

– Management of misplaced IUCD

– Laparoscopic sterilization camps

– Complications of IUCD use

– Barrier methods

– CuT

– Puerperal sterilization

Minipill

Pneumoperitoneum

Nirodh

Cu T Insertion

– Selection of a woman for oral contraceptive pills

– Benefits of oral pills

– Contraindications for CuT insertion

– Saheli

– Pomeroy's method of tubectomy

– Contraindications for OC pills

– Chemical contraception

– Laparoscopic tubal ligation

MTP

LQ

1. Discuss the various medical and surgical methods of MTP in the 2nd trimester of pregnancy.

SN

- Ist trimester MTP
- IInd trimester MTP
- Menstrual regulation
- Methods and complications of Ist trimester MTP
- MTP Law/MTP Act
- Suction evaculation
- Ethacridine Lactate

GENITAL PROLAPSE

LQ

1. What are the supports of the uterus? How would you manage an old lady with prolapse of uterus?
2. Describe the anatomy of the pelvic floor? How will you manage a case of 3° uterovaginal prolapse?
3. What are the sign and symptoms of utero-vaginal prolapse? How will you manage 3° prolapse in a 30 year old multi-para?
4. Describe in brief the supports of the uterus. Give the management of a case of 3rd degree utero-vaginal prolapse in a 40 year old female.
5. Enumerate the causes of uterovaginal prolapse. Describe briefly its prevention.
6. Define the classification of prolapse. Briefly outline the management of a second degree prolapse in a 25 year old woman with one child.

SN

- Enterocele
- Supports of the uterus
- Complications of vaginal hysterectomy
- Aetiology of uterine prolapse
- Cystocele repair

– Treatment of prolapse
– Supports of the uterus

UROGYNAECOLOGY

LQ

1. Describe the aetiology, diagnosis and outline the management of a Vesicovaginal Fistula (VVF).
2. Describe urinary incontinence in the female. What are the causes of Vesicovaginal fistula?

SN

– Bonney's test
– Stress incontinence

MINOR OPERATIVE PROCEDURES

LQ

1. Discuss the indications and complications of D&C.
2. What are the complications of Laparoscopy? How will you prevent them?

SN

– Pneumoperitoneum
– Indications of laparoscopy in gynaecology
– Endometrial biopsy

HYSTERECTOMY

LQ

1. Enumerate the indications for abdominal hysterectomy. What are the common post-operative complications following this operation?

Index

Index

379